AF574078

The Ocular Fundus

A Photographic Documentation Atlas with Diagnostic and Therapeutic Guidelines

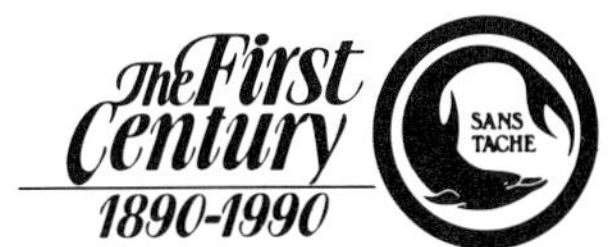

Dr. Med. Horst Huismans
Nordenham, Germany

The Ocular Fundus

A Photographic Documentation Atlas with Diagnostic and Therapeutic Guidelines

ENGLISH TRANSLATION BY
Manfred R. Tetz, M.D.
Department of Ophthalmology
University of Heidelberg
Heidelberg, Germany

David J. Apple, M.D.
Professor and Chairman
Department of Ophthalmology
Medical University of South Carolina
Charleston, South Carolina

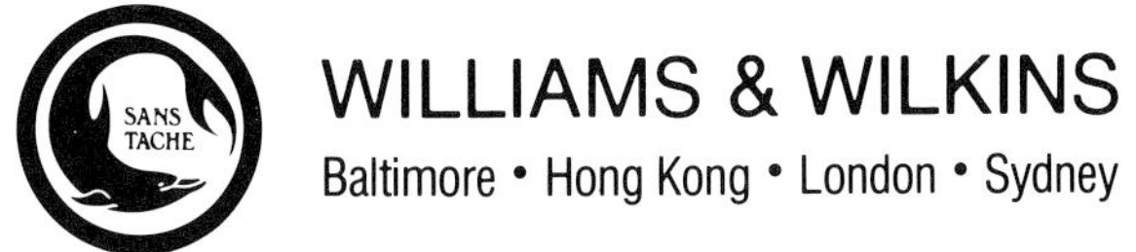

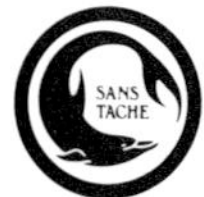

Editor: Carol-Lynn Brown
Associate Editor: Victoria M. Vaughn
Copy Editor: Klementyna L. Bryte
Designer: Norman W. Och
Production Coordinator: Barbara J. Felton

Williams & Wilkins
428 East Preston Street
Baltimore, Maryland 21202, USA

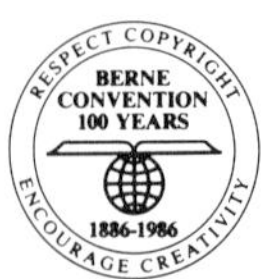

Accurate indications, adverse reactions, and dosage schedules for drugs are provided in this book, but it is possible that they may change. The reader is urged to review the package information data of the manufacturers of the medications mentioned.

Printed in the United States of America

First Edition 1986, originally published in German by S. Karger, Munich, under the title *Der Photographierte Augenhintergrund*

Library of Congress Cataloging in Publication Data

Huismans, Horst.
The ocular fundus.

Translation of: Der photographierte Augenhintergrund.
Bibliography: p.
Includes index.
1. Fundus oculi—Diseases—Atlases. 2. Fundus oculi—Atlases. I. Apple, David J., 1941- . II. Tetz, Manfred. III. Title. [DNLM: 1. Eye Diseases—atlases. 2. Fundus Oculi—atlases. WW 17 H899p]
RE545.H8513 1988 617.7′4 88-127
ISBN 0-683-04255-6

90 91 92 93 94
1 2 3 4 5 6 7 8 9 10

Foreword

The Ocular Fundus by Dr. Horst Huismans, my colleague of many years at the Münster University Eye Clinic, presents an impressively enriching addition to ophthalmological literature.

The author has been successful in making difficult material graphic and vivid and in exhibiting a clear instructional style. Very high quality color illustrations taken from years of medical practice deliver to the reader an overview and summary and give orientation and direction in determining conditions of the retina and fundus.

Of special interest are the numerous sequential photographs of various illnesses, which serve to build an understanding of pathological changes in the fundus of the eye. These changes are discussed in the text as well, enabling the reader to make proper diagnoses.

A large bibliography supplements the figures and makes it simple to do further research about universal medical relationships.

As with the great success of his textbook, *Animal Parasites of Human Eyes (Tierische Parasiten des menschlichen Augues),* I would like to wish this new work a rapid circulation and good reception by our associates in ophthalmology and related specialties.

Professor Dr. Dr. h.c. Fritz Hollwich
Past Director of the Münster University Eye Clinic
Munich, Spring 1986

Preface

This atlas provides a photographic documentation of many common and some rare ocular fundus patterns as seen from the practitioner's viewpoint. All photographs are from the author's practice. In contrast to other well-known publications on these topics, the major emphasis of this atlas is to offer a practice-oriented description of various diseases. Therefore, we have included clinical case histories of the patients whose fundi are presented. The literature list is very detailed and will allow for further study of certain diseases if such is warranted.

As a pictorial guide to the normal and pathological fundus, this atlas should be a guide for all ophthalmologists. It introduces physicians practicing in such medical specialties as general medicine, internal medicine, and neurology, as well as medical students, to pathological changes of the ocular fundus.

Horst Huismans
Nordenham
Spring 1986

Acknowledgments

Valuable contributions in the preparation of this English translation of Dr. Huisman's atlas were made by James W. O'Neil, M.D. (Charleston, SC) and Steven O. Hansen, M.D. (Salt Lake City, UT) who read the manuscript and made suggestions and corrections. Lou H. Allred, my administrative assistant, was the coordinator who organized the translation from transcribing the tapes and incorporating corrections from Dr. Tetz in Germany, my group in South Carolina, and the editors in Baltimore. She worked many, many hours in proofreading, researching, and double-checking facts to make the book as accurate as possible. We are grateful for the professional expertise of the editors and book production staff at Williams & Wilkins who have had exceptional patience in helping to make this project successful.

David J. Apple, M.D.

Contents

Foreword v

Preface v

Overview

Anatomy and Physiology of the Retina and Choroid 1

Retinal pigment epithelium 1
Microscopic structure of the sensory retina 1
Macula lutea 1
Optic disc 3
Vascular supply of the retina 3
Vascular supply of the prelaminar optic nerve 3
Vascular supply of the retrolaminar optic nerve 4
Carotid artery examination methods 4
Normal anatomy and physiology of the optic nerve vasculature 4
Choroid 4
Visual system 5

Ophthalmological Examinations 7

Indirect ophthalmoscopy 7
Direct ophthalmoscopy 7
Chromatoophthalmoscopy 8
Infrared fundus photography 8
Ophthalmodynamography 8
Ophthalmodynamometry 9
Retinal fluorescein angiography 9
Doppler sonography 10

Light Reflexes of the Fundus 12

Vodovozov's classification 12
Normal light reflexes 12
Pathological light reflexes 12

Specific Disorders

Developmental Anomalies 13

Macular colobomas 13
Colobomas of the retina and choroid 13
Bridge coloboma 13
Optic disc coloboma 13
Medullated retinal nerve fibers 13
Epipapillary glial membrane 14
Optic pit 14
Duplication of the optic disc 14
Enlargement of the optic disc 15
Hypoplasia and aplasia of the optic disc 15
Congenital central glial dysplasia of the optic nerve head 15
Persistent Bergmeister's papilla 15
Persistent hyaloid artery 16
Cilioretinal arteries 16
Opticociliary artery or vein 16
Fundus changes in ametropic eyes 16
Myopia 16
Refractive myopia 16
Index myopia 16
Axial myopia 16
Hyperopia 18
Refractive hyperopia 18
Index hyperopia 18
Axial hyperopia 18
Staphyloma-like ectasia of the posterior fundus 18
Ectopia of the macula 19
Primary ectopia 19
Secondary ectopia 19
Pseudoectopia 19

Diseases of the Retina and Choroid 33

Arterial hypertension 33
Retinal vessels 33
Fundus changes 33
Retinal artery occlusion 35
Central retinal artery occlusion 35
Common causes of embolic occlusion 35
Rare causes of embolic occlusion 35
Branch arteriolar occlusion 36
Retinal vein occlusion 37
Central retinal vein occlusion 37
Branch retinal vein occlusion 38
Venous stasis retinopathy 38
Neovascular glaucoma 39
Effects of diabetes mellitus on eye tissue 39
Diabetic retinopathy 39
Ocular changes caused by diabetes 40
Hemoglobin A_{1c} in diabetes mellitus 40
Arteriosclerotic chorioretinopathy 40
Low-vision aids 41
Correlation of arteriosclerotical changes with analogous vascular changes in other organs 42
Juvenile macular degeneration 42
Best's disease 42
Stargardt's disease 43
Sorsby's pseudoinflammatory dystrophy of the macula 44
Choroidal nevi 44
Drusen of Bruch's membrane 44
Central sclerosis of the choroid 45
Angioid streaks 45
Eales' disease 46
Proliferative retinopathy 47
Epiretinal membranes 47
Coats' disease 48
Secondary Coats' disease 49
Behçet's syndrome 49
Central serous chorioretinopathy 50
Circinate retinopathy 50
Septic retinitis 51
Choroiditis 51
Disseminated choroiditis 52
Central localized choroiditis 52

Chorioretinitis 52
Jensen's juxtapapillary retinochoroiditis 52
Chorioretinitis of the optic disc 53
Central hemorrhagic choroiditis 53
Toxoplasmic retinochoroiditis 53
Congenital toxoplasmic infection 53
Late ocular recidivation 53
Acquired toxoplasmic infection 54
Chorioretinitis associated with listeriosis 54
Toxocariasis 55
Acute larvae infection 56
Chronic larvae infection 56
Echinococcus granulosus infection 56
Cytomegalic inclusion disease 57
Subacute sclerosing panencephalitis 58
Tapetoretinal and Tapetochoroidal Degenerations 59
Retinitis pigmentosa 59
Atypical pigment degenerations of the retina 60
Retinitis pigmentosa without pigment 60
Hereditary diseases mimicking retinitis pigmentosa 60
Fundus albipunctatus 60
Fundus flavimaculatus 60
Fundus pulverulentus 61
Reticular dystrophy of the retinal pigment epithelium 61
Pseudoretinitis pigmentosa 61
Choroideremia 61
Gyrate atrophy 62

Diseases of the Optic Nerve 126

Optic neuritis 126
Prelaminar optic neuritis 126
Retrolaminar optic neuritis 126
Multiple sclerosis 127
Toxic optic neuritis 128
Hereditary optic neuropathy 128
Papilledema 128
Mild beginning papilledema 129
Fully developed papilledema 129
Chronic atrophic stage of papilledema 129
Pseudotumor cerebri 131
Optic disc drusen 131
Papilledema associated with iridocyclitis 133
Acute ischemic optic neuropathy 134
Temporal arteritis 135
Optic atrophy 136
Optic nerve head changes associated with glaucoma 138
Glaucomatous cupping of the disc 138
Diagnostic criteria for glaucoma 139
Intraocular pressure and risk factors 139
Staging of glaucomatous excavations 139
Acute glaucoma: Hints for the non-ophthalmologist 139

Tumors of the Retina and Choroid 160

Retinoblastoma 160
Endophytic growth of retinoblastoma 161
Retinoblastoma as a hereditary disease 161
Malignant melanoma of the choroid 161
Benign choroidal tumors 162
Metastatic choroidal tumors 162
Arteriovenous hemangiomas in the elderly 162
Wyburn-Mason syndrome 162
Choroidal metastases 163

Fundus Changes Associated with Pregnancy 168

Eclamptic amaurosis 168
Retinal detachment during pregnancy 169
Optic neuritis during pregnancy 169

Fundus of Infants and Children 173

Fundus of the premature newborn 173
Fundus of the full-term newborn 173
Fundus of children 173
Retinopathy of prematurity 173

Contraceptive Drugs 175

Ocular complications associated with contraceptive drugs 175
Extraocular complications associated with contraceptive drugs 175

Traumatic Fundus Changes 178

Birth trauma 178
Congenital retinal hemorrhages 178
Congenital papilledema 178
Commotio retinae 178
Contusio retinae 178
Traumatic retinopathy 178
Retinopathia sclopetaria 179
Choroidal rupture 179
Choroidal detachment 179
Light or radiation trauma of the macula 180
Optic nerve trauma 180
Traumatic optic atrophy 180
Hematoma of the optic nerve sheath 181
Traumatic disruption of the optic nerve 181
Foreign body embedded in the optic disc 181

Retinal Detachment 188

Primary retinal detachment 188
Secondary retinal detachment 189
Macular holes 189

Fundus Changes Associated with Blood Disorders 193

Leukemic retinopathy 193
Fundus associated with paraproteinemia 193

The anemic fundus 193
Acute hemorrhagic anemia 193
Chronic hemorrhagic anemia 193
Pernicious anemia 194
Hemolytic anemia 194
Fundus changes associated with coagulative disorders 194
Primary polycythemia 195
Secondary polycythemia 195
References 199
Suggested readings 210
Index 211

Anatomy and Physiology of the Retina and Choroid

The normal eye is composed of three primary layers (Fig. 1). The outer layer, or tunica fibrosa, consists of the sclera and the cornea. The uvea, or tunica vasculosa, is the middle layer of the eyeball and consists of choroid, ciliary body, and iris. This atlas focuses on the inner layer, or tunica interna, which is composed of the pigment epithelium and retina. This is the tunic that is normally examined during funduscopy.

The vital retina consists of a smooth, translucent layer that is approximately 0.2-mm thick at the equator and approximately 0.5-mm thick at the posterior pole in the peripapillary region. The posterior portion of the retina is sensitive to light and is therefore called the pars optica retinae. The peripheral portion of the developing two-layered neuroectodermal optic cup, which later forms the epithelia of the ciliary body and iris, is not sensitive to light, hence the name pars ceca retinae.

The pars optica retinae is composed of a layer of receptor cells and a layer of different types of cells that transmit and modify visually induced electrical impulses. The receptor cell layer contains 3–4 million cones that are responsible for photopic vision, for highly discriminatory central vision, and for color vision. Seventy-five million rods are responsible for peripheral vision and vision in low illumination. The inner nuclear layer is composed of cells responsible for the transmission of visual stimuli. The different neurons in this layer are bipolar cells, horizontal cells, amacrine cells, and multipolar or mega-ganglion cells. The nuclei of the Müller cells are also in this layer and provide structural support for the retina. These cells form vertical columns between the nerve fiber bundles. The footplates of the Müller cells form the interface between the retina and the vitreous body (the so-called internal limiting membrane). Outwardly, the apical aspect of the Müller cells terminates in the region of the external limiting membrane of the retina, which is composed of zonular adherence cell junctions.

Another name for the photoreceptor layer of the retina is the neuroepithelial layer. The layer that transmits and modifies visually induced electrical impulses is sometimes designated as the cerebral layer. The optical portion of the retina extends from the optic nerve head to the ora serrata. The latter structure is situated 3–4 mm anterior of the equator of the globe. It has sawtooth-edged peripheral margins. The part of the retina anterior to the ora serrata, the pars ceca retinae, forms the epithelia of the ciliary body and iris. The retina is firmly attached to the underlying pigment epithelium only at the ora serrata and the optic nerve head. It is postulated that intraocular pressure transmitted through the vitreous cavity helps to hold the sensory retina to the pigment epithelium (Waldeyer, 1957).

Retinal Pigment Epithelium

The pigment epithelium has a tenuous attachment to the adjacent photoreceptor layer. It reflects light toward the photoreceptors and mediates metabolic processes between the choriocapillaris and the rods and cones. The blood vessels of the pigment epithelium also nourish the photoreceptor layer and participate in production of rhodopsin.

Microscopic Structure of the Sensory Retina

The retina does not contain sensory nerves. The following layers are found in the normal retina (listed from the outside to the inside toward the vitreal space):

1. Rod and cone layer (photoreceptors);
2. External limiting membrane (formed by cell junctions between photoreceptors and the terminal optical processes of Müller cells);
3. External nuclear layer (nuclei of the rods and cones);
4. Outer plexiform layer (synaptic processes between bipolar cells and photoreceptors);
5. Inner nuclear layer (nuclei of bipolar, horizontal, amacrine, and Müller cells);
6. Inner plexiform layer (synaptic processes between bipolar cells and ganglion cells);
7. Ganglion cell layer;
8. Nerve fiber layer;
9. Internal limiting membrane.[1]

Macula Lutea

The macular region covers an area approximately 5-mm square that is slightly oval horizontally. The distance between the central portion of the macula (fovea centralis retinae) and the temporal margin of the optic nerve measures approximately 4 mm. The macula lutea consists of a lipid-soluble xanthochromatic (yellow) pigment, hence the name. Examination with a red-free light provides the best view of this structure.

[1] The so-called middle limiting membrane is not a true membrane. It delineates the row of synapses between the rods and cones and the dendritic processes of the bipolar cells.

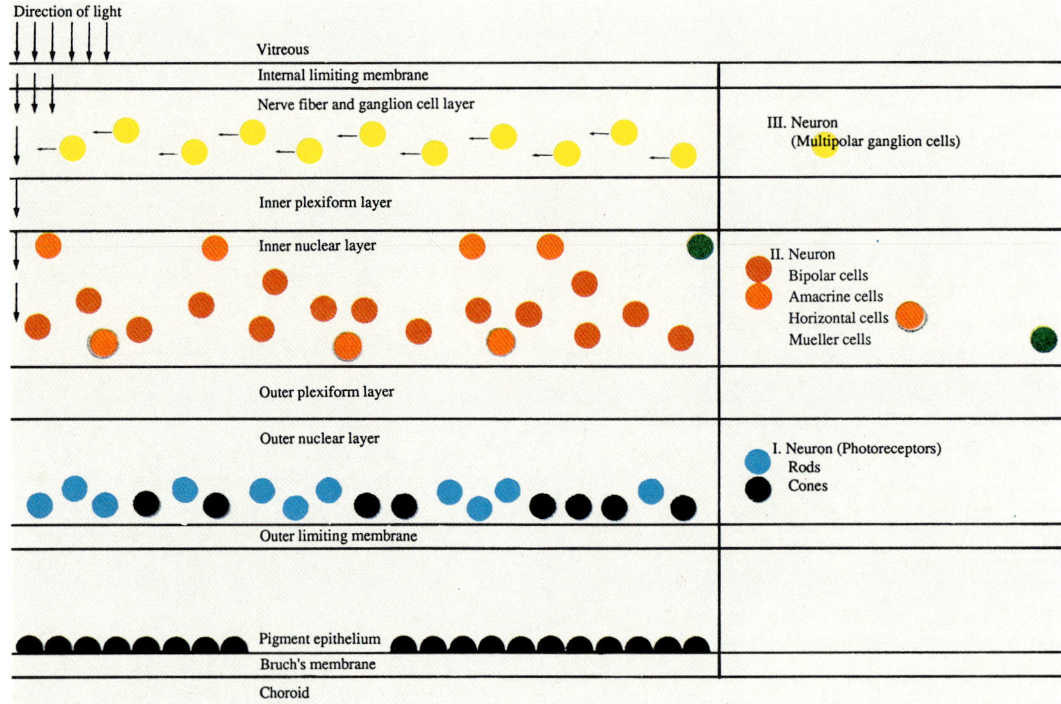

1

Figure 1. Schematic drawing of the histological organization of the retina.

Table 1. The Visual System: Optic Pathways[a]

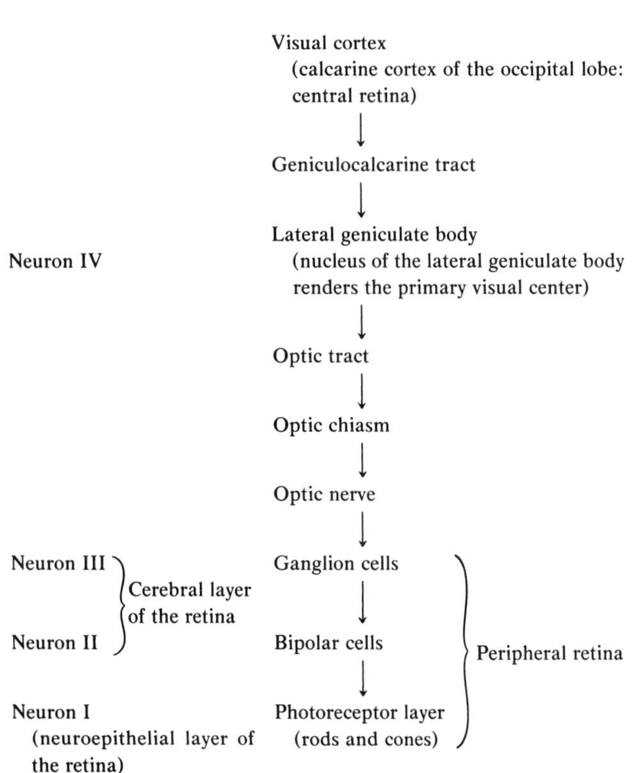

		Visual cortex (calcarine cortex of the occipital lobe: central retina) ↓	
		Geniculocalcarine tract ↓	
Neuron IV		Lateral geniculate body (nucleus of the lateral geniculate body renders the primary visual center) ↓	
		Optic tract ↓	
		Optic chiasm ↓	
		Optic nerve ↓	
Neuron III	Cerebral layer of the retina	Ganglion cells ↓	Peripheral retina
Neuron II		Bipolar cells ↓	
Neuron I (neuroepithelial layer of the retina)		Photoreceptor layer (rods and cones)	

[a]The optic pathways consist of the parastriate area (secondary visual cortex); striate area (primary visual cortex); and the peristriate area (secondary visual cortex).

The macula is the optical center of the retina. However, its location is not in a direct line with the posterior pole of the eye. In other words, the optical axis and the anatomical axis are offset in slightly different locations.

Cones make up the majority of photoreceptors in the macular region, which are more elongated and slender than the cones of the extramacular region. In the macular region bipolar cells, ganglion cells, fibers of the outer plexiform layer (Henle's fiber layer), and Müller cells are displaced circumferentially. These cells show an oblique orientation (as viewed sagittally in histologic sections) that causes thickening of the marginal zone and a central thinning of the retina, forming the fovea centralis retinae. The innermost part of the fovea, where the retina is thinnest, is called the foveola.

The fovea centralis retinae measures approximately 1.0–1.5 mm in diameter. This part of the retina provides the best visual acuity. The peripheral retina contains fewer and larger cones that provide peripheral vision with low optic resolution.

Some distinct pathologic features related to the anatomic organization of the macula can be seen during retinoscopy. One such feature is the so-called cherry-red spot of the macula. This spot is usually associated with a central retinal artery occlusion. The foveola does not contain axons. For that reason, the choriocapillaris becomes visible since it receives its blood supply from the choroidal circulation and is not affected by a central retinal artery occlusion. Normally, the edematous area surrounding the fovea prohibits a normal view of the choriocapillaris.

A common pathological alteration of the macula is a star figure, which is caused by the deposition of exudates in Henle's fiber layer or by a venostasis evoked by several different etiologies. Since the normal anatomy of Henle's fiber layer shows an oblique extension of the photoreceptor axons, transudates and exudates are usually deposited between the fibers, which produce the star-shaped configuration that is seen clinically.

The papillomacular or axial bundle is formed by the axons in the retinal nerve fiber layer. These fibers originate from the ganglion cells of the macular region and course into the temporal portion of the optic nerve head. As the fibers reach a point approximately 15 mm posterior to the eye, they are situated within the core or central axis of the optic nerve.

Optic Disc

Synonyms: Papilla, Mariotte's spot or blind spot (absolute visual field defect caused by the optic nerve head).

Location: The optic nerve is 3.5–4.0 mm from the central fovea on the nasal side, slightly beneath the horizontal meridian.

Size: Jaeger (1983) used Littmann's (1982) method to determine the true size of the optic nerve head. He found an average disc size of 1.896 mm in emmetropic eyes (lowest value 1.33 mm, highest value 2.3 mm). In hyperopic eyes (1–7 diopters) an average disc size of 1.673 mm was found (lowest value 1.29 mm, highest value 2.09 mm). In myopic eyes (1–16 diopters) the average value was found to be 2.017 mm (lowest value 1.51 mm, highest value 2.38 mm) (see Fig. 43).

Color: The color of the optic nerve head is influenced by physiological paleness in newborns and small children, the amount of blood filling, the number of existing capillaries, the depth of the excavation, and the appearance of the gray-white lamina cribrosa sclerae. The temporal half of the disc is usually lighter than the nasal half. The nasal nerve fibers of the retina course radially toward the optic disc. The nerve fibers originating from the macula (maculopapillar bundle) course toward the temporal side of the optic disc. A lack of larger vessels and capillaries in this area causes paleness.

Shape: The optic nerve head is oval with its longest extension vertically. A horizontally oval optic nerve head is often associated with a tilted disc and high myopia, or is found in highly astigmatic eyes.

There is a physiological excavation at the site of the optic nerve head, and the central retinal artery and vein emerge from this cup. Several variations of this physiological excavation have been reported. Elschnig (1900, 1907) differentiated: (*a*) small funnel-shaped excavations; (*b*) nearly cylindrical lateral excavations; and (*c*) cup-shaped large and centrally located excavations. The maximal depth of the physiological excavation is 1 mm. The maximal size of the physiological excavation should not exceed two-thirds of the disc diameter. The physiological (nonpathological) excavation is never a marginal one (see "Diseases of the Optic Nerve, Optic Nerve Head Changes Associated with Glaucoma").

Vascular Supply of the Retina

The arterial blood supply of the retina is provided by the central retinal artery and the choriocapillaris.

Central Retinal Artery. The central retinal artery is a true artery with a diameter of 0.0902 to 0.112 mm (Badtke, 1937). The central retinal artery derives from the ophthalmic artery, which is the first branch of the internal carotid artery. The central retinal artery is an end artery, i.e., there are no collateral vessels. It supplies the inner half of the retina, enters the optic vesicle approximately 10–15 mm posterior to the globe, and reappears on the optic disc. There are four primary fundus branches, named for their location within the retina: superotemporal and superonasal branches, and inferotemporal and inferonasal branches. In some patients, side branches supplying the macular region can be found. These branches are named for the area in which they appear, e.g., superior macular arteriole, media macular arteriole, or inferior macular arteriole. Many individual variations can be found of the central retinal artery and its division into several branches when reappearing from the central optic nerve head excavation.

Choriocapillaris. The choriocapillaris is responsible for the blood supply of the retinal pigment epithelium and the external half of the retina.

Venous Outflow of the Retina. The venous outflow of the retina is provided by the central retinal vein and its branches.

Vascular Supply of the Prelaminar Optic Nerve

The superficial vessels supplying the optic nerve head are derived from the central retinal artery. Nutrition for the prelaminar region of the optic nerve head is supplied by centripetal and recurrent aterial branches of the peripapillary choroid.

The lamina cribrosa sclerae receives its nutrition via vessels derived from the short ciliary arteries. In addition, its blood supply is provided by Zinn's circle and small aterioles from the pia mater. In this region the central retinal artery does not have branches. The number of short posterior ciliary arteries forming Zinn's circle varies markedly (Hayreh, 1975).

Vascular Supply of the Retrolaminar Optic Nerve

The retrolaminar region of the optic disc is supplied by peripheral centripetal vessels of the pia mater. The vascular supply of the optic nerve does not depend on the central retinal artery, and therefore the nutrition of the optic nerve is not affected by destruction of this vessel (Francois, 1975).

The blood supply for most of the intraorbital optic nerve is provided by a vascular network that covers the nerve along its entire length. This arterial vascular network receives most of its blood supply from branches of the internal carotid artery (ophthalmic artery and anterior cerebral artery). Before it enters the optic nerve, branches of the central retinal artery and short ciliary arteries also contribute to the blood supply of the intraorbital optic nerve.

Francois and Neetens (1969) disagree with Hayreh (1969) in his claim that there is an additional axial vascular system within the optic nerve. According to the findings of Francois and Neetens, nutrition for the optic nerve is provided by deep perforating branches of the leptomeningeal vascular network. In one-fourth of cases, they found one arteriole that received its blood supply either from the ophthalmic artery or the preneural part of the central retinal artery. All intraneural vessels show various anastomoses with the capillary network. However, numerous variations of the blood supply of the optic nerve have been described. As stated by Francois (1975), "There is no prototype."

Carotid Artery Examination Methods

Several noninvasive procedures can be used to examine the carotid artery and its branches. These methods include sonography (Fig. 7), ophthalmodynamography (Hager) (Fig. 8), and ophthalmodynamometry (Bailliart). Fluorescein angiography is a very useful addition to these techniques.

Normal Anatomy and Physiology of the Optic Nerve Vasculature

The four major branches of the central retinal artery and vein often branch within the physiological excavation of the optic disc. The four branches are located in the superotemporal, superonasal, inferotemporal, and inferonasal retinal quadrants. Side branches that extend toward the macular region are common and are named according to location, e.g., superior or inferior macular arteriole or venule. Sometimes a nasal arteriole or venule can be observed. Among the four major branches of the retinal vessels, approximately 10 small vessels can be seen that cross the optic disc margin. Fundoscopically, it can be difficult to determine whether these vessels are arterioles or venules. The number of these vessels is decreased when the optic nerve has undergone atrophic changes. With severe optic nerve atrophy these vessels are sometimes completely absent. In histological sections the arteries and veins are found within the nerve fiber layer. The arteries can be seen immediately underneath the internal limiting membrane. The veins are situated between the nerve fibers.

The retinal arteries belong to the group of elastic arteries and therefore closely resemble brain arteries. They are different from arteries found in the human limbs, which are of the muscular type. Only the central retinal artery and its immediate main branches are real arteries. All other retinal arterial vessels are arterioles.

Morphologically, the arteries and arterioles can be distinguished from the retinal veins because the arteries are smaller, show brighter central reflexes, and are bright red. The color of the veins is dark red.

Spontaneous Pulsation of the Retinal Veins. In approximately 70% of all people a so-called "vein pulsation" can be found. This pulsation can be seen in the optic disc excavation or, at times, closer to the papillary margin. This phenomenon is explained by a periodically occurring collapse of the veins during the systolic period of the heart action. The pulsation of the vein can be observed when the pressure within the retinal veins and the intraocular pressure are equally high. Although several authors claim that the presence of a venous pulsation rules out an intracranial pressure elevation, this is not invariably true (Huber, 1956). The phenomenon of a spontaneous vein pulsation can be evoked by applying mild external pressure on the globe.

Spontaneous Pulsation of the Retinal Artery. Pulsation of the central retinal artery (pressure pulsation) is always pathological. It can be found when the intraocular pressure exceeds the diastolic pressure of the central retinal artery. This may be caused by insufficient aortic valves, by an aortic aneurysm (clinical hallmarks: dilated pupil and central retinal arterial pulsation in the right eye and Horner's syndrome (mistic pupil) in the left eye), by orbital tumors, and during an attack of acute glaucoma. This phenomenon can be evoked by massive external pressure onto the globe, e.g., such as is used during ophthalmodynamometry.

Choroid

The choroid, or tunica vasculosa, extends from the optic nerve disc to the ora serrata and continues into the vascular stroma of the ciliary body. Neither the retina nor the choroid contain sensory nerves. The background color of the fundus largely depends on the pigmentation and blood flow of the choroid. Histologically, the choroid has four main layers:

1. Bruch's membrane (lamina elastica);
2. Choriocapillaris;
3. Medium vessels (Sattler's layer) and large vessels (Haller's layer);
4. Suprachoriodal layer.

Bruch's Membrane (Lamina Elastica). *Synonyms:* Lamina basalis, lamina vitrea.

Bruch's membrane is the basement layer, which is approximately 2 μm thick. It is situated between the retina and the choroid. The adjacent inside layer is the retinal pigment epithelium, and the outside layer is the choriocapillaris. By light microscopy Bruch's membrane consists of two visible layers: (*a*) the basal membrane of the retinal pigment epithelium (lamina basalis); and (*b*) the lamina elastica, which consists of fibroelastic connective tissue of the choroid and is the endothelial basement membrane of the adjacent choriocapillaris. Histologically, Bruch's membrane can be divided into five distinct layers: (*a*) The basement membrane (lamina basalis interna) is subjacent to the pigment epithelium. (*b*) Directly external to this is a layer of collagen (fibrosa interna). (*c*) This is followed by a core of elastic tissue (lamina elastica). (*d*) The fourth layer consists of a second thin layer of collagen (lamina fibrosa externa). (*e*) The fifth and outermost layer is a basement membrane (lamina basalis externa) elaborated by the endothelial cells of the choriocapillaris. Anatomically, only the outermost layer of Bruch's membrane (lamina basalis externa) can be considered a part of the choroid since this is the basement membrane of the choriocapillaris.

Choriocapillaris. The dense vascular network of the choriocapillaris provides the vascular supply for the external retinal layers (pigment epithelium and photoreceptor layer) since these layers do not contain blood vessels. The choriocapillaris is embedded in a thin network of connective tissue.

Medium Vessels (Sattler's Layer) and Large Vessels (Haller's Layer). The medium vessels (Sattler's layer) are located toward the inside of the globe, and the large vessels (Haller's layer) are located toward the outside. In reality these two layers, situated in a stroma consisting of collagen and elastic fibers with associated melanocytes, are a system of arterial anastomoses that receive blood from the choroidal vascular system, including Zinn's circle and the long and short ciliary arteries. The venous outflow of this system consists primarily of four to six vortex veins that pass obliquely through scleral channels or emissaria into the ophthalmic vein.

If the retinal pigment epithelium is homogeneously and densely pigmented, neither the choroidal vessels nor the intravascular spaces can be seen. By ophthalmoscopy, the fundus appears red or brown-red. However, the vascular network of the choroid can be seen if the number of pigment cells in the pigment epithelium are decreased and the melanin-containing cells of the choroid are darkly pigmented. In brunets, the intravascular spaces appear dark (tigroid fundus); in blonds, the intravascular spaces appear yellow-red. The pigment content of the cells and choroidal melanocytes is decreased or totally absent in albinos (fundus albinoticus). Fundus coloration also depends on age, differences in the light source used for examination, and the grade of fundus reflexes (Figs. 2-5).

Suprachoroidal Layer. This layer is composed of delicate connective tissue with large intercellular spaces. The major nerves and vessels that transverse the sclera pass through the suprachoroid. This layer also serves a protective function as the choroid and sclera slide on one another during movement or distortion of the globe. This space is opened during a cyclodialysis operation for the treatment of glaucoma.

Visual System

Four different neurons are involved in receiving and transmitting images to the cortical visual center (Table 1). Neuron I is composed of the photoreceptor retinal layer. Neuron II is composed of bipolar cells. Ganglion cells make up neuron III of the retina. The optic nerve contains approximately 1 million nerve fibers that are subdivided into approximately 800–1000 bundles by septa. These nerve fibers perforate the lamina cribrosa sclerae. Posterior to this structure, the nerve fibers are covered with a myelin sheath. The nerve fibers from the nasal half of the retina cross over but the temporal fibers remain on the same side. Posterior to the chiasm, these axons form the optic tract and continue toward the primary visual center in the lateral geniculate body. Some fibers in the optic tract exit before reaching the lateral geniculate body and go to the midbrain and synapse in the pretectal and superior colliculus areas where they contribute to pathways of the afferent pupillary reflex.

The nerve fibers of the optic tract, as they enter the lateral geniculate body, synapse with neuron IV of the visual tract and form the geniculocalcarine tract (also called the optic radiation), which courses to the occipital cortex. The occipital cortical area is immediately adjacent to the calcarine fissure.

Hollwich (1958, 1966), among others, demonstrated that the light perceived by the retina is not only transformed into visual information (optical function), but also forms other tracts, such as the one that transmits stimuli to the hypophyseal system of the midbrain. These fibers interact with the autonomic nervous system.

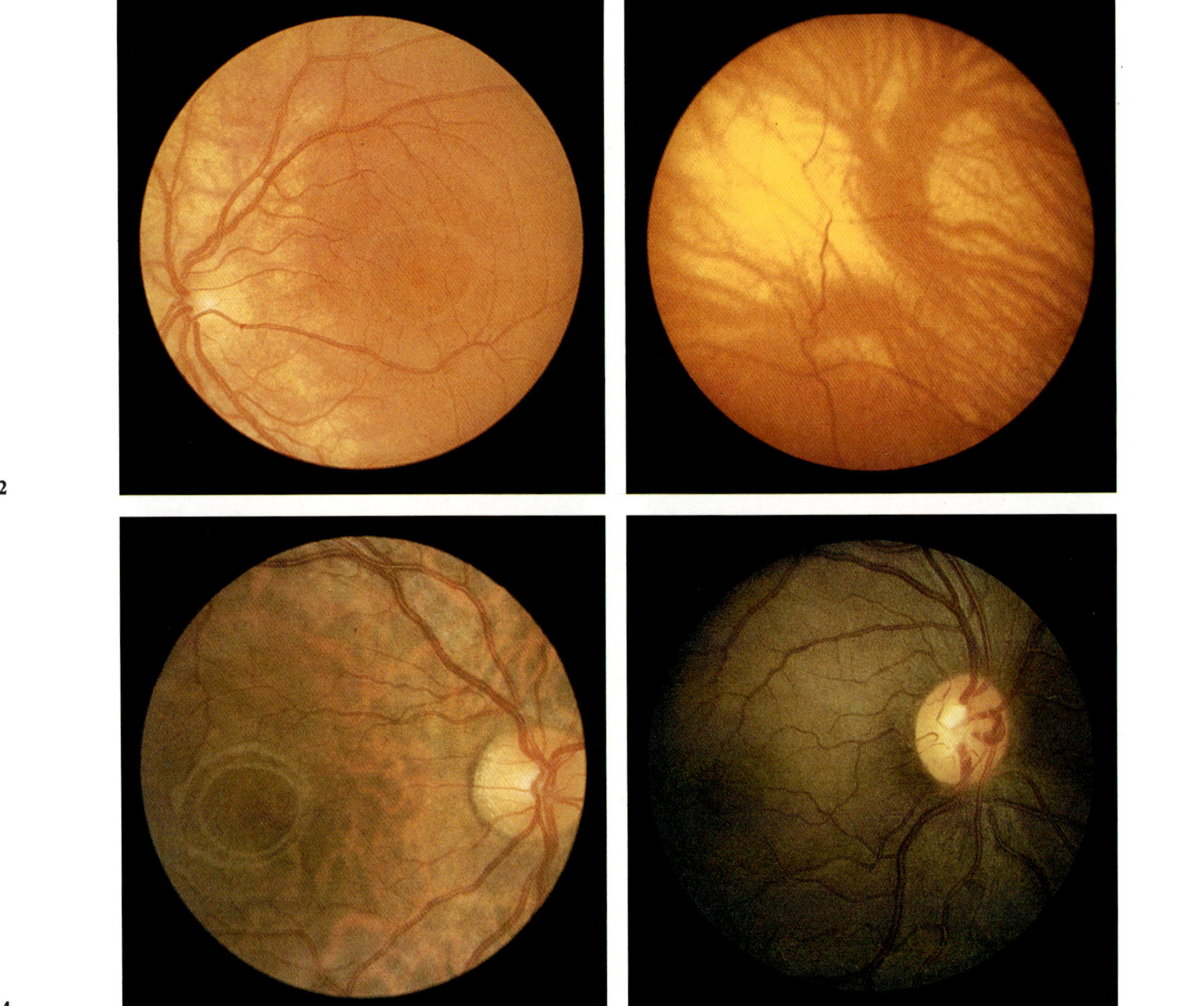

Figure 2. Fundus of the left eye of a 14-year-old blond male patient.

Clinical Findings

The eye was emmetropic. The optic disc was barely discernible and blended almost homogeneously into the peripapillary area. The optic disc had a small central excavation caused by a thinning of the pigment epithelium and choriocapillaris. Larger choroidal vessels were seen against the white sclera, and bright intervascular spaces were also present. The posterior pole is a normal color. The slightly ectopic macula is easily seen, outlined by the normal circular macular reflex. A slight sickle-shaped foveal reflex is visible. The retinal vessels is normal; superior and inferior macular arterioles is easily seen.

Figure 3. Equatorial retinal area showing a vortex vein in the lightly pigmented fundus of a blond patient.

Figure 4. Right eye of a 16-year-old male patient with a tigroid fundus (fundus tabulatus).

Clinical Findings

Refraction in both eyes was +0.75 diopters sphere. The optic disc shows a central excavation and stands out compared with the surrounding area. The tabulated or tigroid appearance of the fundus is caused by reduced pigment within the retinal pigment epithelium. In contrast, the suprachoroidal area is heavily pigmented. The light red choroidal vessels contrast sharply with the darkly pigmented intervascular spaces. The fundus is more homogeneously colored at the posterior pole. Three reflexes can be seen: a tiny sickle-shaped foveal reflex, a circular macular reflex, and an oval perimacular reflex, which is most obvious horizontally. However, the latter reflex is not always visible. The retinal vessels are normal. The hallmark of a senile tigroid fundus associated with arteriosclerosis is the presence of dark intervascular spaces that sharply contrast with the white-yellow choroidal vessels.

Figure 5. Right eye of a 22-year-old black male patient with a normal fundus.

Clinical Findings

The eye is ametropic. The optic disc shows a small central excavation. This fundus is an example of the broad variability possible in normal vascular branching patterns. The homogeneous dark fundus pigmentation does not allow a direct view of the choroidal vessels. The optic nerve fibers are partially visible. The usually circular outer reflex of the macula is shaped like a half-moon in this eye. The macula is slightly ectopic.

Ophthalmological Examinations

Indirect Ophthalmoscopy

In 1850 von Helmholtz invented the ophthalmoscope. Improvements in this device include a powerful light source and an additional biconvex plus lens that are still found in modern indirect ophthalmoscopes.

Examination Methods. Patients can be examined in a sitting, standing, or laying position. Depending on the examiner's arm length, the distance between the patient and the physician is approximately 14–15 cm (16–20 inches). The examiner holds the lens between the thumb and index finger of the left hand, while the fourth and fifth finger are resting upon the patient's forehead, brow, or temple. The lens is held at a distance of approximately 7–8 cm in front of the patient's eye.

A one-handed technique is widely used in Europe. The ophthalmoscope is held in the examiner's right hand while he or she looks above the superior margin of the light source in the direction of the light bundle. Another light is directed via the lens into the patient's eye. An inverted image that is enlarged four to five times of the patient's retina is created approximately 35–40 cm in front of the lens. The examiner must adjust to this inverted image to get a clear view of the patient's retina.

In the United States a similar technique is used, but one that has the advantage of providing a binocular view of the retina. The binocular ophthalmoscope has a built-in prism system that brings both eyes into coaxial view with a light source shining from the middle of the examiner's forehead. Distorting reflexes can be eliminated by tilting the lens in different directions. Minor adjustments can be performed easily by axial displacement of the lens.

Examination Sequence. To standardize an examination the author recommends describing the appearance of the optic disc in terms of color, shape, size, margins, excavations, and vascular pattern. It is useful to have the patient looking in the direction of the examiner's right ear while the right eye is examined, and vice versa for the left eye. The macular region and the posterior pole can be examined best when the patient looks directly into the light source. To examine the peripheral parts of the retina, the patient is asked to move his or her eye in a slow circular pattern while looking upward (to the left) and downward (to the right). Close scrutinization of the peripheral retina is possible only in mydriasis.

Direct Ophthalmoscopy

To obtain a clear view of the fundus a direct ophthalmoscope with a bright light source is necessary.

Examination Methods. Direct ophthalmoscopy is most easily performed while the patient is in a sitting position. However, for a severely ill or older patient, the examination can be performed when the patient is in a supine position.

The examiner uses his or her right eye to examine the patient's right eye, and his or her left eye to view the patient's left eye. The ophthalmoscope is held perpendicular and is supported by or leaned against the orbital rim of the patient's eye. The patient is asked to look with both eyes at the far distance target to eliminate accommodation. The examiner should also eliminate as much accommodation as possible. The ophthalmoscope is positioned approximately 15 cm in front of the patient's eye, and the light beam is directed into the pupil from a slightly temporal position. Following the red fundus reflex, the examiner approaches the front of the patient's eye to a distance of 2–3 cm. To adjust refractive errors in either the patient's or the examiner's eye, the refractive power of the ophthalmoscope can be changed by the Rekoss dial to move the lenses of different refractive power. Such an adjustment in lens refractive power provides a clear picture of the patient's fundus that is useful in determining different levels of fundus lesions, e.g., the elevation of a malignant melanoma. A 3-diopter change signifies a 1-mm change in depth or elevation.

Direct ophthalmoscopy provides an upright image view of part of the fundus at an approximate ×16 magnification.

Examination Sequence. Details of the fundus should be viewed in a systematic fashion: optic disc, retinal vessels, posterior pole with macula, retina details, and differences in elevation or excavation.

Drugs Commonly Used to Dilate and Constrict the Pupil. Some commonly used parasympatholytic, sympathomimetic, and parasympathomimetic drugs are listed in Tables 2 and 3. A physician should always limit use of these drugs and closely follow patients who are using them.

Table 2. Parasympatholytic (Mydriatic) Drugs

Generic Name	Trade Name	Manufacturer	Duration
Tropicamide	Mydriacyl (0.05%)	Alcon	4-6 hours
Tropicamide	Tropicacyl (0.5-1.0%)	Akorn	4-6 hours
Homatropine hydrobromide	Isopto Homatropine (2%)	Alcon	1 or more days
Homatropine hydrobromide	I-Homatrine 5% Ophthalmic Solution	Americal	1 or more days
Cyclopentolate hydrochloride	AK-Penlolate (0.5-1.0%)	Akorn	1-2 days
Cyclopentolate hydrochloride	Cyclogyl (0.5-1.0%)	Alcon	1-2 days
Cyclopentolate hydrochloride	Pentolair 1% Solution	Pharmafair	1-2 days

Table 3. Sympathomimetic (Mydriatic) Drugs and Parasympathomimetic (Miotic) Drugs

Generic Name	Trade Name	Manufacturer	Duration
Sympathomimetic			
Phenylephrine hydrochloride	AK-Dilate (2.5-10%)	Akorn	3 or more hours
Phenylephrine hydrochloride	Mydfrin (2.5%)	Alcon	3 or more hours
Phenylephrine hydrochloride	Dilatair Solution (2.5%)	Pharmafair	3-6 hours
Phenylephrine hydrochloride	Neo-Synephrine (2.5-10%)	Winthrop Pharmaceuticals	3-6 hours
Parasympathomimetic			
Pilocarpine hydrochloride	Pilocar (0.5-2%)	Iolab Pharmaceuticals	4-8 hours
Pilocarpine hydrochloride	Isopto Carpine (0.5-2%)	Alcon	4-8 hours
Pilocarpine hydrochloride	I-Pilocarpine (1%)	Americal	4 or more hours
Pilocarpine hydrochloride	Akarpine (0.5-2%)	Akorn	4-8 hours

Chromatoophthalmoscopy

Synonym: Ophthalmochromoscopy.

This diagnostic method is based on the principle that different wavelengths of light vary in penetration into layers of the fundus. This test allows for an in-depth analysis at different fundus layers. For example:

Short wavelength light (blue and light blue) is primarily reflected on the external limiting membrane of the retina.

Intermediate wavelength light (green and yellow) is reflected inside the retina.

Long wavelength light (orange and red) primarily penetrates into the choroid and is partially reflected at this site. Other wavelengths of the spectrum are reflected by the sclera.

Chromatoophthalmoscopy also provides additional information in the differential diagnosis and prognosis of various types of macular degeneration (for more detail see Vodovozov, 1978, and Jaeger and Käfer, 1979).

Infrared Fundus Photography

Infrared fundus photography is a special application of chromatoophthalmoscopy that is helpful in the diagnosis of ophthalmological tumors. Naumann (G. O. H. Naumann, personal communication) believes that this method is especially useful in the evaluation and observation of melanocytic lesions of the choroid. Dark melanin pigment can often be differentiated from relatively light blood-related pigment by the difference in color.

With infrared-sensitive film and normal illumination, pigment of the choroid appears blue-violet, and pigment of the retinal pigment epithelium appears yellow-brown. In a normal fundus the blue-violet color of choroidal pigment is not visible; it becomes visible if the pigment epithelium is rarified. The yellow-brown retinal pigment epithelium color is easily discernible at sites where the retinal pigment epithelium is thinned by the sharp contrast of the bright scleral background (Jaeger and Käfer, 1979). The author has found that storing vacuum-sealed infrared film or film-loaded cameras in a refrigerator preserves the quality of the film.

Ophthalmodynamography

The "infraton" ophthalmodynamograph, developed in 1956 by Hager and Otto, allows noninvasive oscillographic monitoring of the ophthalmic artery (Fig. 8) to study the vessel's pulsation and determine systolic and diastolic pressure.

Examination method. The ophthalmic arterial pulses are simultaneously monitored with the pulse of the upper arm. The probe is applied to the bony orbit and thus is in indirect contact with both the eye and orbital tissues. The systemic pressure is monitored at the brachial artery by means of a microphone. The Korotkoff sounds are recorded at the antecubital fossa. The pressure in the orbital pressure chamber and the blood pressure cuff are raised via electronic and pneumatic systems. The initial orbital pressure level should be 20 mm above the initial measured systolic blood pressure in the brachial artery. However, a pressure of 190 mm Hg should not be exceeded within the pressure chamber applied to the eye.

The pressure is slowly decreased via a built-in nozzle. During the pressure decrease, automatic impulses for the systolic and diastolic pressure are printed out. Simultaneously the multiple lead system provides an oscillogram of the ophthalmic artery and the Korotkoff sounds of the brachial artery.

The pulsation volume (*PV*) is determined by comparing the maximum peak of the oscillations with the calibration amplitudes. The following formula is used:

$$PV = (A_p/A_e) \times 50\ \mu l$$

where A_p is the mean of the largest amplitudes of the ophthalmic oscillogram (in mm), and A_e is the mean of the calibration amplitudes (in mm) with a calibration volume of 50 μl.

The criteria for the systolic and diastolic pressure in the ophthalmic artery and the brachial artery are determined in the following manner:

Ophthalmic Artery. Systolic criterium: first significant registered pulsation or first significant major pulsation. Diastolic criterium: largest pulse amplitude and transition of the round, flattened minimum of the pulsation curve into an inverse peak.

Brachial Artery. Systolic criterium: first registered Korotkoff sound. Diastolic criterium: last registered Korotkoff sound.

For additional information see Hager (1963b) and the instruction manual that comes with the device (Boucke-Electronic, Tuebingen, West Germany).

Physiologically the pressure in the ophthalmic artery is equally high or only 5–10 mm Hg lower than the arterial pressure in the brachial artery. The pulsation volume is usually between 70 and 220 μl.

This examination method has proven to be very useful especially in the diagnosis of occlusions of the carotid artery.

Ophthalmodynamometry

In 1917 Bailliart suggested that, while visually observing the pulsation of the central retinal artery, the blood pressure within the opthalmic artery can be determined by using a dynamometer. This device is used to create measurable external compressions of the globe. In 80% of cases a presumed diagnosis of a carotid artery occlusion can be verified (for details see Weigelin and Lobstein, 1963). Huismans (1981) described the use of the binocular ophthalmoscope (table-mounted device manufactured by Rodenstock) in combination with a specially developed adapter for the Müller dynamometer. This setup enabled the author to perform examinations without assistance.

Retinal Fluorescein Angiography

In vivo staining of the retinal vascular system (Fig. 6) has several practical diagnostic applications in modern ophthalmology (Wessing, 1973):

1. The vascular system, including capillaries, becomes visible, and structural changes in the microvasculature may be observed.
2. Permeability and leakage from fundus vessels can be observed.
3. Measurement of circulatory time and estimation of flow volume is possible.
4. Fluorescein angiography of vessels permits an indirect assessment of not only microvascular structures but nonvascular structures. For example, one can diagnose defects in the pigment epithelium because a direct view of the fluorescein-containing choroidal vessels is possible. In the normal eye, the choroid is masked by the retinal pigment epithelium. It is only visible during fluorescein angiography as a diffuse background fluorescence. Defects in this background fluorescence can be caused by dense pigment clumps within or overlying the pigment epithelium, such as those caused by preretinal or retinal hemorrhages or nevi.

Examination Method. 5–10 ml of sterile 10% fluorescein sodium solution are rapidly injected intravenously (within 2–3 seconds). The angiographic findings are documented by means of a specially equipped fundus camera with appropriate filters. A newer method is video angiography of the retina (Richard, 1984). A single shot or a series of shots are taken, up to the total number of exposures on the film, in rapid succession between the 6th and 30th second, then at longer intervals up to the 5th minute.

Sequence of Angiography. Shortly after the fluorescein dye is injected, a background illumination occurs (background mottling). The dye then enters the central retinal artery (arterial phase). An axial filling of the arteries is followed by complete arterial filling after an interval of 1.0–1.5 seconds. The second or capillary phase follows. Fluorescence shows at the posterior pole and in the peripapillary region, and fluorescence in the choroidal vessels increases. Individual variations in the timing of these phases are possible.

The third or venous phase is marked by an outflow of dye via the venous system. Fluorescence can be observed when the dye enters the macular venules. Initially, a laminar flow occurs in the large veins. Normally it takes between 4 and 5 seconds for the fluorescein dye and the venous blood to mix totally, indicating complete filling of the venules.

The so-called late phase occurs after 20-30 seconds when the fluorescein dye almost disappears from the retinal vessels except for a residual diffuse choroidal fluorescence that gradually disappears. Fluorescence can be seen in the optic disc area, especially at the margins, for 1 hour or longer.

In newly formed or diseased vessels the fluorescein dye may leak from intravascular compartments and can be observed within the surrounding tissues. Normal retinal circulation time is defined as the interval between the arterial filling and the beginning of the venous filling phase (approximately 8 seconds).

Relative Contraindications and Side Effects of Fluorescein Angiography. Relative contraindications are pregnancy and preexisting disease such as severe cardiovascular diseases and renal dysfunction. Complications or side effects caused by the fluorescein dye, such as headache, nausea, vomiting, or fainting, can be found in 5-20% of all cases (Enzmann and Ruprecht, 1982). Younger patients are most often affected. Acute side effects resolve within a few seconds after the injection, and in general all the symptoms disappear rapidly after 1 minute. Occasionally, a yellowish brown discoloration of the conjunctival skin and/or mucous membranes of the mouth or lips may appear a few minutes after injection of the dye. These side effects resolve within approximately 6 hours.

Rarely, more severe side effects such as pruritus, erythema, urticaria, hypertension, bronchospasm, or cardiac arrhythmia may occur. Anaphylactic shock is a life-threatening side effect that may occur in 0.1-0.5% of patients. Obtaining a complete medical history is important in the prevention of this serious complication. Precautions are indicated in patients with known allergies, hay fever, extrinsic asthma, bronchial asthma, and neurodermitis (Table 4).

Table 4. First Aid Items for Fluorescein Angiography

Antihistamine, such as clemastine fumarate (Tavist) (preferably prepared for intravenous injection)
Calcium (oral)
Epinephrine hydrochloride (1 ml/1000, injection)
Isotonic sodium chloride solution (two 5-ml vials)
Theophylline (injection)
Bronchodilator aerosol (β_2-adrenergic agonist)
Prednisolone (1000 ml, injection)
Lactated Ringer's blood plasma expander solution (two 500-ml, intravenous)
Intubation equipment, including several sizes of tracheal tubing
Oxygen equipment (respiration)
Intravenous catheter (several different sizes)

Doppler Sonography

Doppler sonography is an objective, noninvasive, percutaneous examination procedure that permits evaluation of the blood flow in extracranial cerebral arteries. In cases in which there is stenosis of the internal carotid artery that occludes more than 50% of the lumen, the accuracy of this method is estimated to be 95% (Botzler, 1982).

The ultrasound probe of the doppler device, which is connected to the skin with a contact gel, emits continuous ultrasonic waves that can be set at a frequency range between 4 and 8 MHz. The same probe also contains a receiver crystal that takes up the rejected ultrasound signals. This setup is used to emit ultrasonic signals onto the red blood cells that pass underneath the probe in the vessel. The signals are reflected from the cells with a corresponding change in frequency. The difference between the emitted and rejected frequencies is proportional to the blood flow rate. The rejected signals are in the audible range, allowing for an evaluation of the flow rate of red blood cells. Additionally, with the appropriate setup, the direction of the flow can be determined and monitored with a one-lead system using a hemotachometer.

For routine examination in the ophthalmologist's office, the test is usually limited to examination of the end branches of the ophthalmic artery (supraorbital artery and supratrochlear artery), the carotid sinus, and the internal carotid artery. The contact gel is applied to the ultrasonic probe (set at 8 MHz), and then the supraorbital artery and supratrochlear artery of the right half of the body are examined. The physiological blood flow direction occurs from the intracranial toward the extracranial side, or in the case of the orbit, from the inside toward the outside. The internal carotid artery and its branches show a higher arterial pressure than the external carotid arteries and its branches. The direction of the blood flow does not change when the homolateral branches of the external carotid artery (superficial temporal artery and facial artery) are compressed. The blood flow remains continuous in the normal direction (orthograde flow). Because the peripheral resistance is decreased when the vessels are compressed, the audible signal from the arteries increases in intensity due to the acceleration of the blood flow. The monitor or hemotachometer shows an increase in amplitude of the pulsation.

If the perfusion of the internal carotid artery is significantly decreased, the hemodynamics of the blood flow change. The blood then flows in a retrograde fashion from extracranial to intracranial vessels. In other words, the blood finds its way into the orbit via collateral vessels of the external carotid artery. If the unilateral branches of the external artery are manually compressed, the direction of the blood flow is inversed again. During doppler sonography the signal decreases in intensity. The hemotachometer shows an inversion of the pulse amplitude associated with a decrease in amplitude size. A reverse in the direction of the blood flow or decrease in the signal obtained from the supraorbital or supratrochlear artery during the external compression are important clinical signs for a distortion in the normal perfusion of the internal carotid artery. Angiography of the carotids may be indicated for further diagnostic verification (Fig. 7).

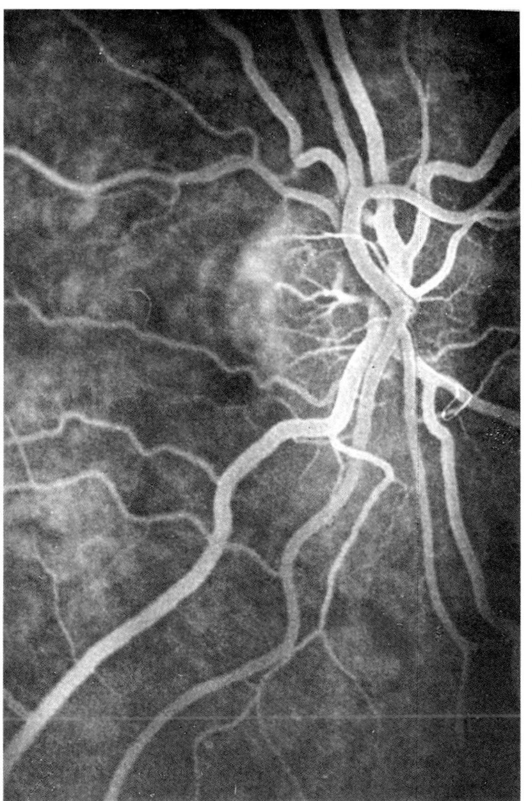

6

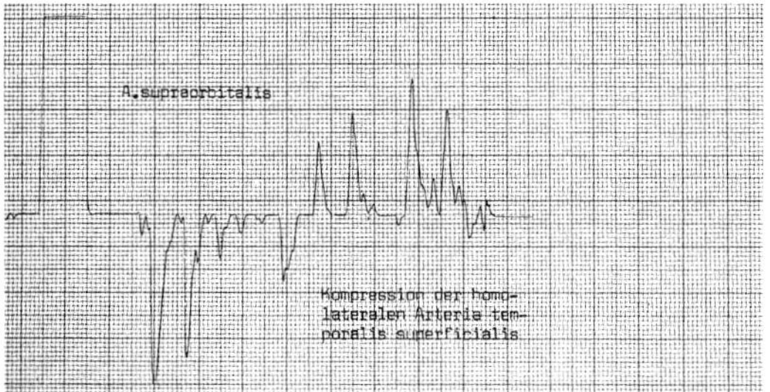

7

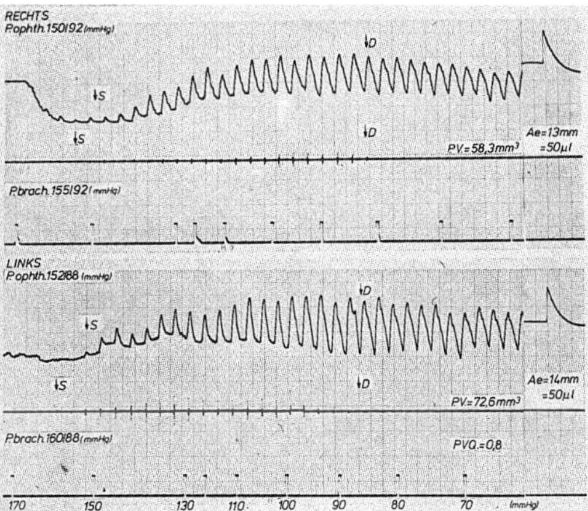

8

Figure 6. A fluorescein angiographic venous filling phase, as seen here, is an example of a vital staining technique used to evaluate fundus vessels. The fluorescein is clearly visible within the retinal arteries and veins.

Figure 7. Hemotachometer printout of the supraorbital artery in the left eye of a 70-year-old male patient with stenosis of the left carotid artery.

Clinical Findings

Visual acuity in the right eye is 20/30, and in the left eye, 20/1000. Ophthalmoscopical examination of the left eye revealed a central retinal artery occlusion with the presence of a cilioretinal artery (see Figs. 68–71). Doppler sonography revealed a normal, orthograde blood flow with an enhanced signal of the supraorbital artery induced by compression of the homolateral superficial temporal artery. At the same time, the hemotachometer showed increased spikes. The blood flow on the left side was inversed (retrograde). A compression of the left superficial temporal artery reversed the blood flow and diminished the acoustic signals of the supraorbital artery. After decompensation of the temporal artery, the signal returned to the original level.

Figure 8. Printout of an ophthalmodynamogram of the left eye of a 68-year-old female patient with acute ischemia of the left optic nerve. The right eye showed an optic atrophy.

Clinical Findings

Visual acuity in both eyes was 20/1000. The blood sedimentation rate showed a value of 92/128 mm. A temporal artery biopsy was negative for temporal arteritis. This case represents a clinical pseudo-Foster-Kennedy syndrome not caused by a stenosis of the carotid artery. The ophthalmodynamogram showed a normal synchronism of arterial pressures in the brachial and ophthalmic artery. The pulsation volume in the right eye was 58.3 µl, and in the left eye, 72.6 µl. The oscillometric index (ratio of pulsation volumes) is therefore 0.8. Values smaller than 0.66 or larger than 1.32 indicate a large difference between the two eyes, which is considered to be pathological.

Light Reflexes of the Fundus

The term "light reflexes of the fundus" was suggested by Vodovozov in 1981. The reflexes that may be seen in an ophthalmoscopic examination include retinal reflexes and reflexes created on the optic disc, Bruch's membrane, or the internal limiting membrane.

Vodovozov's Classification

Normal Light Reflexes

1. The physiological foveolar reflex is created in the excavation of the foveola, which acts like a concave mirror. A missing or attenuated reflex can be interpreted as either a flattening or elevation of the foveola.

2. The ring-like macular reflex is created by the light reflected on the surface of the thickened rim of the fovea.

3. Intramacular, paramacular, or perimacular reflexes are not always visible. The so-called paramacular reflex, found just peripheral to the macular reflex, is created by the concave surface of the retina in this area ("ditch reflex"). The perimacular reflex is created by a slight, ring-shaped elevation of the retinal surface just outside the paramacular region. The intramacular reflex can only be found if the central fovea is elevated and cylinder shaped.

4. Dot or fleck reflexes, found in areas close to retinal vessels, are created on the surface of the external limiting membrane. These reflexes are shaped irregularly and are found most often in the eyes of younger people.

5. Gunn's dots are small yellow spots that are most commonly seen in the peripapillary region. These dots correlate clinically to the Müller cell footplate attachment to the inner limiting membrane.

6. In rare cases, vertical linear reflexes situated between the optic disc and the macular region can be seen.

7. Reflexes on vessels are usually a normal observation. However, pathological vascular reflexes, including "copper wire" or "silver wire" reflexes, represent alterations of the vessel walls, seen in such conditions as arteriosclerosis.

Pathological Light Reflexes

1. Fan-shaped reflexes, found between the foveola and the macular reflex (triangular reflex), are created by changes in the normal morphology of the central fovea, e.g., retinal edema or myopic changes.

2. Focal reflexes are usually ring-shaped and can be found surrounding an elevated retinal lesion or on its most elevated point. Sometimes focal reflexes are the only signs of a beginning lesion.

3. Papillary reflexes can be found either adjacent to, or on, the optic disc. According to Vodovozov (1965), such reflexes are diagnostically significant in early or beginning papilledema. In a beginning papilledema, a semilunar or sickle-shaped reflex can be seen right at the papillary margin. This reflex increases in size toward the optic disc as the papilledema progresses, and it is close to the border of a peripapillary retinal edema. Another example of a peripapillary reflex is the so-called "Weiss reflex," found in myopic eyes.

4. Linear reflexes show either a double contour or have a radial appearance, and may be found in retinal scars. They appear bright and extend radially from the focus. Double contour linear reflexes, usually in pairs, can be found after blunt trauma with associated retinal edema and folds.

5. Stationary reflexes can be found in central fibroproliferative retinal degenerations. The "cellophane macula" described by Gass (1970) belongs in this group.

6. Metallic reflexes (tapetal reflexes) may appear as a shining gold or silver reflex. The gold reflex is found in the macular area, and the silver reflex is seen usually more peripherally. In some cases, such reflexes are the only signs of tapetoretinal degeneration.

7. Crystal reflexes are created by the edges or facets of crystals deposited in the retina. A typical example is the cholesterol crystals that are deposited in the retina and retinal vessels during the course of several different diseases.

Developmental Anomalies

Macular Colobomas

Synonym: Dysplasia of the macula.

This entity has been the topic of many controversial discussions since it was first described by von Ammon in 1852. Some authors believe that a macular coloboma in the fetal eye is caused by an intrauterine or postpartal chorioretinitis or retinochorioiditis (toxoplasmosis infection, syphilis, tuberculosis). Others postulate that colobomas are caused by birth trauma. Another group interpreted this anomaly as a mesodermal or neuroectodermal malformation. Elschnig (1907) suspected an active proliferation of the embryonic optic cup walls in an abnormal direction. Badtke (1958), basing his theory on histological findings, believed that atypical gaps within the retina may be caused by malclosure of an embryonic ocular fissure that is situated in an atypical location.

Heredofamilial cases of colobomas of the macula have been observed (Clausen, 1921; Schott, 1921; Vogelsang, 1936; Evans, 1937). Combinations of this malformation with other anomalies such as microencephaly, microophthalmus, and skeletal and organ anomalies or dysplasias have been described (Sorsby, 1935).

Based on morphological differences, Mann (1927) divided macular colobomas into three different groups: (*a*) pigmented macular colobomas, (*b*) nonpigmented macular colobomas, and (*c*) macular colobomas associated with atypical vessels. She suggested the term "macular dysplasia" should be reserved for true developmental colobomatous defects (Fig. 14).

Colobomas of the Retina and Choroid

In the normal development of the eye, the lips of the embryonic ocular fissure fuse between the 4th and 6th week of gestation. The developmental defect that is termed a coloboma ensues if this normal closure is incomplete. The defect may involve any portion of the embryonic optic cup along its inferonasal aspect and may affect the iris, ciliary body, retina and choroid, and optic nerve. Alterations may occur separately or in various combinations that range in size from a minimal focus such as a crescent or conus, to an extension over the entire length of the embryonic ocular fissure. Genetic transmissions have been observed, and in some cases, colobomatous defects are associated with other bone or organic anomalies (pelvis-shoulder dysplasia syndrome, Gruber's syndrome, Schimmelpennig-Feuerstein-Mims syndrome, Wiedemann's syndrome).

Ophthalmoscopical Appearance. In typical cases the defect is oriented inferonasally. Normally the tapering end of a colobomatous defect affecting the fundus is oriented toward the optic disc and sometimes involves the optic disc. The margins of the defect, which is often parabolic in shape (Fig. 9), are well demarcated and darkly pigmented. The coloboma surface has a yellow grayish-white discoloration. The vessels within the lesion have a rarified, atypical appearance, and a concavity or staphylomatous defect may be present. Choroidal vessels and the retinal pigment epithelium are usually absent, which explains the color imparted by the overlying sclera. Bilateral defects are seen occasionally (Figs. 9–11).

Bridge Coloboma

A bridge coloboma (rudimentary coloboma) represents a defect in which a normal fundus can be seen between the colobomatous erosions. The intervening retina and choroid are not affected (Fig. 10).

Optic Disc Coloboma

Ophthalmoscopically, an optic disc coloboma often shows an inferior conus (Fuchs' coloboma) or presents as an enlarged or deformed optic nerve (tilted disc syndrome) (Figs. 12 and 13). Peripapillary atrophy of the retina and choroid may be present. No visible central vessels are seen at the gray-green to gray-violet optic nerve head because the vessels branch out in the optic nerve before reaching the head. The atypically coursing vessels are located close to the optic disc margin. Functional visual deteriorations depend on the size and location of the defect.

Medullated Retinal Nerve Fibers

The myelinization of the visual tract occurs in a centrifugal manner and is complete up to the lamina cribrosa by the 9th month of gestation. Sometimes the maturation continues into the 1st month of extrauterine life. Myelinated nerves may be seen in the retinal nerve fiber layer anterior to the lamina cribrosa, which leads to the condition termed "medullated retinal nerve fibers" (Figs.

15-20). Nerve sheath maturation does not progress beyond the 1st year of life. It is estimated that the incidence of medullated nerve fibers is approximately 5%. In patients with a descending optic nerve atrophia that may be associated with a demyelinizing disease such as multiple sclerosis, medullated nerve fiber can recede or disappear. Other causes for this phenomenon include optic neuritis, glaucomatous optic atrophy, or papilledema.

Usually medullated optic nerve fibers are a harmless anomaly that does not affect visual function significantly. However, if the area subtended by the medullated nerve fibers is very large, visual field defects may be present.

Ophthalmoscopical Appearance. Medullated nerve fibers usually extend from the margin of the optic disc peripherally. The fibers are white and feathery in appearance and are often bright and shiny. Sometimes medullated fibers can be observed that have no connection to the optic disc. The retinal vessels are commonly masked by these fibers.

Epipapillary Glial Membrane

This entity, also referred to as persistent Bergmeister's papilla, has a hazy or veil-like appearance. It is caused by proliferation of the glial sheaths of the hyaloid artery. This harmless anomaly usually develops during the 2nd embryonic month.

Ophthalmoscopical Appearance. The epipapillary or peripapillary membrane that characterizes this condition is usually delicate, gray-white, and translucent. It may partially cover the optic disc margin and peripapillary vessels (Fig. 21).

Optic Pit

This malformation is sometimes termed congenital excavation of the optic disc (Figs. 22-24). It should be distinguished from typical colobomas of the optic disc in which the lesion is situated in the inferonasal quadrant above the site of the embryonic fissure (Duke-Elder, 1964; Kranenburg, 1960).

Ophthalmoscopical Appearance. In addition to the physiological optic disc excavation that contains the emerging central retinal vessels, an optic pit typically consists of one or more pathological excavations that may be as deep as 10 diopters (approximately 3 mm). These lesions are usually gray, gray-brown, or gray-green. Most optic pits are situated in the temporal or inferotemporal quadrant.

In as many as 30% of cases, an associated serous or exudative separation of the sensory retina from the pigment epithelium occurs in the macular region (Kranenburg, 1960). Some authorities believe that the fluid is derived from the vitreous cavity and flows via the colobomatous defect into the subretinal space.

The development of a lamellar hole partially involving the macular area and associated with a congenital excavation of the optic disc was described by Huismans (1979a). Tillmann and Antoniadis (1973) reported an extremely rare case of a peripheral retinal detachment associated with an optic pit.

Duplication of the Optic Disc

Duplication of the optic disc is extremely rare and is probably caused by a malocclusion of the fetal fissure of the optic cup or fetal optic nerve stalk. Existence of this anomaly has been proven microscopically and histologically in autopsy eyes. True duplication of the optic nerve disc has been described. Other reports have described only the presence of aberrant nerve fiber bundles or isolated duplication of the optic nerve. The left eye is affected more often than the right eye. In a few cases, a duplication of the bony optic nerve channel was seen by roentgenogram (x-ray). Usually the existing optic nerve channel was normal size.

Juxtapapillary colobomas can resemble optic disc duplication. Similarly retinal foci caused by congenital toxoplasmosis or other embryopathies have to be considered in the differential diagnosis. Duplication of the optic disc may be combined with other malformations such as epipapillary membranes, retinochoroidal colobomas, iris colobomas, and nystagmus.

Ophthalmoscopical Appearance. In an otherwise healthy eye, a smaller, equally large, or larger accessory optic disc may be found. Such lesions are most often located inferior to the regularly shaped optic disc. An accessory optic disc may be in contact with the original disc or totally separated from it. Marginal pigmentation of the accessory disc can vary widely.

In contrast to the optic disc pseudoduplication that can be found with colobomatous defects, this anomaly is a true duplication of the vessels. In the colobomatous eye there is a typical vascular pattern of major arterial branches that curve around the margin of the coloboma and disappear and/or reappear out of the colobomatous excavation.

Functional Loss. Functional loss with optic disc duplication depends largely on the location of the anomaly. Central visual acuity is not necessarily affected. Visual field testing usually reveals an absolute scotoma that corresponds with ophthalmoscopical findings.

Enlargement of the Optic Disc

Synonym: Megalopapilla.

According to Franceschetti and Bock (1950) the average optic disc measures 1.62 ± 0.015 mm in diameter (see also Jaeger, 1983). With congenital megalopapilla, these measurements are much larger than normal; often the optic disc diameter is twice as large as seen in a physiologically normal optic disc. This anomaly, first described by Bock in 1949, can occur both unilaterally or bilaterally. According to Duke-Elder (1976), megalopapilla is caused when excessive mesectodermal or glial tissues migrate into the optic nerve stalk during fetal development. Megalopapilla is not necessarily associated with an enlargement of the optic foramen (Figs. 25 and 26).

Hypoplasia and Aplasia of the Optic Disc

Aplasia is defined as a complete absence of the optic disc and the central retinal vessels. This anomaly is extremely rare. Hypoplasia of the optic disc is seen more often. It usually occurs bilaterally, but in unilateral cases, the affected eye often has poor visual acuity. Orthoptic training is not indicated. Hypoplasia has been observed in combination with such other malformations as microphthalmus, coloboma, cyclopia, microcephalus or hydrocephalus, anencephalus, and encephalomeningocele.

Ophthalmoscopically, the optic disc is decreased more than one-third in size and shows a gray-white discoloration, although the vessels may appear normal. In some cases, the hypoplastic optic disc is surrounded by an irregularly pigmented anulus. Von Szily (cited by Aichmair, 1968) observed three different forms of this disease: optic disc hypoplasia with a circular appearance (Fig. 27), hypoplasia with forward differentiation of the optic disc anlage, and an extremely rudimentary optic disc with an atypical structure, shape, and margin.

In some cases, a roentgenogram reveals a smaller foramen opticum on the affected side. Diagnosis of this condition can be verified by an objective evaluation of the optic disc size using Littmann's method.

Congenital Central Glial Dysplasia of the Optic Nerve Head

Synonym: Morning glory syndrome.

Congenital central glial dysplasia of the optic nerve head was identified by Handmann in 1929. It is thought to be caused by an incomplete closure of the embryonic fissure with prolapse of tissues into the colobomatous defect. (Apple and Rabb, 1985).

Ophthalmoscopical Appearance. The optic disc is normal in size and is surrounded by a broad, irregularly pigmented tissue anulus. Sometimes this circle is incomplete and shaped like a half-moon. Pau (1980) described this condition as a peripapillary staphyloma of the sclera because the optic disc is dislocated posteriorly. The excavation is funnel- or cylinder-shaped. The optic disc margins are well-defined and have a gray-green discoloration. The central excavation and vessels are missing, replaced by a homogeneous, dense mass of white tissue from glial proliferation. The vessels of the optic nerve, which may be decreased in diameter, originate close to the papillary margin. It is not rare to observe additional cilioretinal arteries or opticociliary veins coursing radially across the disc margin.

Kindler (1970) compared the congenital central glial dysplasia of the optic nerve head, as described by Handmann, with an optic disc anomaly he termed the "morning glory syndrome." The pink-colored optic disc is extensively enlarged, and a funnel-shaped or cylindrical staphyloma of the sclera is typically observed. Central vessels and the normal physiological, pink excavation are replaced by a central gray-white tissue mass. The vessels are affected the same way in both conditions, and in both conditions, the peripheral retina is normal. The central retina shows pigment irregularities, cystic anomalies, and/or features that closely resemble central serous retinopathy. Both entities have been reported in combination with other anomalies, such as congenital ptosis, microcornea, congenital cataract, persistent hyaloid artery, persistent hyperplastic primary vitreous, and excessive myopia. Sometimes a congenital hypoplastic malformation of the kidneys associated with chronic, progressive renal insufficiency is found. Hereditary transmission has been described. Most ophthalmologists today agree that the anomaly described by Handmann and Kindler's morning glory syndrome are variations of the same malformation.

Persistent Bergmeister's Papilla

This anomaly, named for Bergmeister (1877), is caused by retention of glial sheath elements composed of undifferentiated hypoplastic tissue. Normal resorption or atrophy of this embryonic epithelial papilla and hyaloid vascular structures is incomplete. Physiologically, this involution should be terminated in the 5th month of gestation.

Ophthalmoscopical Appearance. The optic disc shows epipapillary or peripapillary delicate, white to green membranes, which give a washed-out appearance to the optic disc margins (differential diagnosis: glioma, papilledema). The hyperplastic tissue sometimes protrudes into the vitreous. The central retinal vessels are usually not visible in the central disc area but reappear at the disc margin. At this site, cilioretinal arteries or opticociliary veins can be seen. The optic disc is not enlarged, but the macula often appears to be incompletely developed.

Persistent Hyaloid Artery

Persistence of the fetal hyaloid artery, which contributes to the nutrition of the vitreous, is caused by an incomplete atrophy of the vessel at approximately the 7th month of gestation.

Ophthalmoscopical Appearance. The optic disc margins appear washed out, and the disc is hyperemic. The arterial trunk arises from the center of the optic disc and grows anteriorly from the optic nerve head toward the crystalline lens. The persistent hyaloid artery appears grayish and usually moves within the vitreous humor. Sometimes a funnel-shaped opening can be seen anteriorly (Figs. 28 and 29).

Complications. Occasionally a nonrhegmatogenous tractional retinal detachment can be found.

Cilioretinal Arteries

This vascular anomaly can be found in approximately 10% of all individuals. The vessels originate from the choroidal vascular system and participate in the retinal blood supply. In central retinal artery occlusions, these extra vessels may help maintain central visual acuity or prevent some visual field deficiencies. However, in eyes in which the macular region is supplied by cilioretinal arteries, occlusion of these vessels can sometimes lead to an irreversible central scotoma.

Ophthalmoscopical Appearance. Cilioretinal arteries are most often curved around the temporal margin of the optic disc, extend toward the central fovea, and run parallel to the maculopapillary bundle (Figs. 30, 66, and 300).

Opticociliary Artery or Vein

The opticociliary artery emerges from the physiological excavation of the optic disc and contributes to the choroidal blood supply. The opticociliary vein collects venous blood from the choroidal system, which is then released into the central retinal vein. Both vascular variations are rare (Figs. 32–34).

Opticociliary veins sometimes also can be found as a secondary neovascularization caused by hemorrhagic secondary glaucoma or papilledema, or associated with trauma (shunt veins).

Ophthalmoscopical Appearance. Opticociliary arteries or veins are easily overlooked (Figs. 31 and 231) (differential diagnosis: cerebral angiomas or aneurysms). The patient has otherwise unexplained neurological symptoms, e.g., unilateral seizures. The presence of numerous cilioretinal arteries, which may be in unusual locations and show multiple curves or aneurysmatic dilations with or without the presence of opticociliary vessels, are highly suspicious for this condition. According to Glees (1956), one cannot conclude that an aneurysm or angioma is located on the same side as the ophthalmological vascular anomalies.

Fundus Changes in Ametropic Eyes

Myopia

Myopia can be caused by several mechanisms:

Refractive Myopia

The anatomic site for refractive myopia is either the cornea (keratoglobus, keratoconus) or the crystalline lens (lenticonus, lens subluxation or luxation, especially into the anterior chamber).

Index Myopia

Transitorial myopia can be caused by an increase in the refractive index of the crystalline lens, e.g., as a side effect of various drugs (without myosis and accommodative spasm) such as sulfonamides, diuretics, and tranquilizers. This condition also occurs in metabolic disorders such as diabetes mellitus.

Axial Myopia

This is the most important type of myopia affecting the fundus. There are two types of axial myopia:

Simple Myopia (Stationary Myopia). This type of myopia is usually not associated with functional disorders or changes in ocular tissues. Mimimal changes may occur, but usually decreased visual acuity is fully correctable. An electroretinogram (ERG) does not show any changes.

Malignant Myopia (Progressive or Excessive Myopia). This type of myopia is usually associated with severe functional changes and tissue alterations. Visual acuity is often markedly decreased, and an ERG shows pathological changes in 75% of cases.

Causes of Axial Myopia. Cohn and Lindner (cited by Müller and Pietruschka, 1976) theorized that extensive work involving small objects held close to the eye during early childhood was to blame for progressive axial myopia ("school myopia"). Steiger (cited by Müller and Pietruschka, 1976) related axial myopia to inherited factors. Badtke (cited by Müller and Pietruschka, 1976) explained myopia as a sequence of a congenital, abnormal increase in retinal growth.

Ophthalmoscopical Appearance. The temporal papillary margin shows a myopic sickle-shaped crescent. Depending on the amount of atropic tissue present, the crescent might appear white (scleral tissue) or grayish-brown (choroidal tissue). The retinal vessels run peripherally, straight from the optic disc.

Progressive myopic choroidal atrophy may cause the fundus to be lighter in color than is seen in healthy eyes. Choroidal vessels become visible, but are partially obliterated in later stages. The intravascular spaces are clearly discernible.

The sickle-shaped temporal crescent may progress to a circular atrophy that involves larger peripapillary areas. Degenerative areas that are round, oval, or spotty may develop. The posterior pole and the peripheral retina may be affected. Peripheral cystoid degeneration, situated between the ora serrata and the equator, may become the site of a later retinal detachment if a full thickness hole develops.

Ruptures in Bruch's membrane, which appear yellow and may be connected like a network, are termed "lacquer cracks." These alterations may lead to tears and hemorrhage in the macular region, finally causing proliferation of the retinal pigment epithelium. After the blood is resorbed, a gray to black spot, up to the size of the optic disc, may be seen (Foerster-Fuchs' spot). Greenish spots are called Stargardt's spots.

Other clinical signs of excessive myopia are supertraction and sclerectasia. Supertraction is created by a nasal elevation of the papillary margins, which causes a hazy, poorly determined papillary margin similar to that seen with the tilted disc syndrome. Sclerectasia is created by an extreme thinning of the sclera. This condition was termed "staphyloma posticum verum" by von Graefe in 1855. A staphyloma is a circumscribed excavation of the sclera and adjacent uveal tissue in the area of the posterior pole. This excavation may appear terraced or have ridges, be several diopters deep, and cover an area of several papillary diameters. The retinal vessels usually course around the margin of the ectatic area (Figs. 35–42).

Vitreous Affects. High myopia is often associated with vitreous liquifaction, haziness, and/or posterior vitreous detachment.

Inversed Location of Symptoms. In some patients the myopic conus is found nasally and is often associated with choroidal atrophy, supertraction, and atrophic areas.

Refractive Error and Progressive Myopia. There is no direct correlation between the amount of refractive error (in diopters) and progression of myopic fundus changes. Axial myopia usually does not increase past the age of 30. With pathological, progressive myopia, however, the anteroposterior axis of the globe can continue to lengthen, with degenerative and atrophic intraocular changes beyond the 3rd decade of life (Table 5).

Table 5. Grading of Myopia According to Refractive Error

Author	Low Grade Myopia	Middle Grade Myopia	High Grade Myopia
	diopters	*diopters*	*diopters*
Gasteiger, 1963	1–6	7–12	>12
Müller and Pietruschka, 1976	1–8	9–12	>12

High Myopia and Papilledema. In myopic eyes, papilledema may develop in a typical or atypical manner. Because myopic eyes have a reduced capability to develop edema, sometimes only a slight nasal papilledema can be seen. Depending on the presence of bilateral atrophic myopic changes, it may be difficult to evaluate an elevated intracerebral pressure by only observing the optic disc in a myopic eye.

High Myopia and Hypertension. The anteroposterior enlargement of the eye leads to stretching and thinning of the retinal vessels. Changes caused by hypertension in myopic eyes may be difficult to judge.

High Myopia and Glaucoma. Locating a glaucomatous excavation within large peripapillary choroidal atrophies caused by myopia may be a problem. The atropic excavations usually cause an enlargement of the blind spot (seen in visual field testing), which adds to the difficulty in diagnosing glaucoma in myopic eyes. However, atrophic changes and functional distortions may be absent in exceptional cases.

Therapy. The main treatment for myopia is optical correction with spectacles or contact lenses. Some trials with antimyopical drugs have been reported.

Hyperopia

There are several types of hyperopia. The following classifications, similar to those for myopia, have been differentiated:

Refractive Hyperopia

Refractive hyperopia may be caused by flat curvature of the cornea, by aphakia, or by lens luxation into the vitreous body. This condition may also be age-related (so-called "senile hyperopia").

Index Hyperopia

A transitory change in the refractive index of the crystalline lens may be caused in diabetic eyes when the patient's blood glucose concentration is lowered with one of the oral antidiabetic (sulfonylurea) class of drugs (e.g., Diabinese, Orinase, Tolinase) or with insulin.

Axial Hyperopia

Axial hyperopia is observed in microphthalmic eyes or in eyes with macular edema, e.g., in cases with central serous retinopathy. This condition is sometimes associated with orbital tumors, which may force the retina into several folds.

Refractive errors exceeding +6 diopters are unusual even in microphthalmic eyes. Only rarely does the refractive error in these eyes exceed +12 diopters.

Ophthalmoscopical Appearance. The optic disc found in highly hyperopic eyes is reddish, and it may appear prominent with nondistinct margins. This condition is sometimes called pseudoneuritis hyperopia. The prominent optic disc caused by axial hyperopic can be mistaken for papilledema, papillitis, and drusen papilla (deeply located drusen). The retinal vessels show normal thickness, increased tortuosity, and broader reflexes. Frequently, vascular curling can be seen (Fig. 43). Hyperopia is usually not associated with choroidal atrophy and functional disorders except for a change in refraction and related problems.

Hyperopia and Associated Diseases. The short axial length in hyperopic eyes associated with a smaller corneal diameter and narrower anterior chamber angle may predispose the eye to development of glaucoma. Furthermore, the increased accommodation that must be used to overcome the hyperopia may lead to development of a convergent strabismus in childhood. This phenomenon is explained by the increased accommodative impulse that is physiologically associated with converging eye movements. Hyperopic eyes may be also weak in the ability to fuse images.

Therapy. Optical correction with spectacles or contact lenses is usually the only treatment needed.

Differential Diagnosis of Tortuous Vessels. The differential diagnosis of tortuous vessels includes cardiac valve anomalies, cardiac insufficiency, polycythemia, sickle cell anemia, hereditary tortuous small retinal arteries with hemorrhage, Riley-Day syndrome, Fabry's disease, cryoglobulinemia, mucopolysaccaridosis type VI (Brailsford-Morquio disease).

Staphyloma-like Ectasia of the Posterior Fundus

Synonyms: Eccentrical posterior sclerectasia, posterior fundus ectasia, staphyloma-like ectasia. Depending on the location of the lesion, a temporal or nasal scotoma may be found during visual field testing.

This entity represents a nonhereditary, rare malformation of the fundus in nonmyopic eyes.

Characteristics

Morphological Criteria. This condition can appear unilaterally or bilaterally, is often symmetrical, and usually is found in the inferior half of the fundus. A sclerectasia, located either temporally or nasally, may vary in the depth of the excavation. The optic disc and macula may be also involved to different degrees.

Functional Criteria. A refractive anomaly, which cannot be corrected fully, and a scotoma may be present. Some ectatic areas may not be discovered with usual perimetrical testing because the test light may not illuminate the posteriorly dislocated staphylomatous excavation. The usually sufficient light intensity of the test dot may be too weak to be perceived in the depths of the cavity (Kommerell, 1969). Bitemporal or binasal scotoma can be corrected. This entity should not be misdiagnosed as a neurological disorder, e.g., as a lesion of the visual system.

Ophthalmoscopical Appearance. Ophthalmoscopy may be difficult to achieve because of so-called "fundus astigmatism." Such astigmatism-like findings represent multiple aberrations of the normal retinal image created by irregularities in the curvature of the fundus. When involved, the optic disc may show blurred margins or appear to be slightly prominent. The central vessels may be dislocated superiorly. The macula may have radial folds superior to the ectatic area. In the ectatic area, which may have different levels, the choriocapillaris may be atrophic, showing several large choroidal vessels and intervascular spaces. The retinal vessels within this area may be normal or elongated and thinned. If hyperpigmentation is present, it may appear in an irregular, scattered fashion (Denden, 1970).

Ectopia of the Macula

Synonym: Heterotropia of the macula.

Three forms of macular ectopia have been differentiated:

Primary Ectopia

This malformation is a hereditary anomaly without functional changes. Ophthalmoscopically, the macula is most often displaced inferiorly or, less often, superiorly. The space is decreased between the macular area and the superoinferior branch of the retinal artery.

Secondary Ectopia

Several retinal disorders may lead to a secondary ectopia of the macula, e.g., inflammatory or traumatic scar tissue formation (Fig. 158).

Pseudoectopia

Pseudoectopia is caused by a rotation of the globe around its sagittal axis. The distance between the macula and the optic disc is normal. The central retinal artery and its branches are also displaced in the direction of the rotation (Vodovozov, 1976a). Pseudoectopia of the macula can be found in hyperopic eyes with concomitant strabismus.

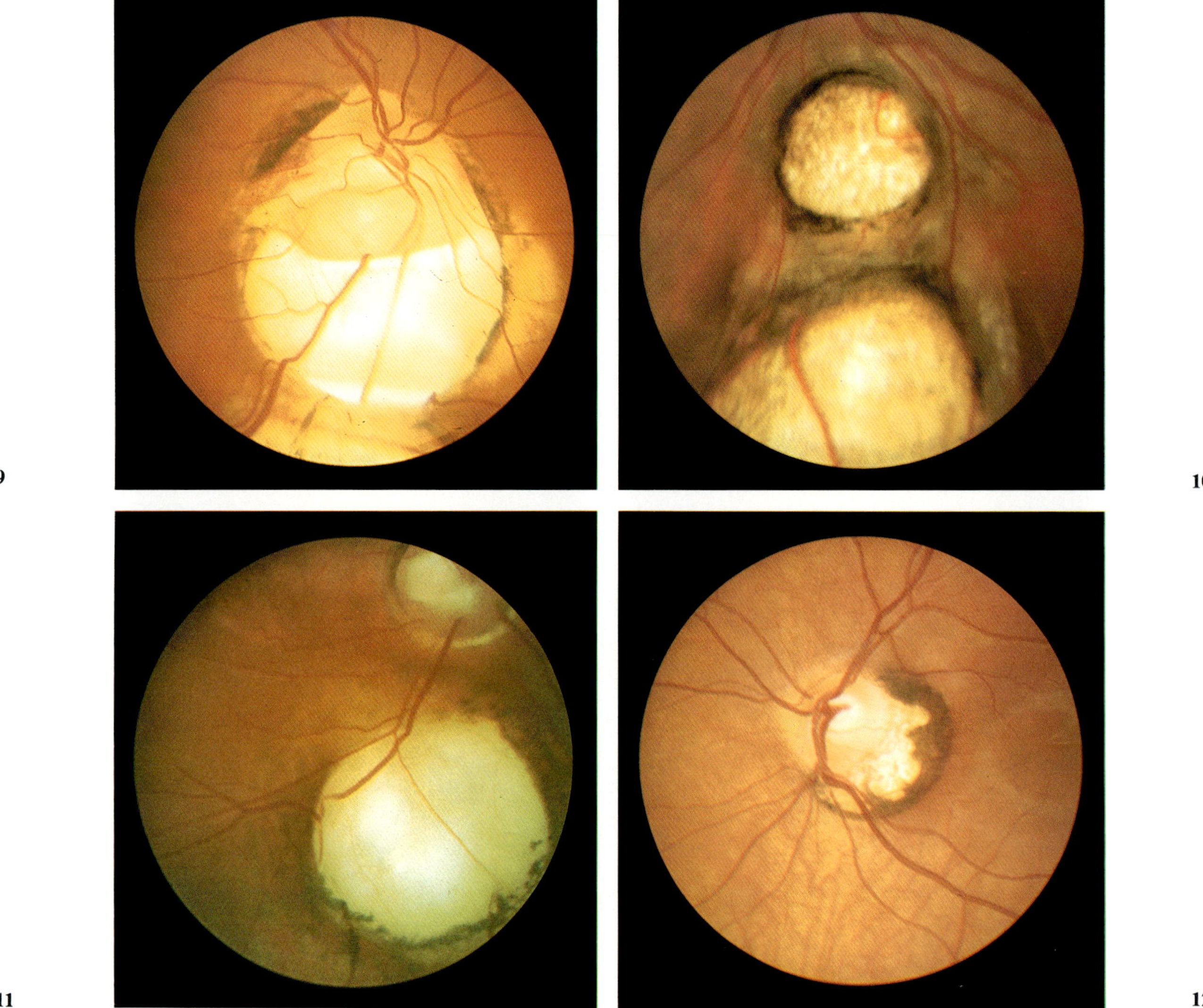

Figure 9. Right eye of a 45-year-old male patient with rudimentary coloboma of the retina and choroid. The optic disc is partially involved in the colobomatous excavation.

Clinical Findings

The right eye could be corrected with +0.25 sphere, −0.75 cylinder, axis 75° to a visual acuity of 20/25 despite the extension and location of this defect. The refractive media were clear. Intraocular pressure was 14 mm Hg. Visual field testing showed an absolute scotoma in an area adjacent to the blind spot that corresponds to the coloboma. Slitlamp examination confirmed the presence of an iris coloboma.

Figure 10. Left eye of a 24-year-old female patient with a bridge coloboma of the retina and choroid.

Clinical Findings

With a refraction of −3.75 sphere, −2.25 cylinder, axis 0°, corrected visual acuity was 20/25. Visual field examination showed a central scotoma and two small absolute scotomas in the peripheral field that matched the location of the colobomatous defects. An atypical microcoloboma (optic pit) was present in both eyes (see Figs. 23-24).

Clinical Course

A light coagulation treatment was performed on the temporal half of the posterior pole after a partial macular hole developed. Following this treatment, visual acuity could be corrected to 20/30.

Figure 11. Right eye of a 31-year-old male patient with a colobomatous defect of the optic nerve associated with a rudimentary coloboma of the retina and choroid.

Clinical Findings

With a correction of +11.25 sphere, −0.5 cylinder, axis 155°, visual acuity could be corrected to 20/25. The refractive media were clear. Visual field testing revealed an absolute scotoma that corresponded to the colobomatous defect. The left eye was emmetropic with normal binocular function.

Therapy

The severe anisometropia was corrected with a contact lens.

Figure 12. Left eye of a 16-year-old female patient with a small colobomatous defect of the optic nerve.

Clinical Findings

Both eyes were slightly myopic (−0.75 sphere), and visual acuity in both eyes was 20/30. Nystagmus was present. The refractive media were clear, and visual field testing showed normal borders. The blind spot was enlarged in the left eye. Mesopic vision and color vision were normal.

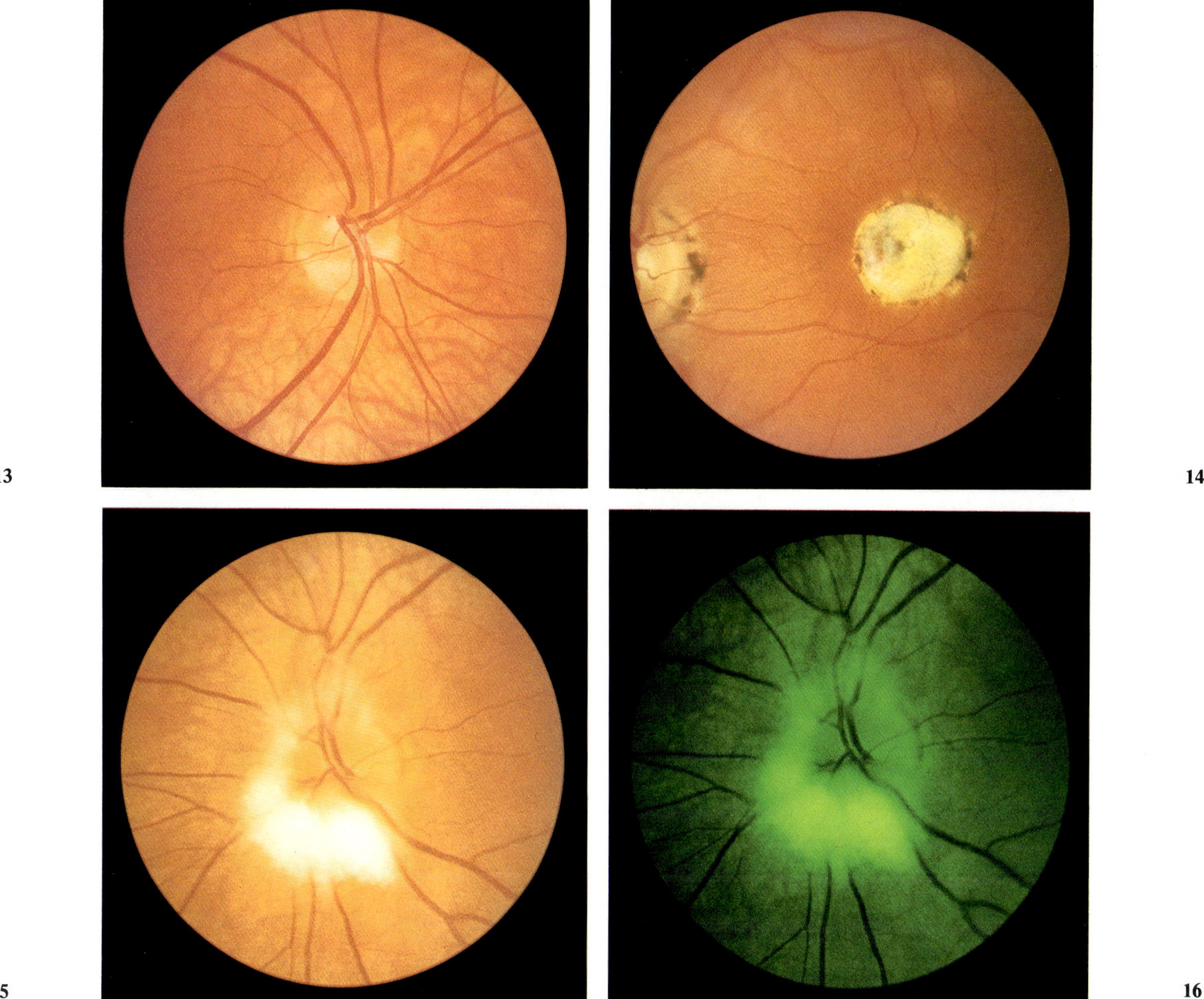

Figure 13. Right eye of a 20-year-old male patient with an inferior conus (Fuchs' coloboma).

Clinical Findings

This eye had a refractive error of +3.75 sphere, −1.0 cylinder, axis 15°. All other ocular findings were normal. An inferior conus or Fuchs' coloboma is believed to represent a rudimentary coloboma.

Figure 14. Left eye of a 37-year-old female patient with a macular coloboma (dysplasia).

Clinical Findings

With a refraction of +8.0 sphere, −1.0 cylinder, axis 160°, visual acuity was corrected to 20/400. A secondary divergent strabismus (exotropia) was present. The refractive media were clear except for peripheral corneal opacities. Visual field testing showed an absolute central scotoma. Ophthalmoscopical examination revealed an oval ectatic lesion that had replaced the macula. The lesion, which was one optic disc in diameter, had no normal structures in the ectatic area. The denuded sclera is visible. The marginal retinal choroidal scar is irregularly pigmented. Very fine radial retinal folds extend from the coloboma into the area surrounding the lesion.

Figure 15. Left eye of a 19-year-old female patient with medullated retinal nerve fibers.

Clinical Findings

A refractive error of +2.25 sphere, −1.0 cylinder, axis 170° was corrected to achieve a visual acuity of 20/50. The eye was amblyopic due to a convergent strabismus (esotropia). The refractive media were clear.

Figure 16. Same eye as in Fig. 15 photographed in a red-free light.

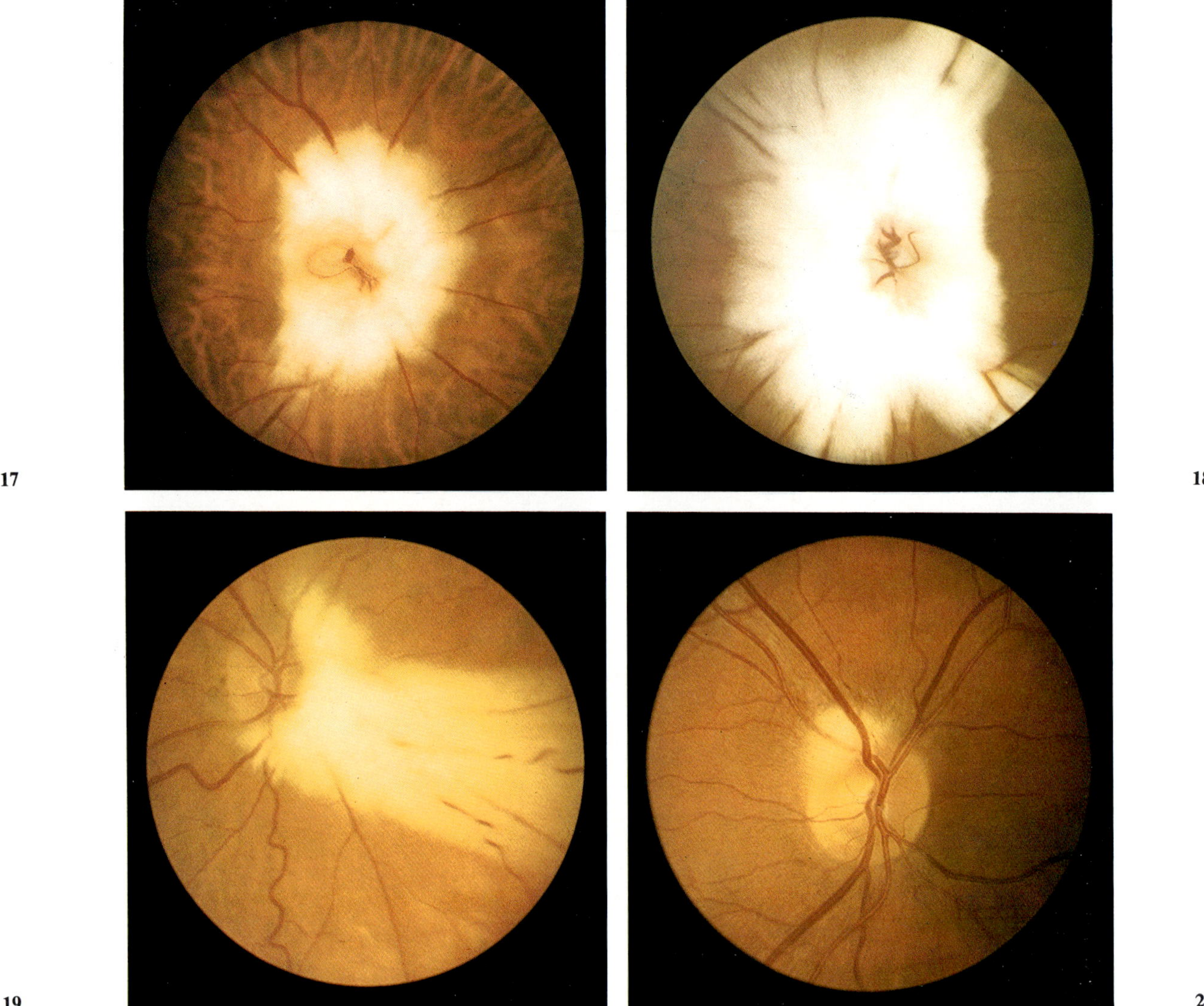
17 18
19 20

Figure 17. Right eye of a 45-year-old female patient with medullated retinal nerve fibers.

Clinical Findings

The eye was slightly hyperopic, requiring a correction of +2.5 sphere. Visual acuity was 20/20, and the refractive media were clear.

Figure 18. Left eye of a 40-year-old female patient with medullated retinal nerve fibers.

Clinical Findings

With a correction of −1.5 sphere, −2.0 cylinder, axis 95°, visual acuity was 20/25. The refractive media were clear.

Figure 19. Left eye of a 60-year-old female patient with medullated retinal fibers with a large extension from the optic disc. Note how the medullated nerve fibers nearly completely mask the retinal vessels (compare to Figs. 15–17).

Clinical Findings

Visual acuity was 20/30 with a correction of −2.5 sphere, −1.0 cylinder, axis 100°. The refractive media were clear.

Figure 20. Left eye of a 50-year-old male patient with medullated retinal nerve fibers that extend like a comet's tail from the optic disc.

Clinical Findings

The eye showed a hyperopia of +4.75 diopters. Visual acuity was 20/20, and the refractive media were clear.

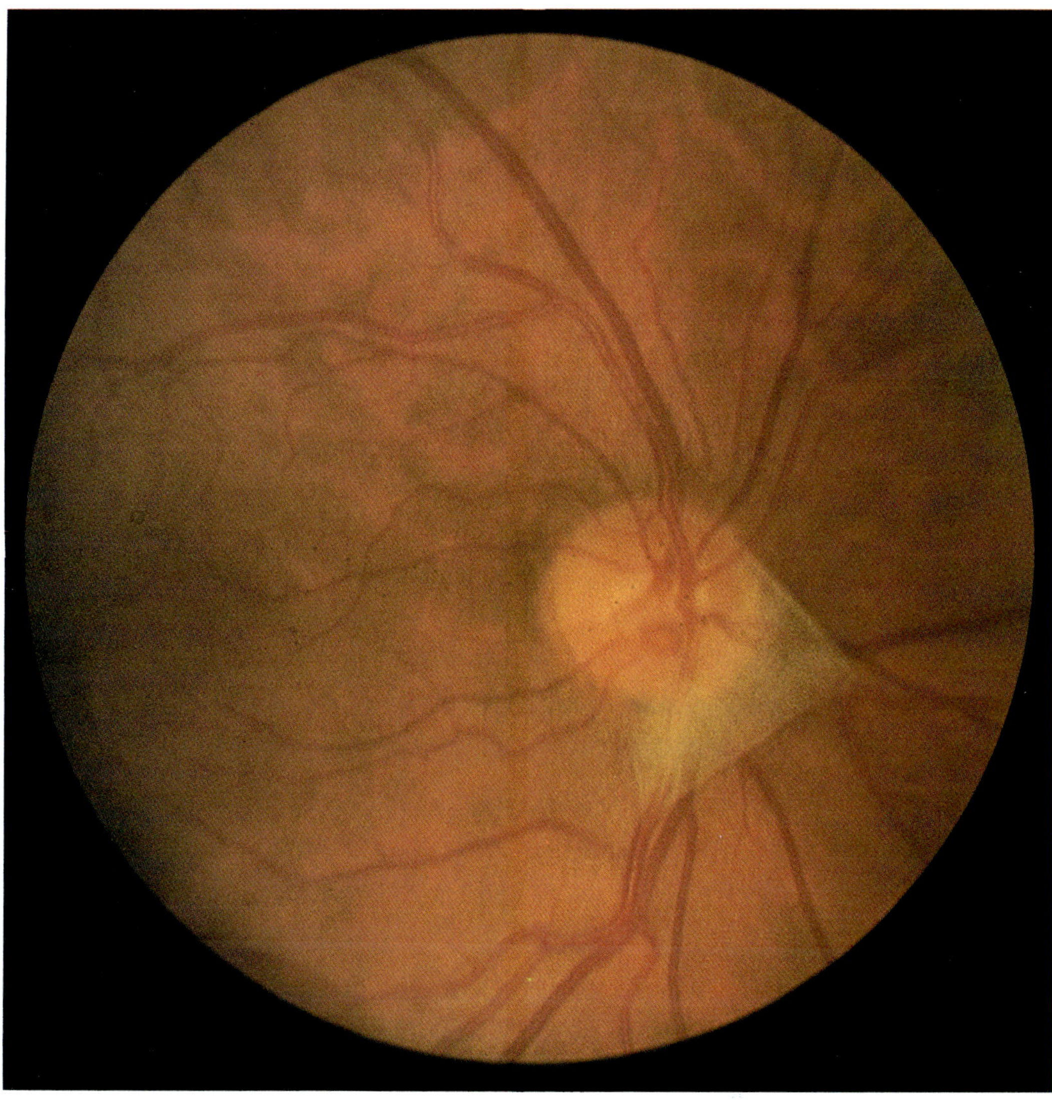

21

Figure 21. Right eye of a 40-year-old male patient with an epipapillary glial membrane.

Clinical Findings

The sail-shaped epipapillary membrane extends inferonasally from the optic disc and partially masks the nasal and inferotemporal vascular trunks. The refractive error in this eye was +1.0 sphere, −1.7 cylinder, axis 0°, and corrected visual acuity was 20/25. The refractive media were clear.

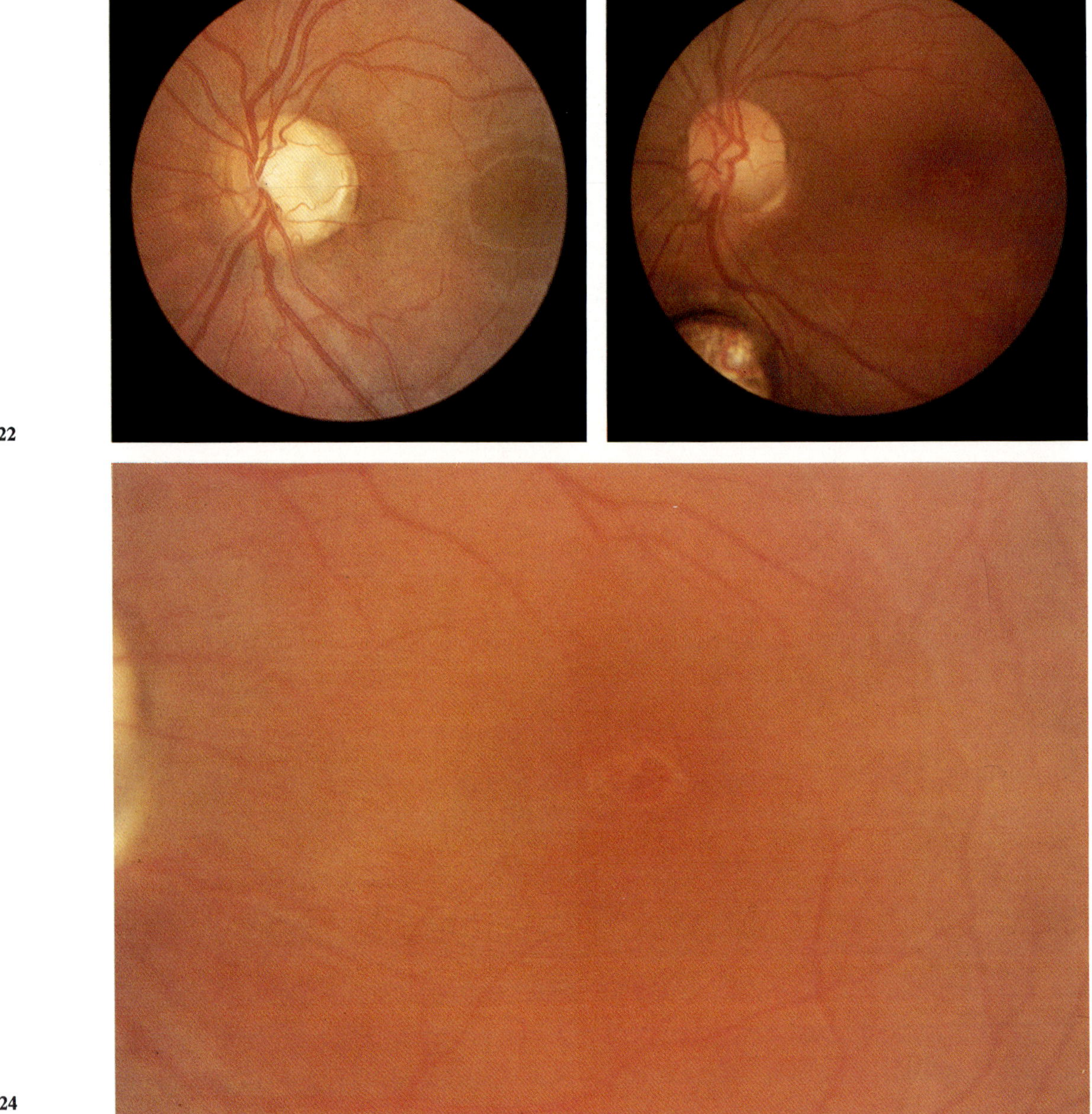

22

23

24

Figure 22. Left eye of an 8-year-old male patient with an atypical microcoloboma of the optic disc (optic pit).

Clinical Findings

The eye was slightly hyperopic (+1.25 diopters) but visual acuity was 20/20. The depth of the excavation was 1.5 diopters, measured ophthalmoscopically.

Figure 23. Left eye of a 24-year-old female patient with a combined developmental anomaly (Fuchs' coloboma and bridge coloboma) of the retina and choroid (see also Fig. 10). This myopic eye developed a partial macular hole (see Fig. 24).

Clinical Findings

The refractive error was −3.75 sphere, −0.25 cylinder, axis 100°, which corrected visual acuity to 20/25.

Clinical Course

The myopia increased a total of 2 diopters between March 1974 and August 1977. Assuming this was based on an axial myopia, the bulbus length must have increased 0.66 mm. The depth of the excavation was 2 diopters.

Figure 24. Same left eye as in Fig. 23 showing the partial macular hole. Best corrected visual acuity achieved following xenon light coagulation was 20/30.

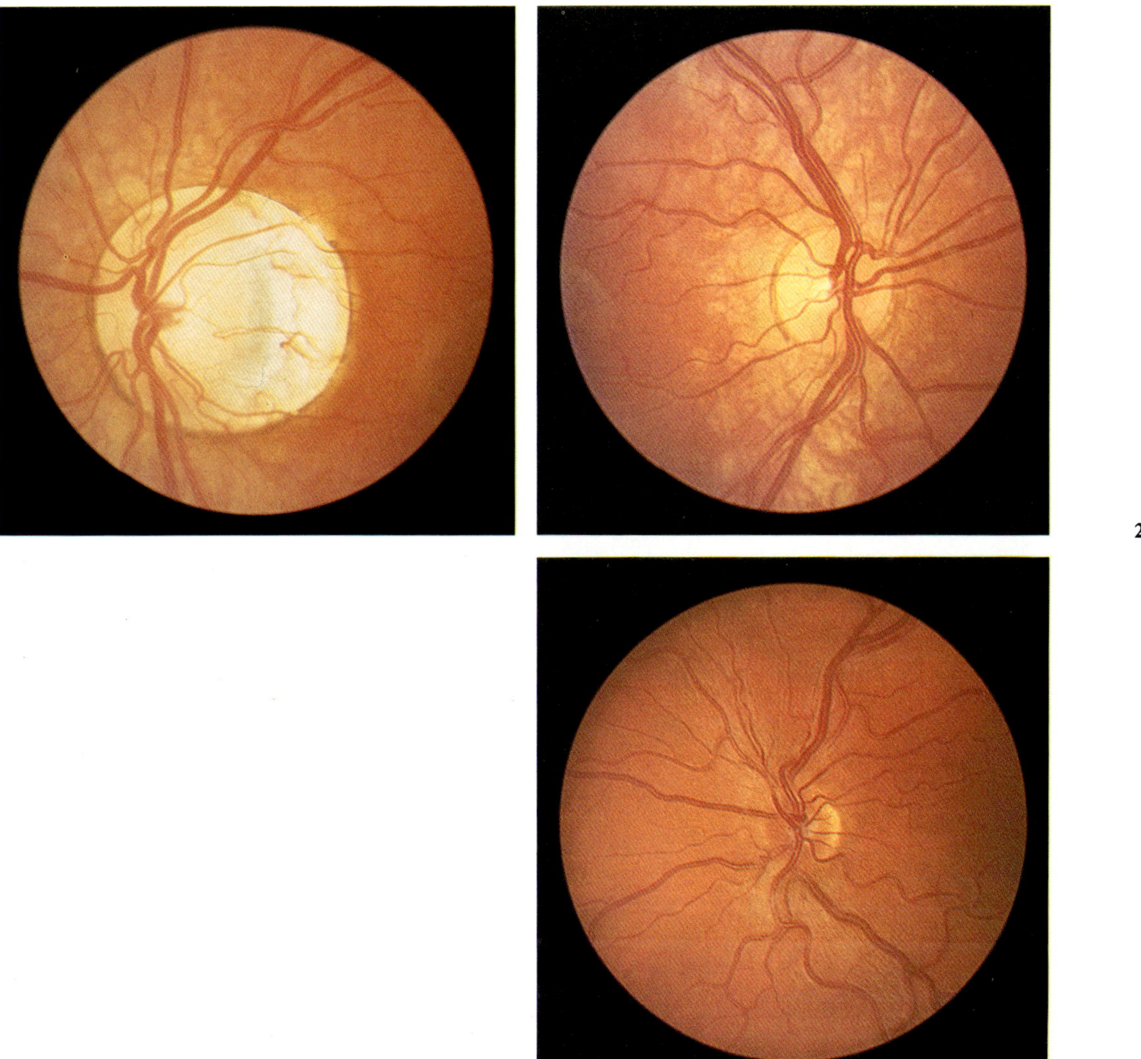
25 26
27

Figure 25. Left eye of a 5-year-old male patient with megalopapilla.
Clinical Findings
The objective refraction revealed nearly ametropic conditions (+0.25 sphere in both eyes). Visual acuity was 20/20 using the illiterate E chart. The refractive media were clear and binocular vision was intact. No nystagmus or distortion of color vision were found. Intraocular pressure was 14 mm Hg. The optic disc diameter in the right eye was 1.4 mm and in the left eye was 3.4 mm including the choroidal conus. Without the choroidal conus, the disc measured 2.52 mm. An x-ray evaluation showed normal symmetrical optic parenchyma in both eyes.

Figure 26. Right eye of the same patient as seen in Fig. 25. The optic disc in this fellow eye appears completely normal.

Figure 27. Left eye of a 14-year-old male patient with optic disc hyperplasia.
Clinical Findings
The objective refraction in both eyes was +4.0 diopters sphere and visual acuity was 20/20 in both eyes. Using the Littmann method, the optic disc diameter in the right eye was 1.4 mm and only 1.15 mm in the left eye. An x-ray examination showed both optic parenchyma had a normal symmetrical opening.

28

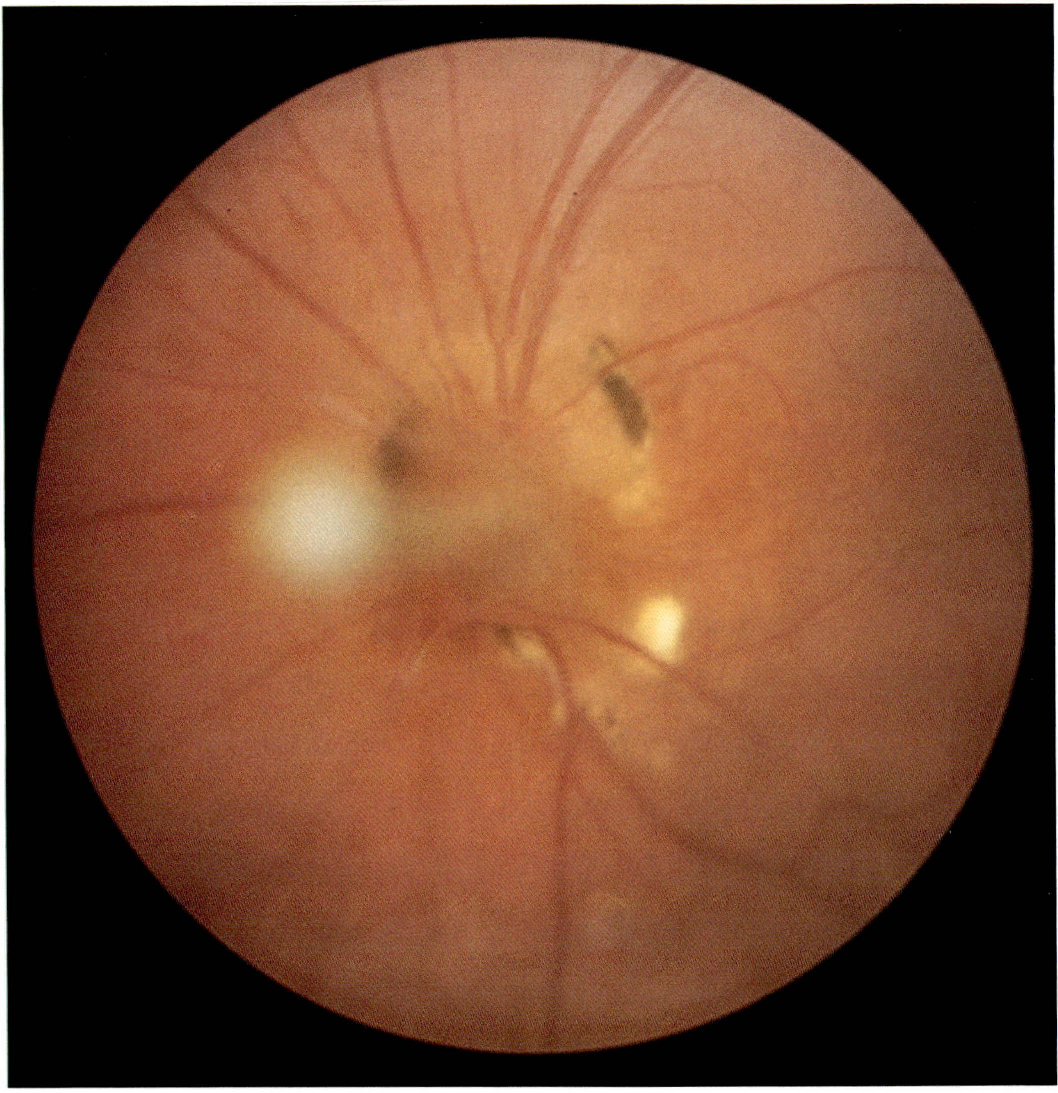

Figure 28. Left eye of an 18-year-old male patient with a persistent hyaloid artery.

Clinical Findings

The best corrected visual acuity achieved with a refraction of −1.25 cylinder, axis 170° was 20/400. This eye showed an esotropia, an anomalous trichromatism, and an extreme deuteranomaly.

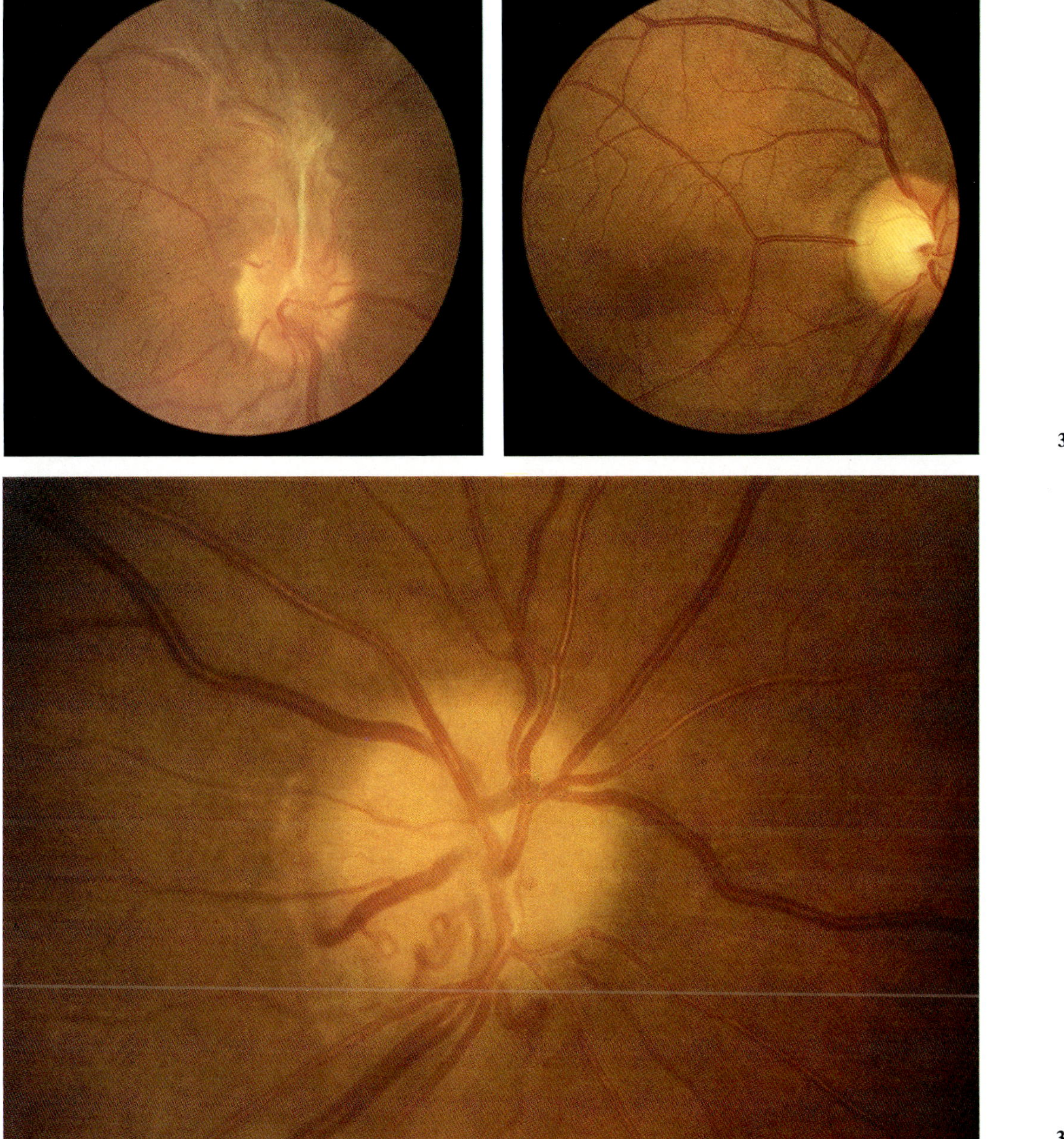

Figure 29. Right eye of a 25-year-old male patient with persistent hyaloid artery.

Clinical Findings

Visual acuity was 20/25 with a correction of +4.25 sphere, −2.0 cylinder, axis 75° in the right eye, and 20/20 in the left eye with a correction of +1.25 sphere. There was normal binocular function and color vision. A falciform retinal detachment was present in the right eye.

Figure 30. Right eye of a 20-year-old female patient with a normal fundus vascular variation.

Clinical Findings

Visual acuity was 20/20. A cilioretinal artery is present with widespread branching toward the macular region. This condition represents one variation of a normal fundus pattern.

Figure 31. Right eye of a 45-year-old female patient with an opticociliary vein.

Clinical Findings

Visual acuity is 20/20. A venous trunk connecting the central retinal vein with the choroidal circulation can be seen temporally (*left*). A neuroophthalmological examination found no abnormalities, and neurological and neuroradiological examinations were also normal. This fundus represents a nonpathological vascular variation.

32

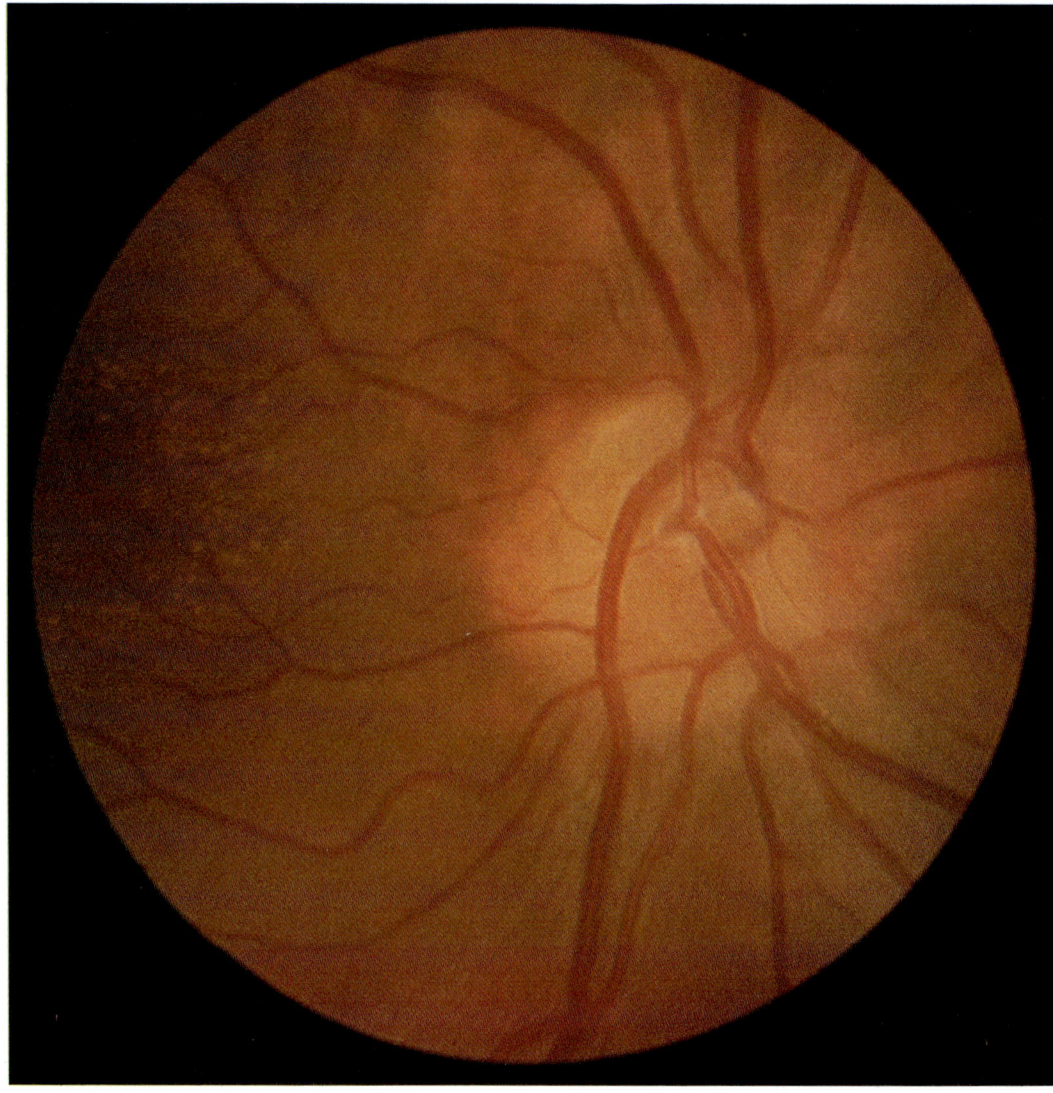

Figure 32. Right eye of a 40-year-old female patient showing venous variation of the central retinal vein, which originates superonasally and has an unusual branching pattern.

Clinical Findings

The eye was emmetropic with a visual acuity of 20/20. Note the presence of macular drusen.

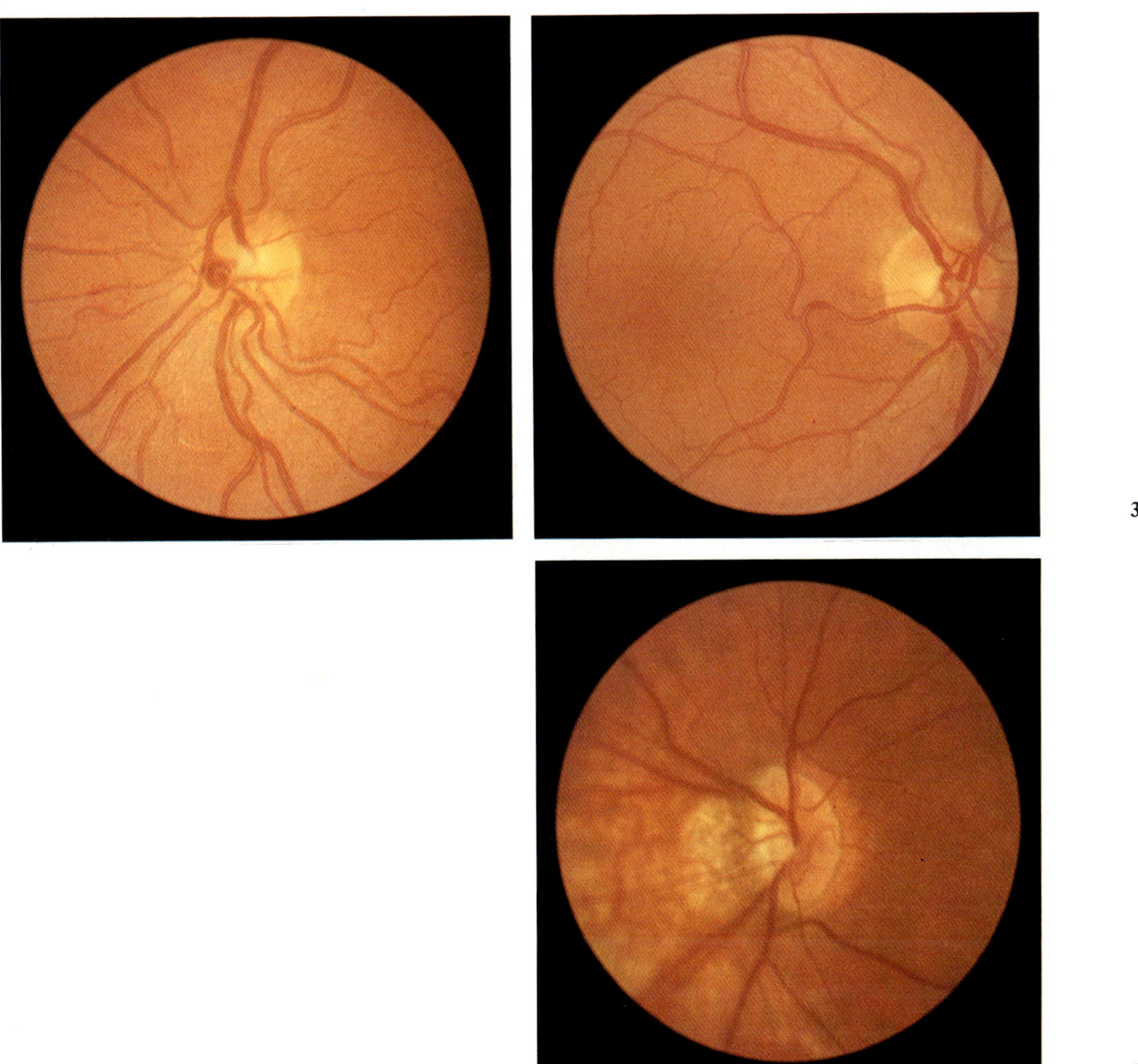

Figure 33. Left eye of a 20-year-old female patient showing a convoluted arterial variation.

Clinical Findings

The eye was moderately hyperopic (+3.0 diopters sphere) and visual acuity was 20/20 with correction.

Figure 34. Left eye of a 33-year-old female patient with macular arteriolar variation (see also Fig. 30). The four major branches of the retinal vascular system are supplemented by a more central macular arteriole.

Clinical Findings

Visual acuity was 20/25 with a correction of +0.5 sphere, −0.5 cylinder, axis 90°. The refractive media were clear.

Figure 35. Left eye of a 20-year-old male patient with malignant myopia (excessive myopia or progressive myopia). The optic disc shows a temporal crescent (conus myopicus).

Clinical Findings

With a correction of −15.5 sphere, −2.5 cylinder, axis 80°, visual acuity was only 20/1000 with an eccentric fixation. The optic nerve enters the eye at an acute angle causing the tilted disc appearance.

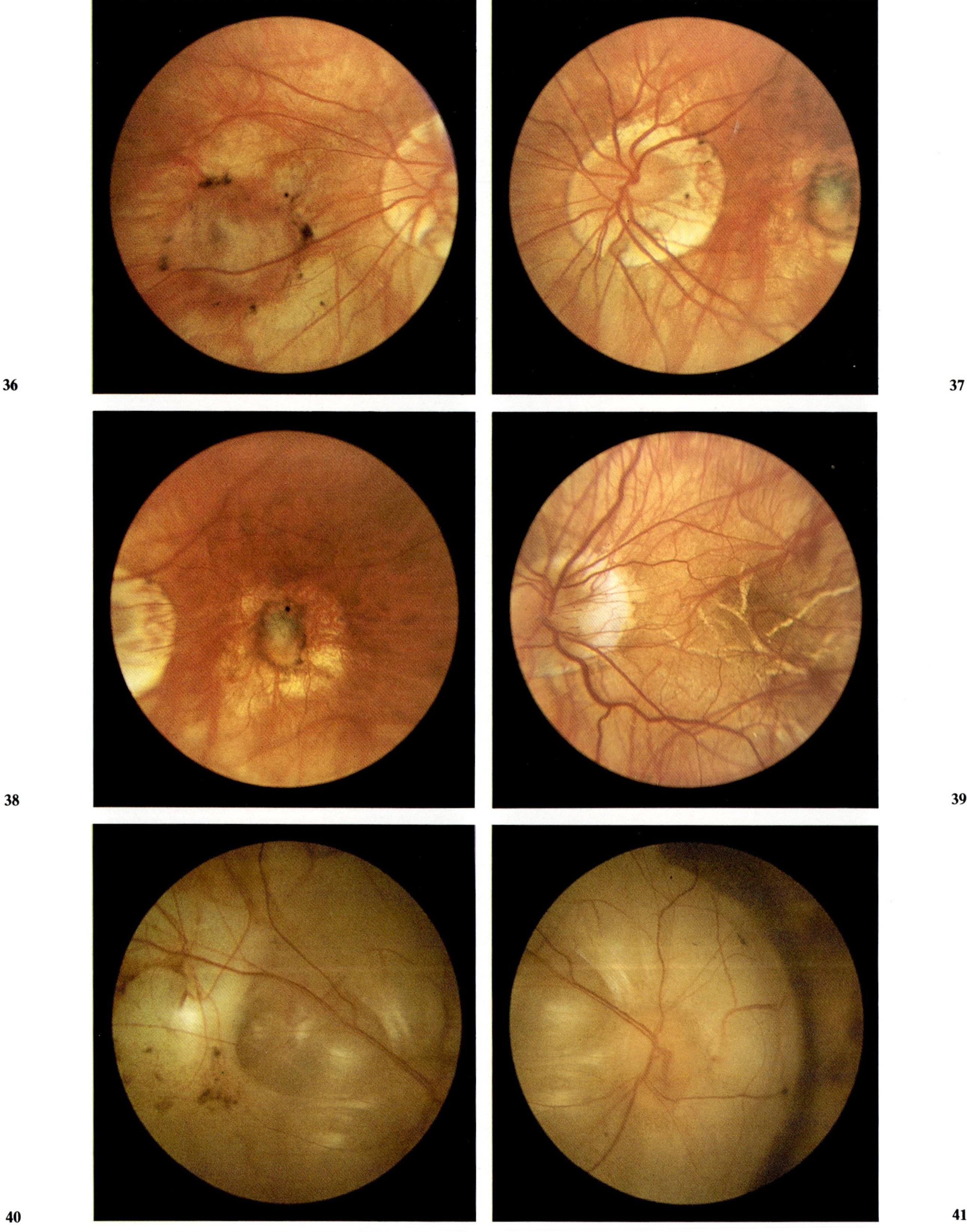

36

37

38

39

40

41

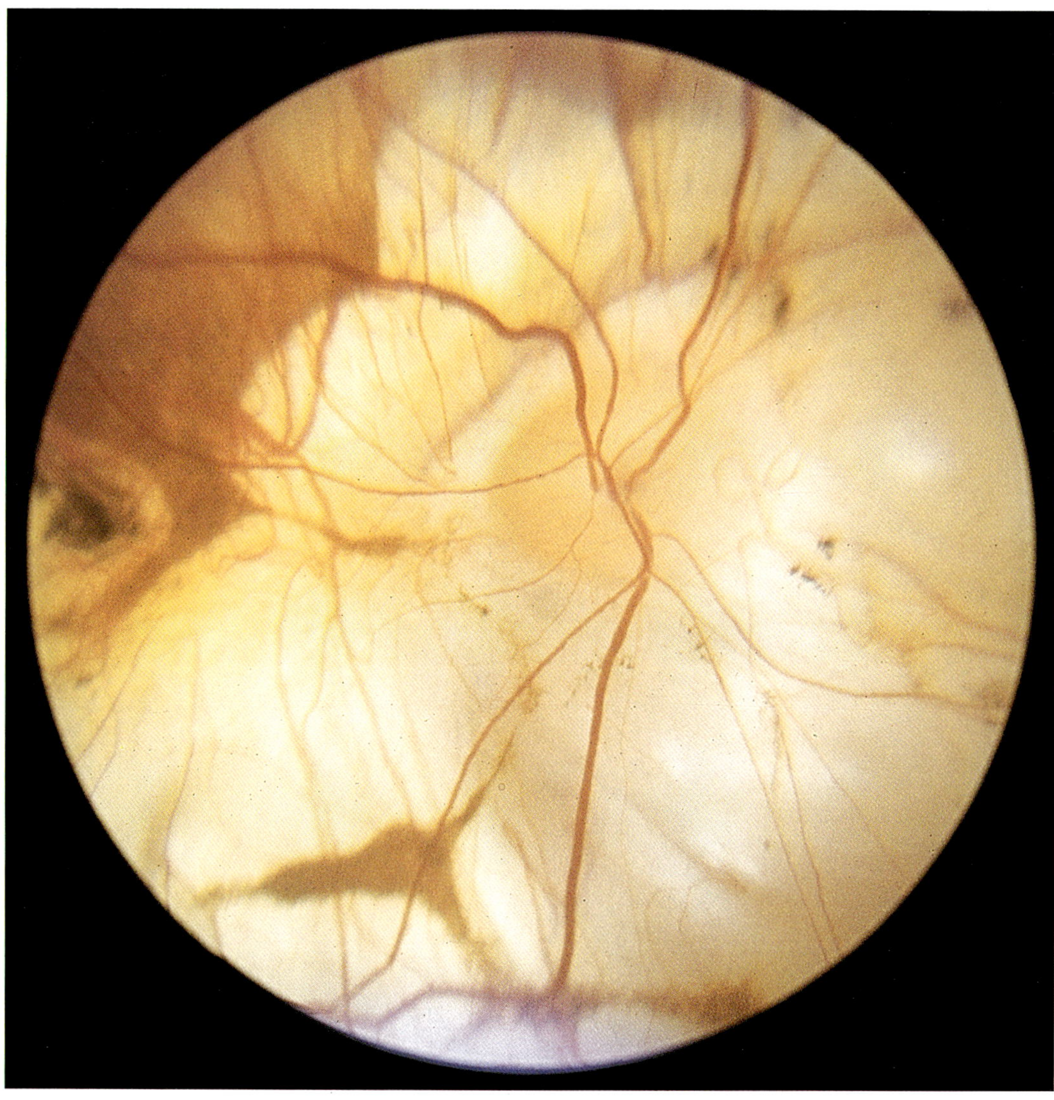

42

Figures 36–38. Right eye (Fig. 36) and left eye (Figs. 37 and 38) of a 26-year-old male patient with malignant myopia. A Purtscher-Fuchs' spot was present in both eyes.

Clinical Findings

The myopic right eye showed a refractive error of −5.0 sphere, −0.05 cylinder, axis 60° with visual acuity of 20/35. The left eye showed a myopia of −18.25 sphere, −0.75 cylinder, axis 85° with visual acuity of less than 20/1000. A hemianopsia was present in both eyes, but color vision was unaffected. Gonioscopy revealed a deep anterior chamber angle. Visual field testing revealed a central scotoma in the left eye. Using an exophthalmometer, a measure of 16-93-18 mm was obtained. The right palpebral fissure measured 8 mm and the left palpebral fissure measured 12 mm.

Figure 39. Left eye of a 25-year-old male patient with ruptures in Bruch's membrane caused by malignant myopia. The entire choroid appears to be thinned and atropic. Several bright lines, indicating ruptures in Bruch's membrane, are visible temporally from the optic disc.

Clinical Findings

The right eye was slightly hyperopic (+1.0 diopters), and the left eye had a refraction of −17.5 sphere, −1.5 cylinder, axis 155°. Visual acuity in the right eye was 20/20, and in the left eye 20/700.

Figures 40 and 41. Right eye of a 73-year-old female patient with malignant myopia. There is a posterior staphyloma present in the posterior pole of this eye.

Clinical Findings

The eye was aphakic and showed a myopia of −15.75 diopters, measured toward the posterior pole. Visual acuity was 20/400.

Figure 42. Right eye of a 78-year-old male patient with malignant myopia. A Purtscher-Fuchs' spot and a large posterior staphyloma involving the optic disc were present.

Clinical Findings

With a refractive error of −20.5 sphere, −1.5 cylinder, axis 150°, the best visual acuity achieved was 20/400. An incipient age-related (senile) cataract was present. Intraocular pressure was 12 mm Hg. Visual field testing revealed a central scotoma with a concentric constriction of the outer borders. Clinically this eye had the appearance of a gyrate atrophy because of the combination of myopic changes seen in the fundus periphery.

43

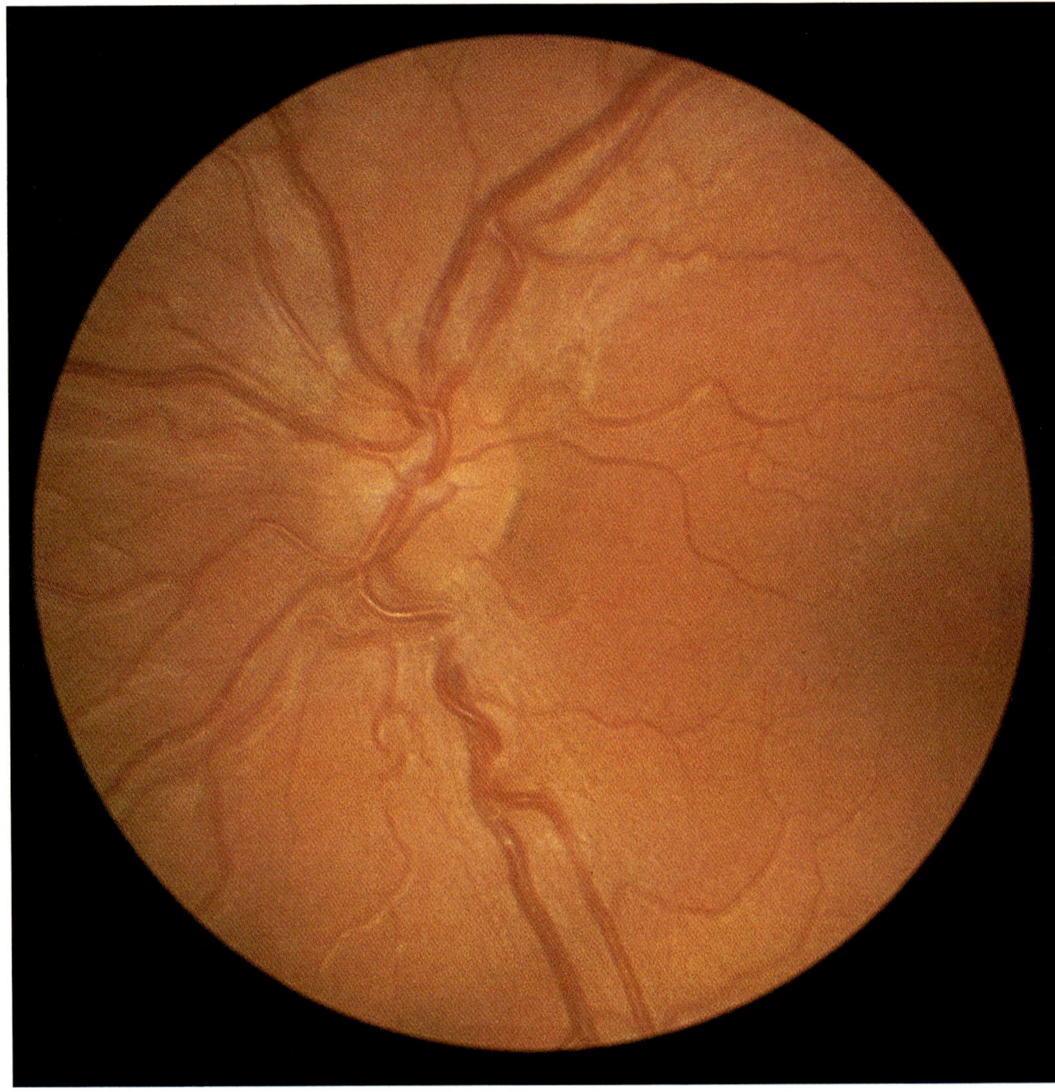

Figure 43. Left eye of a 12-year-old male patient showing tortuosity of the retinal vessels in a hyperopic eye.

Clinical Findings

Under cyclopedic conditions, the refraction was +4.0 sphere in both eyes, and visual acuity was 20/20. No other functional distortions were noted. The macula is slightly ectopic. The optic disc appears small. Using the Littmann formula (to determine the sizes of different fundus structures) the anterior corneal curvature had a radius equal to 7.9 mm ($r_1 = 7.9$ mm). The optic disc diameter measured 4 mm on the negative film ($s = 4$ mm). The constant of the fundus camera that is related to the angle of the optic disc is 1.37. Depending on the ametropic status of the eye, the Littmann curves have to be applied to evaluate the ratio q, which indicates the ratio between the object (optic disc) and the observation angle. For an ametropia of 4 diopters ($A = 4$ diopters), this ratio was found to be 0.272 ($q = 0.272$). Therefore, in this case, the Littmann formula renders the following diameter for the optic disc: $s \times 1.37 \times q = 4 \times 1.37 \times 0.272 = 1.49$ mm.

Diseases of the Retina and Choroid

Arterial Hypertension

Fundus examination is a unique, noninvasive means of directly viewing and evaluating blood vessels within the human body. For this reason, ophthalmoscopy of fundus vessels has been used in the diagnosis and follow-up of hypertensive patients. There are several classifications of hypertensive changes, some of which are the result of close cooperation between ophthalmologists and internists. Some of the most common classifications are listed in Tables 6–11.

At one time it was believed that the state and progression of a hypertensive disease in other parts of the body could be judged by retinal vascular changes. The ophthalmoscope does allow the examiner to see a part of the peripheral vascular system, but it is now known that this does not allow conclusions to be drawn about hypertonic changes in all peripheral arterial and capillary systems. Fundus changes do not always directly correlate with changes in other organ systems (brain, kidneys, heart) (Rintelen, 1957). However, based on several autopsy series, in some cases with severe pathological cerebral and renal vascular diseases, a correlation with existing retinal vascular anomalies was found.

In both the early and late stages of hypertensive retinopathy, an exact judgment of the fundus may be difficult because hypertensive and arteriosclerotic vascular changes may appear simultaneously. Extensive experience is necessary to interpret such fundus changes. Normal variations, the current refraction, and the patient's age have to be taken into consideration. As Rintelen (1957) correctly stated, it is crucial to correctly diagnose the ocular fundus by correlating the patient's history and clinical findings. One should not try to interpret a finding in the ocular fundus that could objectively also be interpreted in a different way.

Retinal Vessels

1. Arteriovenous (Fig. 2) and venoarterial (Fig. 44) crossings are physiological observations. In 70% of cases, the arteries course superiorly over the veins; in 30% of cases, veins pass in front of, or anterior to, the arterioles (Jensen, 1936).

2. Arteriovenous crossing changes (Fig. 45) (Gunn's sign) are not created by a compression of retinal vessels. Any apparent thinning of the vessels just before and after the crossing indicates sclerosis of the vascular adventitia (von Sallmann, 1937; Seitz, 1968). Thickening of the adventitious tissue prevents a clear view of the vessel contours.

Anatomically, arteriovenous crossings show a specific structure. The arterial and venous channels share a common adventitial sheath, and portions of the vascular wall may be also shared. Some components intertwine to form a small arteriovenous vascular network (Seitz, 1968).

Arteriovenous crossing changes may be indicative of arteriosclerosis or hypertensive disease, or a combination of both conditions (Figs. 52–58).

3. Parallel Gunn's sign (Fig. 46) appears as a segmental thinning of arterioles or venules when these vessels are closely adjacent to each other.

4. Guist's sign (Guist, 1931) (Fig. 47) is described as a corkscrew-like perimacular torsion of the venules.

5. Vascular spasms, segmental irregularities, and diameter changes (Fig. 51) are caused by a loss in transparency of the vascular wall and adventitial tissue. However, these changes are not definite proof of lumen constriction.

6. Copper wire arteries and vascular axial reflexes (Fig. 48) are broadened and appear reddish gold. The arteries may be engorged and approximate the thickness of the veins. This phenomenon is most often found in younger hypertensive patients.

7. Omega branching (Fig. 49) is found at the site where an arteriole separates into two branches. The branches are widened and the smaller vessels are slightly dislocated to the side, simulating the Greek letter "Ω."

8. Silver wire arteries and reflexes (Fig. 50) are associated with more advanced sclerotic changes and are caused by a diminution in the reflex of the red blood column. These changes are a sign of arteriosclerosis.

9. Arcuate arteriovenous (AV) crossings (Salus' sign (Salus, 1935)) (Fig. 51) are a deviation of the venous channels. The venule curves around the engorged proximal end of the thickened arteriole.

Fundus Changes

More severe forms of hypertension not only cause changes in the retinal vessels, but also in the various layers of the retina. Such alterations include:

1. Hemorrhage (Fig. 59) can be identified by the different topographical shapes in the retinal layers. Small punctate foci and larger dot and blot hemorrhages are usually located within the granular cell layers. Linear,

flame-shaped, or radial hemorrhages assume these typical shapes because extravasated erythrocytes are deposited between the nerve fiber axons. Preretinal hemorrhages that cover extremely large surface areas and extend into the vitreous humor are located in front of the internal limiting membrane. These hemorrhages may resemble an inverted "Napoleon's hat."

2. Cotton wool exudates (cytoid bodies or soft exudates) (Figs. 59, 64 and 65) are white to yellow-white exudations with blurred margins, which are named because of their resemblance to tufts of cotton or wool. Such exudates represent areas of ischemia and edema in the nerve fiber layer caused by microvascular occlusions (Fig. 60). The nerve fibers undergo a bulbous dilatation at the site of ischemic damage or infarction. The axoplasmatic flow in either direction is extremely reduced or interrupted. Cotton wool exudates may be reversible.

3. Hard exudates (Figs. 64 and 65) are true exudates that appear yellow-white, are usually smaller than cotton wool spots, and have very distinct margins. A macular star figure is a classic example. Hard exudates may also be reversible.

4. Retinal edema appears as grayish edematous spots in the retina, which can become greatly enlarged in cases of serous retinal detachment.

5. Papilledema (Figs. 61-63) is caused by engorgement of the papillary capillaries and retinal venules. Extreme papilledema can be observed in patients with vascular diseases.

6. Prethrombosis may occur when stasis and vascular engorgement lead to perivascular hemorrhages, especially at AV crossing sites (see also "Retinal Artery Occlusion" and "Contraceptive Drugs").

Table 6. Blood Pressure Classification of Kropp et al. (1970)

Stage 0	No vascular abnormalities (normal juvenile fundus)
Stage 1	Normal caliber arterioles, peripapillaries slightly pronounced, and irregular vascular reflexes
Stage 2	Arteriole caliber within low normal range, thickening and dulling of vessel reflexes
Stage 3	Partial spasm of major arterial branches and arterioles, slight changes in vascular walls

Table 7. Blood Pressure Classification of Keith et al. (1939)

Stage 1	Minimal narrowing or sclerosis of arterioles
Stage 2	Generalized or localized narrowing of arterioles, increasing sclerosis, thickening and dulling of vascular reflexions
Stage 3	Angiospastic retinopathy, arteriolar spasms, pronounced sclerotic changes of arterioles, retinal edema, exudates, hemorrhages
Stage 4	Same as Stage 3 with papilledema

Table 8. Classification of the German League for Aggressive Treatment of Hypertension (1980)

	Ophthalmoscopical Appearance		
	Retinal Arteries	Retina	Optic Disc
Fundus hypertonicus[a]	Mild to severe vascular changes	Normal	Normal
Fundus hypertonicus[b]	Severe vascular changes	1 to many lesions	Normal or with papilledema

[a] Formerly fundus hypertonicus I and II.
[b] Formerly fundus hypertonicus III and IV.

Table 9. Classification of Arterial Hypertension According to Severity of Organ System Involvement

Stage 1	No objectively verified lesions
Stage 2	At least one of the following indications of organic involvement or complications is present:
Heart	Hypertrophia of the left ventricle (physical examination, thorax x-ray, ECG)
Fundus	Generalized or localized spasm of the retinal arteries
Laboratory test results	Proteinuria and/or slight increase in the plasma and creatinine concentration
Stage 3	Symptoms or signs of hypertensive organic complications:
Heart	Insufficiency of the left ventricle
Brain	Cerebral, cerebellar, or brainstem hemorrhage, hypertensive encephalopathy
Fundus	Retinal hemorrhages and exudates, with or without papilledema (papilledema is pathognomonic for malignant hypertension)
Other possible complications in Stage 3	
Heart	Angina pectoria, myocardial infarction
Brain	Intracranial arterial vascular occlusion
Vessels	Dissecans aneurysm, arterial occlusion disease
Kidneys	Functional losses

Table 10. Range of Adult Blood Pressure (Bock, 1978)

Normal	
Up to 140/90 mm Hg	
Borderline	
Systolic	140-160 mm Hg
Diastolic	90-95 mm Hg
Special forms	
Unstable	Blood pressure fluctuates from normal to high
Stable	Blood pressure always increased above 160/95 mm Hg
Malignant	Diastolic blood pressure always increased above 120-130 mm Hg

Table 11. Modified Hypertensive Classification of Thiel (1963)

Hypertensive Retinopathy[a]
- Early stage
  - Optic disc: normal
  - Arteries: copper wire reflexes, curved courses, omega branching
  - Arterioles: normal
  - Veins: Gunn's sign, Guist's sign, moderate curling of midsized and small veins, stasis hemorrhages prior to arteriovenous (AV) crossings, varicose dilatations between AV crossings
  - Venules: corkscrew, curving, prominent
  - Retinal parenchym: pronounced dark-red color (red hypertension) (Volhard, 1931)
- Late stage
  - Optic disc: peripapillary capillary ectasis
  - Arteries: usually nasal branches are affected first, decrease in arterial curling, pronounced localized or generalized thickened vessel walls that prohibit a direct view of the normally visible blood column, gray-whitish spots
  - Retinal parenchym: punctate hemorrhages that may be isolated or in groups (final branches of arteries or veins), edematous spots, whitish-yellow dots (which may be garland-shaped) of focal degeneration, mild pigmentary distortion in the central fovea as a sequela to earlier hemorrhages, pigmentary bone-like distortions in peripheral retina, depigmentation of choriocapillaris
  - Optic nerve: distortion in the normal optic nerve blood flow leading to ischemic papilledema (acute ischemic neuropathy); rarely, optic nerve fiber degeneration caused by relative or absolute sclerotic artery occlusion within optic nerve, leading to vascular optic nerve atrophy

Hypertensive Retinopathy[b]
- Early stage
  - Optic disc: hyperemia (venous stasis), edema, blurring of disc margins indicating beginning ischemia
  - Arteries: generally thinned arterial spasms, small bright vascular reflexes
  - Arterioles: extremely thinned
  - Veins: Gunn's sign, Guist's sign, Salus' sign (arcuate AV crossings), moderate curling of midsized and small veins, stasis hemorrhages prior to AV crossings, varicose dilatations between AV crossings, engorged and tortuous, venous stasis
  - Venules: corkscrew, curving, prominent, extremely thinned
  - Retina: light red color (pale hypertension) (Volhard, 1931), fine flame-shaped or splinter-shaped retinal hemorrhages, cotton wool exudates
- Late stage
  - Optic disc: increasing edema leading to the final appearance of a fully developed vascular papilledema
  - Arteries: silver wire reflexes, angiospastic thinning, localized or generalized
  - Arterioles: extremely thinned, hardly visible
  - Veins: thinned (if pressure in the cerebral vascular system is not raised)
  - Venules: often thinned
  - Retina parenchym: isolated punctate or dot-shaped hemorrhages, peripapillary and macular edema, ischemic discolorations, hard exudates (macular star figure), preretinal hemorrhages, serous retinal detachment

[a] Formerly Stages I and II of cardiovascular benign essential hypertension (fundus hypertonicus).
[b] Formerly Stages III and IV of renal malignant hypertonia (angiospastic retinopathy).

Retinal Artery Occlusion

Synonym: Ischemic retinopathy.

Central Retinal Artery Occlusion

In 1859, von Graefe first described the characteristic ocular appearance of a central retinal artery occlusion. Embolic occlusion or embolus are terms often used to describe not only an embolic occlusion of the central retinal artery but also central retinal artery spasms that occur mainly in younger patients during migraine attacks. The ophthalmoscopical appearance of both entities is similar or sometimes identical.

Common Causes of Embolic Occlusion

In most cases, the embolism originates from ipsilateral plaques in the carotid artery and its branches, and it may consist of aggregations of platelets or cholesterol derived from arteriosclerotic plugs. Thrombosis also may develop with arteriosclerosis, arteriolosclerosis, endangiitis obliterans, temporal arteritis, or periarteritis nodosa.

Rare Causes of Embolic Occlusion

Rarely, the embolic occlusion may originate because of endocarditis, myocardial infarction, neoplasms, infections, inflammation, trauma, retrobulbar or optic nerve sheath hematoma, gas gangrene, or fungi. Such an occlusion may also occur iatrogenically, caused by a lavage of the maxillary sinus, from a diagnostic air injection into the cerebrospinal fluid or manipulations of a pneumothorax, and after abortions involving lavage of the uterus with a soap solution. Fat emboli can develop after fractures of long bones and severe soft tissue and thermal injuries. Both air and fat emboli may lead to transitory central blindness caused by a cortical anoxic lesion in the occipital portion of the brain. If there is no retinal involvement in cases with such transitory blindness, the prognosis is often favorable.

Embolic occlusions have been observed after paraffin injections (oil occlusions), subcutaneous injection of crystalline steroids into facial skin or as a peribulbar or retrobulbar injection, or injections into the nasal conchae. Occlusions are also caused by such functional disorders as severe migraine. An overdose of the antimigraine drug, dihydroergotamine, can also be causative in some instances. Hereditary metabolic conditions such as Tay-Sachs disease, Gaucher's disease, Niemann-Pick disease, or disseminated lipogranulomatosis (Farber's syndrome), or intoxication with ethyl alcohol, lead, quinine, or cyanide can also produce emboli.

Clinical Appearance. Central retinal artery occlusions are illustrated in Figures 66–77.

Amaurosis Fugax. The patient may report a transitory visual loss. Two-thirds of all such patients suffer from an acute prodromal painless visual loss, which often occurs in the early morning hours. In some patients, a sickle-shaped temporal band is spared within the visual field. Pupillary reaction to light may be decreased. The vascular occlusion is usually located at the lamina cribrosa.

Ophthalmoscopical Appearance. The entire retina appears pale and edematous except for the so-called "cherry-red spot" in the macula. At that site the retina is not edematous and a normal transmission of the red reflexes of the choroidal circulation is evident. The optic disc appears pale with blurred margins. Sometimes isolated hemorrhages can be observed close to the occlusion site. Retinal veins appear normal, but retinal arteries are extremely thin and lack normal blood filling in some areas. In some cases, segmental areas that are infused with blood are faintly visible. This phenomenon is created when aggregations of erythrocytes cluster in several segments, which are interrupted by segments in which there are no red blood cells ("box-car effect"). The sluggish flow of blood is so slow that the individual erythrocytes can be seen (sludge phenomenon). Sometimes this phenomenon can be evoked artificially by applying a slight exterior pressure on the globe.

Clinical Course. The initially gray-colored edema increases within the first few hours and later changes to milky white. After approximately 3 weeks, the red fundus reflex is reestablished. Often, however, the arteries will remain thin and the optic disc pale, leading to optic atrophy.

Histopathological Findings. The intercellular contents of ganglion cells and axons undergo a hydropic swelling approximately 50 minutes after development of a vascular occlusion. Between 1 and 5 hours later, ganglion and bipolar cells within the inner nuclear layer undergo irreversible damage, which consists of severe intracellular edema leading to nuclear and cellular membrane disintegration. Approximately 16 hours later, a coagulated necrosis of the inner retinal layers occurs (Daicker, 1977).

Prognosis. In most cases the prognosis is very poor, especially if the ischemia was caused by an embolism. If the occlusion was incomplete, later improvements may be possible even several weeks after onset.

Therapy. There is no commonly accepted therapeutic regimen. Ocular treatment must be followed by treatment of the underlying disease. For treatment of hypertension, the author suggests:

1. Sublingual dose of 5 mg of nitroglycerin.
2. Injection of (*a*) 500 mg of acetazolamide (Diamox); (*b*) 5 ml of pentoxifylline (Trental); and (*c*) 1000 mg of prednisolone.
3. Intravenous infusion of 250 ml of 25% mannitol, followed by a subsequent infusion of 500 ml of Dextran 40. (Precaution: Dextran may cause a severe anaphylactic reaction in some patients. To test a patient's reaction to this drug, a slow intravenous injection of 20 ml of Dextran 1 should be given first, before Dextran 40 or 70. Use of Dextran 40 or 70 is contraindicated if any adverse reactions occur during the initial test injection. Even if no reactions ensue from the test injection of Dextran 1, it must be repeated if Dextran 40 or 70 is not given within 48 hours.)
4. In some cases an anterior chamber tap (paracentesis) may be indicated.
5. If fibrinolytic therapy is considered, the reader is referred to Leydhecker and coauthors (1978) for management of, and contraindications for, this treatment. Because the risk of hemorrhage is not predictable, some conditions have to be ruled out before starting fibrinolytic therapy:

Contraindications (from an internist's viewpoint):

Arterial hypertension: blood pressure >200/100 mm Hg;
Severe arteriosclerosis (usually found in patients 65 years old or older);
Severe diabetes with fundus changes and/or previous apoplectic insults;
Malignant or inflammatory ulcerative lesions (e.g., in the gastrointestinal system);
Advanced hepatic cirrhosis;
Recent operative or diagnostic manipulations on major blood vessels (within 3–14 days);
Severe renal insufficiency during the first 3 months of pregnancy;
Congenital or acquired disorders of the hemotopoietic system.

Contraindications (from an ophthalmologist's viewpoint):

Arterial occlusion occurred more than 6 hours before any treatment could be started;
Central retinal visual acuity is not affected.

Branch Arteriolar Occlusion

One or more arterial branches may be affected, but most often the occlusion is located in an arteriole close to the optic disc.

Ophthalmoscopical Appearance. The appearance of an arteriolar branch occlusion is similar to that seen with a central retinal artery occlusion. However, edema involves only that part of the retina supplied by the occluded vessel. A distinct line can be seen between the edematous retinal area and the normal retina. If the branch occlusion occurs in close proximity to the papillary margin, the optic disc margin will be blurred in that area. A visual acuity affection, varying from mild to severe, may occur. Sector visual field defects involving only one quadrant are common.

Retinal Vein Occlusion

Central Retinal Vein Occlusion

Synonyms: Hemorrhagic retinopathy, apoplexia retina.

In 1878 von Michel termed this condition "central retinal vein thrombosis." Since that time, histopathological studies have shown that a central retinal vein occlusion is rarely caused only by a primary thrombosis. Focal arteriosclerotic or hypertonus-induced alterations of the central retinal artery may extend onto the adjacent vein in the lamina cribrosa and compress the venous lumen. Intima and endothelial proliferations can lead to occlusion of the vein, which may be located in the lamina cribrosa or, more frequently, at a site posterior to the laminar region. The central retinal vessels are anatomically and functionally constricted at this site.

Etiology. Central retinal vein occlusions are most often associated with arterial or arteriosclerotic and/or hypertensive distortions and alterations of the retinal vascular walls. In a few cases, such occlusions are associated with rheologic dysfunctions (dysproteinemia, polycythemia, sickle cell anemia, leukemia), metabolic disorders (alterations in the metabolism of lipids, purines, and carbohydrates), orbital tumors, cavernous sinus fistulas, or thromboses. Other rare causes of this disease are subarachnoidal hemorrhages, peritoneal dialysis, oral contraceptives, tuberculosis, syphilis, inflammatory vascular diseases (sarcoidosis, Behçet's disease), cystic fibrosis (mucoviscidosis), chronic glaucoma, thrombosis of the carotid artery, Takayasu's disease (pulseless disease), and intoxication (carbon monoxide, benzene, aniline).

A thrombosis of the central retinal vein occurs much more frequently than an embolic occlusion. A thrombosis is usually unilateral, and there is a better overall prognosis than with an embolic occlusion.

Clinical Appearance. The patient often complains about flickering images and sometimes reports "veils" or "haze" in the affected eye. In contrast to the acute visual loss associated with a central artery occlusion, visual acuity decreases slowly with a central vein occlusion. Therefore, patients usually consult an ophthalmologist later, and by that time visual acuity has often decreased to 20/1000 or less. However, this poor visual acuity is not prognostic for the final visual outcome because late improvements may occur.

Ophthalmoscopical Appearance. The optic disc margins appear blurred and may be prominent, indicating a hemorrhagic edematous process. The retinal veins are engorged and tortuous, and the diameter of the arteries may be decreased. The deep-red color of the affected area identifies an obstruction in the outflow of blood.

Initially scattered hemorrhages can be observed, followed by multiple hemorrhages that occur along the vessels extending into the peripheral retina. Typically, peripapillary linear flame-shaped or radial hemorrhages are located in the nerve fiber layer and conform to the alignment of the Henle's fiber layer. Diffuse dot-shaped or punctate hemorrhages are usually located within the inner plexiform or inner nuclear layer. Subretinal or preretinal hemorrhages are less common. Resorption of the extravasated blood may take up to 1 year (hemorrhagic retinopathy). Sometimes retinal vessels are masked by extensive hemorrhage or associated retinal edema. In 6% of cases, soft exudates (cotton wool spots) develop. Hard exudates, composed of lipids from degenerated ganglion cells, may form as an isolated lesion or a macular star figure. In circinate retinopathy, the lipids are deposited within the superficial retinal layer.

Visual acuity depends largely on the development and severity of cystoid macular edema, which can resolve within weeks to months. However, it may persist and further decrease visual acuity. Long-standing macular edema may progress to cystoid macular degeneration or macular retinoschisis and formation of a macular hole may ensue.

In some cases, areas of hyperpigmentation are the only residual signs of the macular edema. The hemorrhages resorb and/or undergo a gliotic transformation. Following this process, vascular abnormalities such as arteriovenous anastomoses, capillary dilatations, and neovascularizations become visible. Dilated capillaries represent an attempt by the vascular circulation to increase perfusion. This increased perfusion of preexisting capillaries must be differentiated from neovascularization, which is characterized by newly formed, but defective, vessels that are prone to hemorrhages. Neovascularization is therefore a destructive, nonreparative process. These newly formed vessels may also be found in the retina or the optic disc (rete mirabile) (Figs. 78–93).

Branch Retinal Vein Occlusion

Most branch retinal vein occlusions result from obstruction of venous flow at arteriovenous crossing sites where the arteriole and venule share a common adventitial sheath. At times the media fibers of both vessels are intertwined (arteriovenous wall network) (Seitz, 1969).

Branch vein occlusions located in the temporal quadrant usually have greater clinical significance than do the less common nasal branch vein occlusions. This is because the temporal venous branches provide the blood supply for the macular region.

Etiology. The etiology of a branch vein occlusion is similar to that of a central vein obstruction. Arterial hypertension and arteriosclerosis are the most common underlying diseases.

Clinical Appearance. The clinical symptoms largely depend on location of the occluded vein. An asymptomatic branch vein occlusion may be accidently found during a routine examination of a hypertensive patient. Usually, a patient will consult an ophthalmologist immediately because of the decreased visual acuity associated with an occlusion of the temporal branches.

Ophthalmoscopical Appearance. Pathological features are similar to those of central vein obstruction. However, the changes are localized in a single retinal quadrant or sector (Figs. 92 and 93).

Complications. A branch vein occlusion may lead to cystoid macular edema, retinoschisis, preretinal fibrosis, neovascularization, and hemorrhagic secondary glaucoma. The prognosis in terms of visual acuity is usually better than that for patients with central vein occlusions.

Therapy. Various etiologies may be involved in the development of a vein occlusion, and therefore no common therapeutic regimen can be recommended. Various therapeutic measures have been suggested in the literature, such as anticoagulants, enzyme inhibitors, and steroids. Fibrinolytic treatment is indicated only if the occlusion is less than 24 hours old and only few retinal hemorrhages are present (Leydhecker et al., 1978). Dilating drugs are contraindicated.

Isovolemic hemodilution is another therapeutic measure. Gallasch (1983) recommended that this treatment consist of drawing 500 ml of the patient's blood on 6 consecutive days. The blood is separated by a centrifuge, and the plasma (approximately 250 ml) is mixed with 250 ml of hydroxyethylcellulose (molecular weight of 450,000) and then reinfused into the patient's circulation. This lowers the hematocrit to approximately 30%.

Based on the author's experience, early in the treatment of a vein occlusion an oral anticoagulant provides good therapeutic results.

In addition, there has been increased interest in argon or xenon laser coagulation as a therapeutic treatment for venous occlusions. There is still some controversy about how long after the occlusion occurs before the coagulation treatment should be initiated. Some physicians recommend early coagulation therapy (within the first 6 weeks after the event). Others recommend starting the therapy 6 months after the occlusion.

Lüllwitz (1978) recommended the following regimen for a temporal branch vein occlusion:

Visual acuity below 20/60: coagulation should be started approximately 3 months after the occlusion.

Visual acuity above 20/60: coagulation should be started 6 months after the occlusion.

Special care should be taken that the dilated capillary beds, which will have developed by that time, be spared from the coagulation treatment. These capillaries drain blood from the occluded areas. Leaving them intact, therefore, will allow for better drainage from the macular region and will lower capillary pressure within the marginal thrombolic retinal areas.

Various coagulation techniques may be used, based on evaluation of each patient. The laser lesions may be applied using a barrier technique or a vessel-parallel technique, or the entire affected area may be coagulated. If a central retinal vein is occluded, it is suggested in the literature that the coagulation therapy should begin 1 optic disc diameter from the optic disc. The perivenous area of all major veins should be coagulated, extending into the midperiphery of the retina.

Venous Stasis Retinopathy

According to Hayreh (1976a, 1976b), this entity is best described as a self-limiting, chronic disease with a good prognosis. This is the major difference between venous statis retinopathy and hemorrhagic retinopathy (central vein thrombosis). A major complication of venous stasis retinopathy is the development of cystoid macular edema, which causes decreased visual acuity. Without systemic corticosteroid therapy (starting doses 40–60 mg daily, slowly tapered to a minimal dose over several months), cystoid macular edema may lead to an irreversible cystoid macular degeneration. Hayreh (1976b) states that therapy with anticoagulants is contraindicated.

Neovascular Glaucoma

Synonym: Hemorrhagic secondary glaucoma.

Neovascular glaucoma represents a threatening complication of central vein thrombosis.

Time Period in Which Neovascular Glaucoma May Develop. Von Graefe (1869) described a period for development of neovascular glaucoma of 2–6 months. Van Beuningen (1967) described an average of 6 months. Raitta (1965) found the period to be 4 months in two-thirds of his cases, 5 to 12 months in one-sixth of his cases, and over 1 year in the remaining one-sixth of cases. Drobec (1982) described a period of 2 weeks to 2 years (144-case study).

Disposition. Especially at risk are patients with hypertension and arteriosclerosis.

Affected Ages. This entity is most often found in patients older than 50 years of age. Neovascular glaucoma is generally unilateral. However, the fellow eye quite often shows simple, chronic glaucoma. The affected eye is painful, and at an early stage the visual acuity is markedly decreased. High intraocular pressure is always present. The average pressure is approximately 50 mm Hg, but pressures as high as 90 mm Hg have been reported.

Frequently neovascular glaucoma does not respond to treatment, and unilateral rubeosis of the iris almost always occurs. In contrast, rubeosis iridis in diabetic patients is normally bilateral. The newly formed vessels associated with neovascular glaucoma follow the intraocular pressure elevation, rather than precede it.

Other Ocular Findings. Other abnormalities associated with neovascular glaucoma include edema of the corneal epithelium, hyphema, anterior chamber flare, posterior synechiae, fibrovascular membranes within the anterior chamber angle, ectropion uveae, secondary cataract, and vitreous hemorrhage.

Effects of Diabetes Mellitus on Eye Tissues

Diabetic retinopathy is one of the most common causes of blindness. Two percent of all diabetics will probably suffer a complete loss of vision. Twenty percent of all people who develop blindness after the age of 50 are diabetic.

Diabetic Retinopathy

The morphological appearance of diabetic retinopathy was first described by Jaeger in 1855. The initial lesion of diabetic retinopathy is a microangiopathy that affects primarily capillaries, arterioles, and venules at the posterior pole (Figs. 94 and 95). Ophthalmoscopically, punctate hemorrhages, isolated or arranged in small groups, may be present. Small microaneurysms of the retinal arterioles can also be found. Hemorrhages and microaneurysms indicate an already advanced stage of diabetic retinopathy.

In later stages, the background retinopathy may advance to a proliferative retinopathy in which newly formed vessels can be seen on the optic disc, as well as in

Table 12. Classification of Diabetic Retinopathy[a]

Stage 1. Simple Diabetic Retinopathy

In this stage, the optic disc, arteries, and arterioles show no morphological changes. The retinal veins are engorged and may have spindle- and/or bead-shaped, dilated areas caused by ectasia of the vascular walls. Isolated microaneurysms are a chacteristic finding. Dot and blot or flame-shaped hemorrhages may supplement the morphological appearance.

Doden (1974) described a characteric omega-shape of the retinal veins in which the vessel shows a dilated area along the arch of the letter's end, with constricted areas at the letter's footplates. Sometimes the constricted areas are connected by another thin vessel. According to Riaskoff (1972), this vascular anomaly may be induced by preexisting cotton wool spots immediately adjacent to the vein. Another case was described by von Stieber (1955).

Stage 2. Exudative Phase of Diabetic Retinopathy

The same morphological changes described in Stage 1 may be present, but are more pronounced. Groups of microaneurysms and more flame-shaped hemorrhages can be seen.

Hard exudates (yellow, waxy). Hard exudates represent extravasated proteinaceous and lipid material. These gray-white to yellow exudates are a polygonal shape with sharp demarcations. Initially, they are isolated but in later stages the lesions appear in groups that may conflux. These exudates are mostly concentrated at the posterior pole and may be deposited in a circinate fashion around the macula.

Soft exudates. Soft exudates (cotton wool spots or cytoid bodies) are actually not true exudates. They are composed of clusters of ganglion cell axons in the nerve fiber layer that have undergone a bulbous dilatation at the site of ischemic damage or infarction. In connection with hypertensive vascular changes, these exudates may indicate Kimmelstiel-Wilson's syndrome.

Stage 3. Hemorrhagic, Proliferative Diabetic Retinopathy

All the changes described in Stage 2 may be present. In addition, proliferation of newly formed retinal vessels leaving the level of the retina are present. Such vessels may occur as a rete mirabilis. Retinal and vitreous hemorrhages are often present. Such hemorrhages become organized and form fibrovascular strands. These strands shrink and cause traction on the retina, ultimately leading to retinal detachment.

Transient retinal detachment caused by light coagulation of the posterior pole in diabetic retinopathy. This entity is a rare complication observed after light coagulation within the temporal retinal vascular trunks. It usually has a good prognosis. The central retinal edema leads to decreased visual acuity 1–2 days after light coagulation. This complication is quite often associated with less pigmented fundi that show lipoid deposition.

Background retinopathy. This term is used synonymously with nonproliferative diabetic retinopathy.

[a]From van Heydenreich (1979).

the midperipheral and peripheral fundus (Figs. 96–107). In this stage both eyes are affected, but not always to the same extent. The capillaries show increased permeability, leading to secondary changes within the retina (edema and exudates) that are most commonly located between the temporal vascular branches. Hard exudates that are initially isolated may conflux and form a macular star figure (circinate retinopathy).

Soft exudates (cotton wool spots) and hypertensive vascular abnormalities are suspicious for Kimmelstiel-Wilson syndrome (intracapsular glomerulosclerosis), which is still a life-threatening complication of diabetes that may lead to complete renal insufficiency. This disease may occur in juvenile diabetics approximately 10 years after manifestation of the disease. This complication sometimes occurs in Type II (adult-onset) diabetics and is often superimposed on an already existing arteriosclerosis. As mentioned previously, the exudative stage of diabetic retinopathy may be followed by a hemorrhagic proliferative phase. Clinically, intermittent retinal and vitreal hemorrhages determine the course of this disease. Proliferative fibrous strands of tissue and fibrovascular scar tissue formation within the vitreous may cause traction on the retina and finally lead to retinal detachment (Table 12).

Ocular Changes Caused by Diabetes

Anterior segment diabetic changes may include chronic blepharitis, hordeolus, and iritis (rare).

Rubeosis iridis is frequently associated with proliferative diabetic retinopathy. Hemorrhagic secondary glaucoma may be observed. A lacy vacuolation of the iris pigment epithelium is a relatively unusual but highly characteristic finding. The basement membrane of the pigmented ciliary epithelium often shows a diffuse thickening.

Lens, Diabetic Cataract. The most common forms of cataract associated with diabetes are subcapsular vacuoles, gray-white opacities, and punctate opacities in the anterior cortical layers ("snowflakes in a cloudy sky" effect). The superficial lens sutures may appear more pronounced. Reversible, star-shaped opacities within the posterior subcapsular cortical material may develop.

Refractive changes in the crystalline lens associated with osmotic changes are well documented and usually consist of a transient myopia during periods of hyperglycemia. A transitory hyperopia may occur with the start of insulin therapy caused by a sudden decrease in the concentration of blood glucose. The refractive index can change quite often during the day depending on the blood glucose concentration, and the accommodative capacity of the lens is often reduced accordingly.

Hemoglobin A_{1c} in Diabetes Mellitus

The glucohemoglobin HbA_1 has become an important parameter in the laboratory diagnosis of diabetes mellitus. Three fractions of this molecule can be differentiated: HbA_{1a}, HbA_{1b}, and HbA_{1c}. HbA_{1c} represents the largest hemoglobin fraction. Normally between 2.9 and 7.1% of hemoglobin is HbA_{1c}. The average in a healthy adult is approximately 4.8%. A fraction of HbA_{1c} exceeding 8% indicates a poorly controlled blood glucose concentration. For the laboratory analysis, 2 ml of ethylenediaminetetraacetic acid (EDTA) or heparinized blood are needed. The test is performed by means of column chromatography.

As the blood glucose concentration is increased, the stable molecule HbA_{1c} is built via a chain of intermittent substances. After its uptake by erythrocytes, HbA_{1c} cannot be metabolized during the life span of the erythrocytes, i.e., for approximately 120 days.

Practical Aspects. Blood glucose concentration and glucose metabolism in a patient can be judged very accurately and retrospectively over a period of at least 4 weeks.

Ateriosclerotic Chorioretinopathy

There are several classifications defining the various stages of hypertensive and arteriosclerotic retinopathy, e.g., the Scheie and the Keith-Wagener classifications. Table 13 presents the clinical classification of Sautter (1961).

Table 13. Arteriosclerotic Fundus Classification of Sautter (1961)

Simple Arteriosclerotic Fundus (Fundus Scleroticus A) (Figs. 108–110)

Vascular alterations are the most prominent finding. The vascular reflexes are enhanced. The vessels are irregularly thickened, which is caused by a partially thickened vascular sclerotic wall. Arteriovenous crossings may be present, and arteriosclerotic plaques, often seen as white deposits at the branches of the arterioles, can be seen. Small vascular branches are constricted and little side branching can be seen. The choroid may appear darkly pigmented in the areas between larger choroidal vessels. The most important complication of these arteriosclerotic changes may be development of a senile macular hole.

Dyshoric foci (age-related or senile drusen) are isolated or grouped dot-shaped areas of yellowish white material in the fovea and its immediate surroundings, which represent hyaline substances within the tissue. The term "dyshoric" describes a clinical condition associated with an alteration or distortion of the blood-retina barrier. This term was described by Schürmann and MacMahon in 1933.

Visual acuity is usually not affected in this stage if no macular hole is present.

Dry Stage of Arteriosclerotic Chorioretinopathy (Fundus Scleroticus B) (Figs. 111–114)

In addition to the vascular changes previously described, the retina is involved. Larger age-related (senile) drusen and lightly depigmented areas within the retina may accrue, mostly at the posterior pole but sometimes in the equatorial and peripheral areas of the retina. Depigmentation and granular and dot-shaped pigmentations may be present, leading to pigment irregularities. Visual acuity may be affected; often the patient describes subjective difficulties with reading.

Exudative Stage of Arteriosclerotic Chorioretinopathy (Fundus Scleroticus C) (Figs. 115–122)

In addition to the changes described previously, retinal edema and retinal hemorrhages can be found (insudation of the macula (Sautter, 1961)). The deeper retinal layers show areas of degeneration and lipid deposition, glial metaplasia, and finally, secondary deposition of cholesterol and calcification (chronic degenerative changes).

Senile pseudotumor of the macula and an elevated macular scar are the end stage of this disease. Synonyms: disciform macular degeneration (Kuhnt-Junius degeneratio maculi luteae disciformis).

Visual Acuity. The peripheral vision is usually intact, but central visual acuity at this stage is completely destroyed.

Fundus Scleroticus D (Figs. 123–125)

In this stage the arteriosclerotic changes basically affect the choroidal vessels. This type of fundus scleroticus therefore may be observed as an isolated entity without involvement of the retina. The choroidal vessels are obliterated, a finding that is most pronounced in the choriocapillaris layer. Ophthalmoscopically, the intervascular spaces of the choroid appear darkly pigmented, whereas the larger choroidal vessels are sclerotic and appear light. This leads to so-called "senile fundus tabulatus." Visual acuity is only minimally affected. Most often people older than 50 years of age are affected by this type of arteriosclerotic chorioretinopathy.

Etiology. Histologically and physiologically, destruction and alterations in the flow of blood products through Bruch's membrane are causative.

Therapy. After systemic alterations in the lipid metabolism, hormone irregularities, or heart and circulatory disorders have been ruled out, a combined treatment with rheologic agents and digitalis may be tried. In addition, a dietary regimen and treatment with vitamins A, B_6, and E may be advantageous. In case of an exudative macular degeneration, irradition of the posterior pole has been suggested (6 × 25 rad).

Wessing (1973) described his findings regarding light coagulation in cases of exudative senile maculopathy. This type of treatment is indicated after the diagnosis of exudative maculopathy is confirmed by fluorescein angiography in the following conditions: (*a*) exudative nonproliferative stages with noncomplicated detachment of the retinal pigment epithelium; (*b*) in cases with localized vascular proliferations; and (*c*) in chronic cases that are in transition to a final scar.

Low-Vision Aids

To improve a patient's vision, a number of eye problems require nothing more than simple magnification. This is especially true with central field losses, macular lesions, and disorders characterized by dimness of vision. Magnification is less useful in cases with extensive peripheral field loss and large central or sector scotomas. To achieve the best results in the treatment of visually handicapped or partially sighted people, it is very important to know exactly the individual status of each eye. A trustful cooperation between patient, ophthalmologist, and a specially trained optician is necessary.

There are a wide variety of hand-held magnifiers and stand magnifiers of different magnifications in the range between ×2 and ×5. Higher magnification spectacles are another visual aid. The best selection of such low-vision aids for each patient requires patience and experience. Individually fitted spectacles are usually much more expensive than other magnifiers. Loupes are a special form of magnifying spectacles that usually provide magnification only up to ×2. Therefore, simple loupes are not adequate for the severely visually handicapped. Higher magnification can be achieved by the use of telescopic devices, which can be mounted within a spectacle frame.

Low-vision aids that incorporate a telescopic device are based on the Galilean or Kepler principle. There are specific indications for both systems. Such magnifying aids may be both monocular and binocular in variable combinations. For distance vision, one can achieve a magnification from ×1.8 to ×3.8; for near vision, the magnification ranges from ×2 to ×8. Such telescopic devices are especially indicated for patients with complete loss of central vision in which the fixation area has shifted to the marginal zone of the affected retina (Aulhorn, 1971). There has to be a high degree of patient compliance and a strong motivation to read because not all patients will accept the markedly reduced field of vision that is rendered by such devices. However, once accepted, often patients are able to read normal size type in books and newspapers.

Telescopic spectacles do not offer any advantage to patients who are visually impaired because of retinal pigmentary degeneration, nor to the patient who has alterations in the refractive media. In the latter case, there is the general disadvantages of a magnified image, i.e., reduced contrast and light intensity, and the disadvantage of having the original refractive alteration magnified as well. Such visual aids are also contraindicated in patients with interruptions and alterations of the visual tract, e.g., in cases of homonymous hemianopsia. In patients with incomplete macular degeneration, magnifying aids are often not successful because a small amount of central vision remains.

In the severely visually impaired patient who still has functioning peripheral vision and whose visual acuity is reduced below 20/200, electronic reading devices, such as the closed-circuit television reader, may be used. Depending on the type of device used, magnifications between ×3 and ×45 are possible. The devices often are offered in combination with a typewriter. Most of the devices currently on the market offer not only positive writing, but also negative writing (white type on a black background), which purportedly reduces blurring effects.

Electronic reading devices are especially advantageous for the visually impaired patient with macular degeneration but without cataracts. Based on the author's observations, even in an advanced stage of glaucoma, patients who do not have a cataract and patients with optic nerve atrophy or tapetoretinal degeneration can achieve astonishing results. A portable view-scan that weighs only 4 kg can even be stored in a briefcase. The magnification is variable and provides eight different levels from ×4 to ×64 magnification. Use of this hand-held camera can be easily learned.

Correlation of Arteriosclerotical Changes with Analogous Vascular Changes in Other Organs

Synonym: Fundus arterioscleroticus with hypertensive changes.

The correlation of vascular changes observed in the retina and vascular changes in other organ systems has been the topic of several investigations. Lund (1980) summarized his findings as follows: once arteriosclerosis of the retinal arteries is present, one can assume that there is arteriosclerosis in other organ systems (kidneys, brain, coronary arteries, aorta). There seems to be a close and nearly linear correlation between retinal involvement and brain vessels. Brain cells are affected in 98.4% of cases if arteriosclerosis of the retinal vessels is present. Therefore, one may conclude that there is no such thing as an isolated retinal arteriosclerosis. On the other hand, arteriosclerosis in other organ systems can not be ruled out if the fundus does not show any arteriosclerotic changes.

Juvenile Macular Degeneration

There are several entities that may affect the macula in younger patients. A clinical classification is presented in Table 14. The diagnosis of these diseases is based on:

1. The ophthalmoscopical appearance (always bilateral and symmetrical occurrence);
2. Examination of visual functions (visual acuity, dark adaptation, color vision, visual fields);
3. Electroretinogram (ERG);
4. Electrooculogram (EOG);
5. Family history and genetic evaluation of the family.

Table 14. Clinical Classification of Juvenile Macular Degeneration[a]

Neuroepithelium Affected Primarily

Stargardt's disease, dominant progressive foveal atrophy, central or pericentral retinitis pigmentosa, progressive cone dystrophy, dominant cystoid macular edema.

Pigment Epithelium Affected Primarily

Vitelliforme dystrophy of the fovea, fundus flavimaculatus, reticular dystrophy of the retinal pigment epithelium (Sjögren's syndrome), butterfly-shaped pigment dystrophy of the fovea, grouped pigmentations of the foveal area.

Bruch's Membrane Affected Primarily

Dominant drusen of Bruch's membrane, dominant progressive foveal atrophy.

Choroid Affected Primarily

Geographic atrophy of the pigment epithelium and choriocapillaris (formerly termed "central irregular choroidal dystrophy"), pseudoinflammatory dystrophy (Sorsby, 1935).

[a] According to François (1979).

Best's Disease

This entity was first described by Adams in 1883. However, this form of dystrophy carries the name of Best, who described it in 1905. Clinically, the course of Best's disease occurs in four different stages of this inherited or early childhood-onset degeneration of the macula. This disease is transmitted as an autosomal dominant trait with reduced penetration and highly variable expression (François, 1979).

This hereditary infantile macular dystrophy is identical to the disease described by von Zanen and Rausin (1950), who called it "kiste vitelliforme congenital de la macule." In the contemporary literature it is often referred to as vitelliforme macular degeneration (Figs. 126–133).

Manifestations have been observed in newborns at 1 week of age. More commonly the diagnosis is made incidentally during an ophthalmoscopical examination of patients between 5 and 15 years of age. According to the literature, late manifestations are most often found in patients between 36 and 48 years of age.

François et al. (1967) differentiated four ophthalmoscopically observed stages.

Stage 1

This vitelliforme stage is characterized by a typical morphological appearance that is termed "un oeuf sur le plat" in the French literature. In the English literature, it is described as an "egg yolk" in the macula. The lesion is sharply demarcated, round, homogeneous, and lacks any vessels. Its diameter measures between 0.5 and 2 disc diameters. One slightly prominent, red or yellow lesion is usually found in each eye. However, sometimes multiple lesions located outside the macular area may be found (most often in adult patients). Possible complications of this stage are bleeding, hemorrhage into the cyst, rupture of the cyst, and development of a macular hole.

Stage 2

Because of gravity, the contents of the cyst separate and heavier parts settle to the bottom, leading to the appearance of pseudohypopyon or pseudocyst.

Stage 3

Scarring and organization of the cyst occur.

Stage 4

End stage pigmented chorioretinal atrophy cannot be differentiated morphologically from other juvenile or senile macular degenerations.

Diagnosis. The diagnosis is confirmed ophthalmoscopically or with an EOG. Normally an EOG does not show any pathological changes in other forms of juvenile or senile macular degeneration. In Best's disease, the retinal pigment epithelium is subnormal or completely absent and, therefore, an EOG represents an important clinical criterion in the differential diagnosis of this disease. The EOG also allows for screening of nonmanifest affected carriers of this disease. Only in rare cases are the ERG waves affected. The amplitude of the B wave may be slightly flattened. Dark adaptation is normal and color vision is usually not affected. Initially, the visual field remains intact, but in late stages a central scotoma develops.

Differential Diagnosis. The differential diagnosis of Best's dystrophy includes all forms of inflammatory central chorioretinitis and, in older patients, age-related macular degenerations.

Good visual acuity, which may continue for several years, is a characteristic of this disease, a fact that can seem to be contradictory to the ophthalmoscopical appearance of the lesion.

Stargardt's Disease

This entity is usually noted in childhood or pubescence, at which time it leads to an optically noncorrectable decrease in visual acuity. Stargardt's disease does not cause complete blindness; however, the central visual acuity is often reduced to 20/200 or less by the 4th decade. Visual acuity may be affected to a different extent in both eyes.

Synonyms: Stargardt's juvenile macular degeneration, Stargardt's syndrome, familial macular cerebral degeneration, central tapetoretinal dystrophy (François, 1979). According to François, this disease, which was originally described by Stargardt in 1909, represents the basic pattern of juvenile macular degeneration. Stargardt's disease is a slow, progressive dystrophy affecting the posterior pole. According to new studies, an inherited enzymatic defect seems to be causative. This defect leads to a primary atrophy of the neuroepithelial layer and pigment epithelium (Figs. 134–136).

Stargardt's disease is usually transmitted recessively, rarely in an autosomal dominant manner. A dominant progressive foveal dystrophy has been described in several families. Sporadic cases have been reported.

Additional Findings. The color vision shows dyschromatopsia in the red-green distinction. Dark adaptation is normal with a biphasic adaptation curve. Interestingly, vision under dim light conditions is usually better than vision in bright daylight. Visual field testing shows normal peripheral borders. The initial relative central scotoma progresses into an absolute scotoma extending over an area of 20–30°. Eventually the blind spot will be integrated into the original scotoma, leading to a centrocecal scotoma. If associated with the peripheral tapetoretinal dystrophy, a ring scotoma may be noted. An ERG may be normal or subnormal; if associated with a peripheral tapetoretinal dystrophy, the normal ERG wave may be eliminated completely. An EOG is usually normal, but it may be subnormal in cases in which Stargardt's disease is associated with a fundus flavimaculatus (approximately 50% of patients).

Stargardt's disease can also be associated with corneal alterations such as keratoconus and corneal dystrophy, auditory disorders (hearing impairment and even deafness), and neurologic disorders (heredocerebellar ataxia or Pierre-Marie's syndrome or Marie's disease), hereditary spinal ataxia (Friedreich's disease), and olivopontocerebellar atrophy (Déjérine-Sottas disease).

Ophthalmoscopical Appearance. Optic disc, retinal vessels, and peripheral retina appear normal. The loss of the foveal reflex is an early symptom. Initially, brown or gray-yellow pigmented microdots may be seen in the macular area. The macular region shows a diffuse punctate pigmentation that eventually covers the entire area. With localized loss of the retinal pigment epithelium, the choroid becomes visible. In late stages, the posterior pole shows a central chorioretinal atrophy with varying amounts of pigmentation. The oval central dystrophic area may horizontally measure between 0.4 and 3 optic disc diameters, with a vertical measurement of up to 1.5 optic disc diameters.

In cases associated with a fundus flavimaculitus, characteristic pericentral yellow spots are present, which may be isolated or grouped in round, linear, or swirl formations. An associated peripheral tapetoretinal dystrophy becomes manifest as a granular pigmentation with a normal disc and vascular status that resembles a "pepper and salt" fundus or a bone spicule-like pigmentation with markedly narrowed retinal vessels and a candlewax-like, yellowish optic disc (ascendent optic nerve atrophy (François, 1979)).

Therapy. No effective therapy is known.

Prophylaxis. Genetic exploration may be helpful; however, sporadic cases that can not be predicted do occur.

Sorsby's Pseudoinflammatory Dystrophy of the Macula

This entity was first described by Hutchinson in 1875 and was investigated in more depth by Sorsby and Mason in 1949. It is usually transmitted as an autosomal dominant trait, but rare cases of autosomal recessive transmission have been reported (François, 1979).

Sorsby's pseudoinflammatory dystrophy of the macula is usually manifested by the 3rd to 5th decade, depending on the families involved. Distorted, blurred vision is the leading symptom.

Other Findings. Color vision testing shows acquired disc chromotopsia in the red-green distinction. Dark adaptation is not affected. The peripheral visual field is always unchanged, but a central scotoma develops early. Both an ERG and an EOG can be normal or subnormal.

Ophthalmoscopical Appearance. The optic disc and retinal vessels are normal. Both eyes are affected symmetrically. Early on, small dots that may accrue become visible in the macular region making it appear speckled or spotted. This early stage is rarely seen ophthalmoscopically. Clinicians are more familiar with a later stage that closely resembles an infectious chorioretinitis, showing central retinal edema, hemorrhages, and exudates. This exudative stage is followed by scar formation within the macular area. The pseudoinflammation slowly, but continually, progresses peripherally by expanding the separate focal lesions. During the various stages fresh pseudoinflammatory foci and sclerotic foci can be seen at the same time. The pigmentation varies markedly.

Therapy. Only symptomatic therapy is known. Rheologic agents may be tried. Visual rehabilitation may be improved by the use of low-vision aids (see "Low-Vision Aids").

Prophylaxis. Genetic exploration may be helpful.

Choroidal Nevi

In this chapter we discuss multiple or grouped lesions, rather than the well-known single or isolated choroidal nevus. Several terms are used synonymously: grouped pigmentation of the fundus, nevoid pigmentation or multiple melanosis of the fundus, melanosis retinae, and grouped nevoid pigmentation of the retina. Choroidal nevi were first described by von Jaeger in 1869. Such nevi represent an inborn anomaly that is not hereditary. The ophthalmoscopical appearance remains the same throughout life (Fig. 140). No functional losses are present, such as decreased visual acuity, distortions in color vision or dark adaptation, or visual field defects. ERG is normal. Histopathologically, the pigment epithelial cells show hypertropic and hyperplastic abnormalities and an irregular distribution and density of pigment granules (Egerer, 1976). This entity represents a benign hypertrophy of the retinal pigment epithelium.

Ophthalmoscopical Appearance. Groups of predominantly monocular dark-gray to black pigment dots are located near the retinal vessels. The density of pigmentation may vary, and the dots are sharply demarcated. Characteristically, the size of the lesions increases toward the periphery. Usually only one sector of the retina is affected; however, the lesions may be found in several separated sectors or scattered over the entire fundus area. The macula is not usually affected. Some exceptional cases with macular involvement were described by Welter in 1927, as well as by Meunier and Boursiun in 1951 (Figs. 137 and 138).

Drusen of Bruch's Membrane

Synonyms: Hyaline dystropy, colloid degeneration, flecked retina syndrome.

Mucopolysaccharide and cerebroside materials are deposited between the pigment epithelium and Bruch's membrane. One has to differentiate between primary and secondary drusen. Primary drusen represent a hereditary hyaline dystrophy. This disease is usually transmitted as an autosomal dominant trait, but an irregular transmission has sometimes been described. Drusen become manifest between the 2nd and 3rd decade of life. Within an affected family, the drusen formation is similar, but between families the formation varies extensively, possibly caused by a varying expression in the dominant inheritance. Several entities belong in the group of dominant drusen diseases, including Tay's disease (central guttata choroiditis), Holthouse-Batten chorioretinitis, Doyne's honeycomb choroidopathy, and familial drusen. According to Franceschetti et al. (1963) and Deutmann (1971), the only difference between these entities is the terminology used to describe them.

Primary drusen most probably represent a presenile or age-related (senile) degenerative hyaline dystrophy of Bruch's membrane.

Secondary drusen are the sequelae of a choroidal inflammation or tumor. They are often found incidentally during a histological examination.

Ophthalmoscopical Appearance. The lesions are located equatorially (age-related form) or in the central fundus area (hereditary form). Characteristically, white to white-yellow foci and small, prominent dots that vary in size and number and are sharply demarcated may be present. These lesions may appear round or polygonal (older drusen) and may accrue, and some drusen may be superimposed over others. The retinal vessels are not affected and cross over the lesions. Some drusen have a crystalline appearance as a sequela of calcification. Typically, hereditary drusen are located nasally from the optic disc. Age-related (senile) drusen are usually associated with other degenerative fundus changes (Figs. 141–144).

Differential Diagnosis. The differential diagnosis of drusen includes fundus albipunctatus, fundus flavimaculatus, or retinitis punctata albescens (progressive albipunctate dystrophy).

Functional Distortions. Central visual acuity remains intact for a long period of time, as does the mesopic visual acuity. Color vision screening may reveal alterations in the blue-green perception. ERG is normal to subnormal. EOG is initially unchanged but in later stages may show subnormal results.

Therapy. No useful therapy is known.

Central Sclerosis of the Choroid

First described by von Jaeger in 1855 (cited in Duke-Elder, 1976), central sclerosis of the choroid was investigated further by Sorsby in 1949. This disease is transmitted as an autosomal recessive trait, or, rarely, as an autosomal dominant trait (François, 1979). The symptoms develop between the 2nd and 4th decades of life and are fully developed after the 5th decade.

Color Vision. The patient most often has a history of an acquired disc chromatopsia in the blue and yellow ranges. Visual field testing always reveals intact peripheral fields with late development of a central scotoma. The ERG and EOG are often pathologic.

Ophthalmoscopical Appearance. The macula shows pigmentary irregularities that may appear as yellowish dots. In later stages, exudates and edema may ensue, and the disease then resembles an exudative macular degeneration. The final stage is characterized by a sharply demarcated round or oval atrophic area that covers 2-4 optic disc diameters. Pigment epithelium and choriocapillaries have vanished and sclerosed choroidal vessels become visible (Fig. 145). The ophthalmoscopical appearance may be mistaken for a late stage of Stargardt's disease.

Therapy. Only symptomatic therapy is possible, i.e., a trial of rheologic agents and visual improvement by means of low-vision aids (see "Low-Vision Aids").

Angioid Streaks

This disease was first described by Doyne in 1889. The term used today, angioid streaks (German: angioide pigmentstreifen), was suggested by von Knapp in 1892.

Elastic tissues are affected primarily in this disease. Therefore, systemic diseases that produce elastic tissue degeneration, such as pseudoxanthoma elasticum, Groenblad-Strandberg syndrome, fibrodysplasia, hyperelastica (Ehlers-Danlos syndrome), senile elastosis of the skin, cardiovascular diseases, and sickle cell disease, often have been associated with angioid streaks. The streaks are usually bilateral and are frequently associated with drusen. The mean manifestation age is between the 3rd and 5th decade of life (Figs. 146 and 147).

Pathogenetically, a primary degeneration of Bruch's membrane causes a secondary rupture that becomes a pigmented lesion. Proliferations of choroidal and choriocapillary vessels may form neovascular membranes that can be the cause of subretinal hemorrhages.

Ophthalmoscopical Appearance. Initially, the optic disc remains normal and is surrounded by a brown to brown-red concentric ring. Strands or streaks extend from this ring centrifugally into the fundus periphery. The streaks resemble vessels, hence the term "angioid streaks." The morphologic appearance is similar to lacquer cracks with an irregular branching pattern and a peripheral decrease in width. Angioid streaks show distinctly brighter margins. Vascular proliferation may be suspected if the streaks undergo color changes and appear gray or white. The posterior pole often shows pigment irregularities. The retinal vessels remain unchanged.

In advanced stages, serous transudates and exudates and subretinal hemorrhages, most commonly within the macular area, may appear. Such lesions undergo fibrotic scarring and their appearance is similar to that seen in disciform macular degeneration (Figs. 117, 119, and 120).

Differential Diagnosis. The differential diagnosis of angioid streaks includes Kuhnt-Junius degeneration (disciform macular degeneration), serpiginous or geographical chorioretinitis (Fig. 148), retinochorioretinitis peripapillaries, choroiditis areata, choroiditis striae, or helicoid peripapillary chorioretinal atrophy (Franceschetti, 1962).

This disease is characterized by a peripapillary retinal choroidal atrophy with flame-shaped extensions toward the fundus periphery. The lesions are not necessarily associated with the course of the retinal vessels. This condition is always bilateral, and the sexes are equally affected. According to Franceschetti (1962), two different clinical courses are possible, a stationary, congenital form and a progressive adult form. The etiology of this disease is unknown, and no hereditary cases have been reported.

Another disease that must be ruled out in a differental diagnosis is pigmented paravenous chorioretinal atrophy (Franceschetti, 1962). Like angioid streaks, this disease also affects both eyes and is characterized by paravenous irregularities, clumped pigmented retinochoroidal degenerations that are always located along the large veins and their branches. The vessels themselves do not show any changes. The etiology of pigmented paravenous chorioretinal atrophy is unknown. Possible causes are congenital anomalies and degenerative or inflammatory processes, i.e., syphilis and tuberculosis. Synonyms for pigmented paravenous chorioretinal atrophy include retinochoroiditis radiata, paravenous retinal degeneration, and congenital pigmentation of the retina.

Therapy. No therapy is known. Symptomatic treatment includes use of vitamins C and E and anabolic steroids.

Eales' Disease

Synonyms: Morbus Eales' periphlebitis retinae, juvenile recurrent vitreous hemorrhages.

Eales' disease is most often found in young men and is usually diagnosed in the 2nd or 3rd decade of life. The etiology of this disease that mainly affects retinal veins remains unknown. Several causes, for example, allergic-hyperergic reactions and hormonal factors, are discussed. One or both eyes may be affected. The active phase of the disease may terminate spontaneously after a period of approximately 3 years. Twenty-five percent of patients have a poor visual prognosis, mostly because of proliferative retinopathy that causes scar formation and traction on the retina. Some cases develop a hemorrhagic secondary glaucoma.

Ophthalmoscopical Appearance. Initially, small inflammatory foci develop in the fundus periphery. Isolated or grouped venous punctate or linear hemorrhages may be present. The punctate hemorrhages most likely develop from extravasation of red blood cells, whereas the linear hemorrhages often indicate rupture of small vessels. The veins surrounding the affected area show increased tortuosity and caliber irregularities that sometimes resemble beading. Localized yellow-white infiltrations are visible within the vascular walls. Some veins have dense vessel parallel sheaths. In the fundus periphery these vascular segments tend to undergo thrombosis that leads to string-shaped scarring (Figs. 149–152).

In advanced stages, after recurrent venous-vitreous hemorrhages have been resorbed, net-shaped anastomoses between adjacent venous branches can be found (rete mirabile). The capillaries are dilated and capillary aneurysms and fan-shaped neovascularization may be present. The vitreous hemorrhages become organized and scar tissue strands form between the retina and the vitreous, often seen as white or gray-white, sail- or veil-shaped strands. These strands may cause a tractional retinal detachment.

In the early stage of the disease, fluorescein angiography reveals peripheral capillary dilatation and microaneurysms and intervascular anastomoses. In later stages, vascular leakage, especially in areas of neovascularization, becomes visible. Such leakage can also be found in areas of ensheathed veins. These retia mirabilia (German: "wundernets") do not usually show fluorescein leakage. Venous occlusions can also be verified with an angiography.

Differential Diagnosis. The differential diagnosis of ensheathed veins includes acute disseminated encephalomyelitis, Behçet's disease, sarcoidosis, Coats' disease, Terry's syndrome (retinopathy of prematurity, retrolental fibroplasia), thromboangiitis obliterans, Winiwarter-Buerger disease, or sickle cell disease.

Laboratory and Other Findings. Findings include increased erythropoiesis, coagulopathy (hyperfibrinolysis and thrombopathy), and increased vascular permeability and fragility. Tuberculosis has been implicated, but a consistent pathogenesis of this condition has not been determined (Apple and Rabb, 1985).

Subjective Symptoms. The patient suffers from intermittent episodes of decreased and hazy vision. The affected eye does not show any external abnormalities.

Doden (1963) differentiated three different types of Eales' disease, based on a study of 1261 eyes in 730 patients:

1. Exudative type (20% of cases) with ensheathed veins, infiltrations in the vascular walls, and preretinal exudates;
2. Hemorrhagic type (55% of cases) with severe recurrent retinal and vitreous hemorrhages;
3. Proliferative type (25% of cases) with extensive neovascularization in retina and vitreous and formation of dense proliferative strands. Fifty percent of patients in this group suffer from retinal detachment caused by proliferative retinopathy.

Therapy. Early light coagulation and vitrectomy are indicated in cases of slowly resorbing vitreous hemorrhages. Use of corticosteroids is not effective.

Proliferative Retinopathy

The older term "retinitis proliferans" was coined by von Manz in 1876; however, the first description of the disease was given by von Jaeger in 1869.

Proliferative retinopathy describes various pathological changes that may be observed in several diseases of different etiologies. Fibrovascular and glial proliferations, in addition to retinal neovascularization that may extend into the vitreous, characterizes the clinical appearance. Proliferative retinopathy may be observed as a sequela of hemorrhage and/or hypoglycemia. A lack of oxygen seems to trigger an insufficent compensatory response.

Ophthalmoscopical Appearance. Ophthalmoscopically, gray-white fibrovascular strands and traction bands, sometimes sail-shaped, can be seen, which originate from retinal areas extending to the vitreous. As the term "fibrovascular" indicates, these strands may be partially vascularized and tend to shrink and exert traction on the retina, leading to tractional retinal detachment. Peripherally located strands may not be discovered for a long time because this condition does not usually produce any subjective symptoms. However, if these fibrovascular changes are located at the posterior pole, and there is almost always a loss in central visual acuity. A pseudoglioma is an extreme and ultimate example of this condition in which the vitreous is completely replaced by fibrous masses.

Proliferative retinopathy can be found in Eales' disease, diabetic retinopathy, hypertension, arteriosclerosis, and after perforating trauma, as well as being associated with chronic infection (e.g., syphilis) (Figs. 153–157).

Therapy. Depending on the extent of vitreous changes, a combined retinal-vitreal surgical intervention may be necessary.

Epiretinal Membranes

Synonyms: Intraretinal fibroplasia with macular degeneration, intraretinal gliosis, macular epiretinal fibroplasia, preepiretinitis or epiretinitis, postcoagulation degeneration, postcoagulative macular degeneration, star-fold retinitis, or central vitreoretinal fibroplastic syndrome.

The true pathogenesis of this disease is still unknown. The changes can be observed in any age group and are sex-independent.

Ophthalmoscopical Appearance. Vodovozov (1981) described stationary reflexes surrounding arterioles, especially in the macular area. These reflexes may be varied with a nummular or lobular appearance, or splint or ring shapes. This early stage in the formation of epiretinal membranes is followed by an edematous insudative phase (Gloor and Werner, 1967). The superotemporal and inferotemporal marginal zones of the macula seem to be most often affected (Fig. 158). The first fibroblastic reactions can be observed while the intraretinal edema is still present. Gray foci with irregular borders appear. The color eventually changes into the white-gray of the proliferative stage. The foci may become sharply demarcated and prominent, or create a flat membrane or preretinal strands that are attached to some retinal areas. Capillaries appear dilated and show caliber irregularities and proliferative changes. Punctate and small linear hemorrhages complete the morphological appearance. No pigmentation is present.

The beginning of the shrinking process leads to severe radial striae formation within the retina. The retinal vessels surrounding these striae may deviate toward the center of the traction. Quite often a macular ectopia develops. Late complications of this disease are cystic macular degeneration, localized retinoschisis, macular hole, and retinal detachment. These changes are most often seen unilaterally.

Predisposing Conditions and Symptoms. Epiretinal membranes occur in a number of conditions, e.g., after retinal photocoagulation or cryotherapy, after blunt or penetrating injuries, after surgical interventions (retinal or cataract surgery), as an idiopathic process in otherwise normal eyes, in ocular inflammatory conditions (iridocyclitis, uveitis, central or paracentral chorioretinitis, Eales' disease, acute glaucoma), or associated with metabolic diseases (proliferative diabetic retinopathy, arteriosclerosis, hypertension).

The patient's symptoms may vary according to the location and extent of the fibrous membrane and the traction that it exerts on other tissues. Macular or perimacular lesions are characterized by a decreased visual acuity that usually develops slowly. The decrease in vision may be caused by or be associated with symptoms such as metamorphopsia, blurred and washed-out contours, and/or vertical diplopia.

Other Findings. In eyes with epiretinal membranes, vitreous changes can be detected by slitlamp examination.

Posterior Vitreous Detachment. Cells and abnormal membranes within the posterior vitreous are quite typical findings.

Visual Field Losses. Depending on the location of the lesion, absolute or relative central or pericentral scotomas may be present. By using Amsler's chart, metamorphopsia can be detected very early.

Fluorescein Angiography. According to Gloor and Werner (1967), a lack of vascular leakage in the affected retinal areas is characteristic. Hiller (1971b), however, showed that there is marked extravasation of fluorescein during the edematous stage with a diffuse staining of the lesion. Defects in vessels related to traction on the retina can also be found. Newly formed capillaries, microaneurysms, and caliber irregularities were described by Hiller (1971b). The author interpreted his results by theorizing that there may be two different forms of this disease, a primary, inflammatory form, in which there is fluorescein leakage, and a primary, degenerative form with no vascular leakage. Once the lesion has been transformed into a solid scar, no fluorescein leakage occurs.

Therapy. The use of corticosteroids has been tried successfully in some cases while the disease is in its early edematous stage. Hiller (1971b) injected retrobulbar dexamethasone, and Liesenhoff (1968) tried subconjunctival injections of prednisolone. Varga and Gáll (1969) recommended light coagulation at the sites where the preretinal membrane is attached to the retina. Bangerter (1970) treated the lesion with irradiation.

Prognosis. The prognosis regarding final visual acuity can vary, and the prognosis for sporadic cases is essentially better than that of operatively caused cases. Visual acuity rarely decreases below 20/200 in either form of the disease.

Coats' Disease

Synonyms: Coats' syndrome, morbus Coats, exudative external retinitis, or primary Coats' syndrome.

Classically, Coats' disease is a nonfamilial, almost always unilateral disease that occurs in the absence of other systemic findings primarily in infants or juveniles. Bilateral affection is exceptional. Green (1967) reported a case of a 13-year-old girl with bilateral disease.

The clinical course is characterized by a slow, lingering onset and extremely slow progression. Spontaneous remissions in the progression of the disease are possible. Major complications of Coats' disease are iritis, complicated cataract, retinal detachment, secondary glaucoma, and phthisis bulbi. Coats (1908, 1912) differentiated three disease groups:

Group 1
Vessels appear normal ophthalmoscopically, but retinal exudates may be present.

Group 2
Vessels exhibit clinically obvious changes such as telangiectasic aneurysms, vascular sheathing, neovascularization, and retinal exudates.

Group 3
This group is now recognized as von-Hippel-Lindau angiomatosis (transmitted as an autosomal dominant trait with incomplete penetrance). Angiomatosis in other organs, e.g., in the cerebellum of the brain, occurs bilaterally in 50% of cases.

The characteristic finding, retinal exudates, in Groups 1 and 2 represents subretinal and intraretinal deposition of cholesterol-containing lipid exudates. These clinically and pathologically evident deposits are whitish yellow, may appear flat, progress to cover a larger area, or form nodules. Quite often large plaques can be found. A macular star figure may be seen in the posterior pole. Peripheral isolated nodular lesions may be mistaken morphologically for a malignant melanoma. Retinal hemorrhages, most often found in Group 2, can become quite massive. Fluorescein angiography can reveal the vascular changes in Group 2, i.e., excessive capillary dilatation, nonperfusing areas, and capillary and larger vessel aneurysms. Usually, true neovascularization is not found. Electron microscopy reveals a loss of endothelial cells and pericytes from the vascular walls, as well as thickening of the basement membrane with deposition of mucopolysaccharides (Figs. 159–162).

Some authors believe that Leber's miliary aneurysms represent an early stage of Coats' disease (Reese, 1956; Pau, 1979a). Coats' disease in combination with tapetoretinal degeneration has been described (Schmidt and Faulborn, 1972; Witschel, 1974; Rix et al., 1982). An association with a congenital muscular dystrophy has also been shown (Small, 1968).

The essential pathogenetic factor is probably a loss of vascular endothelial cell tight junctions (zonular occludens), leading to a breakdown of the blood-retina barrier. Blood fluids and lipids cross this barrier and are deposited within the vessel walls and in the perivascular interstitial tissues. According to François et al. (1956), Coats' disease represents a primary angiomatosis.

Therapy. Xenon laser coagulation of affected vessels and microaneurysms is recommended. However, coagulation and isolation of lipid deposits is not recommended. If a retinal detachment covers a whole quadrant, a combined globe shortening operation and interscleral diathermia and light coagulation may be helpful. No comprehensive drug treatment is known, but treatment of the symptoms may be advantgeous.

Secondary Coats' Disease

According to Reese (1956) and Manschot and De Bruijn (1967), the terms "Coats' disease" or "morbus Coats" should be used only for cases of exudative retinopathy and retinal vascular anomalies in childhood. These terms should not be used if the disease is observed in adults (Figs. 163-166). Coats' disease or secondary Coats' disease has been described in adults (Apple and Rabb, 1985).

Behçet's Syndrome

Synonyms: Morbus Gilbert-Adamantiades-Behçet, Behçet's disease, recurrent hypopyon-iritis, uveo-encephalitic syndrome, oculobuccogenital syndrome, or aphthous ulcers.

The possible connection of ocular and skin symptoms were suggested by Gilbert in 1920 and 1925, and by Adamantiades in 1931, before Behçet in 1937 described the entity that bears his name. The etiology of this disease is unknown. Several etiological factors such as virus infection, tuberculosis, venereal disease, staphylococcal infections, leptospirosis, and immunological disease have been considered as causative. Etiological connections to erythema multiforme exudativum and to Stevens-Johnson syndrome may be possible.

Behçet's syndrome is manifest in most patients between 15 and 35 years of age, and men are affected primarily. Geographically, an increased incidence of Behçet's disease is seen in such Mediterranean countries as Greece, Italy, and Turkey. There is also an increased incidence in Japan.

Histopathologically, inflammatory and degenerative vascular changes with edematous intima, perivascular round cell infiltrates, and fibrinoid necrosis have been described.

General Clinical Appearance. During an inflammatory episode the patient feels very ill and shows such general symptoms as loss of appetite, fatigue, fever, sweating, myalgia, arthralgia, and thrombophlebitis migrans. Inflammation in other organ systems complicates the course of the disease (esophagitis, gastric and colon ulcers, urethritis, orchitis, and epididymitis). Complications of the central nervous systems can be life-threatening, including the so-called "neuro-Behçet" meningoencephalitis, cranial nerve palsy (affecting the III, IV, VI, and VII nerves), brainstem syndrome that may advance to a lethal bulbar paralysis, hemiplegia, and ataxia. Psychic alterations also have been described.

Characteristic laboratory findings include an extremely increased sedimentation rate, leukocytosis with left shift, and eosinophilic leukocytosis.

Clinical Appearance. Only in rare cases are all of the major symptoms present at the same time. Some symptoms may be noted months or years prior to the onset of the generalized disease. The most common symptoms are skin and eye lesions, i.e., the so-called "oculobuccogenital triad," iritis with recurrent hypopyons, and ulcerations (aphthae) of the oral mucosa and genitals.

Skin and Mucosa Lesions. Aphthae of the oral mucosa and buccal mucosa, appearing as isolated or disseminated multiple lesions, is characteristic. The lesions are painful, but disappear within a short time, making the differential diagnosis difficult in cases with only simple ulcers. Genital lesions soon progress from erythematous affections to deep ulcerations. Other possible skin lesions are papulopustular, papulovesicular, and furunculous erythema. The skin is often hyperreactive after injections.

Eye Symptoms. At a relatively late stage of the disease, iritis with recurrent hypopyons that may be hemorrhagic can develop. The disease usually begins in only one eye, but the second eye may become involved years later. The inflammatory reaction may affect the posterior uvea and cause focal posterior uveitis. At times posterior uveitis is the first symptom. Most often a round to oval lesion with washed-out borders and measuring 1-3 optic disc diameters is found. This lesion may be gray-yellow to gray-green. In other cases, the effects on retinal vessels in the form of periarteritis, periphlebitis, and phlebitis determine the clinical picture. In some cases, a severe intraocular hemorrhage may be the first symptom. Other ocular manifestations include ulcerated keratitis, episcleritis, scleritis, papillitis with transformation into optic nerve atrophy, exudative retinal detachment, complicated cataract, and secondary glaucoma (Figs. 167 and 168).

Therapy. Some success in the treatment of this disease has been achieved with salicylates, adrenocorticotropic hormone (ACTH), corticosteroids, gamma globulin, blood transfusions, and immunosuppressive agents. Topical therapy consists of subconjunctival injections of corticosteroids and atropine, and use of cortisone drops or ointments.

Prognosis. The prognosis for final visual acuity is extremely poor and binocular blindness seems to be an unavoidable ultimate complication. In addition, Behçet's disease can be life-threatening, especially if the central nervous system is involved.

Central Serous Chorioretinopathy

Central serous chorioretinopathy was first described in 1866 by von Graefe, who termed it "central recurrent retinitis." The etiology of this disease remains unknown. Several etiologic factors have been discussed such as infections and toxic or allergic-hyperergic reactions. Other possible causes are angioneurotic diathesis, degenerative or inherited alterations of Bruch's membrane and of the pigment epithelium, and psychic and psychosomatic disease.

Central serous chorioretinopathy usually becomes manifest between the 3rd and 5th decade of life. Men are most often affected. Recidivations are extremely common.

Clinical Appearance. The visual acuity is markedly affected. Due to the elevation of the macula, the eyes become slightly hyperopic (up to 1.5 diopters). Metamorphopsia, micropsia, and alterations in color vision for yellow, blue-green, and red are among the symptoms.

Ophthalmoscopical Appearance. Early stages of the disease are characterized only by lack of the normal foveal reflex. After 1-2 weeks, a demarcated, elevated edema, up to 3 diopters, develops within the posterior pole. In the third to fourth week, subretinal, punctate, yellow-white precipitates within the edema become recognizable. The optic disc and retinal vessels appear normal during the entire course of the disease (Figs. 169-171).

Fluorescein angiography has shown three different types of macular lesions:

Type 1

Dot or punctate areas of vascular leakage with an obvious leakage source occurs in 2/3 of all cases. Leakage up to 1/4 optic disc diameter in size through Bruch's membrane is most often located around the margin of the serous detachment some distance from the foveola. A serous exudate, located between the neuroepithelium and pigment epithelium, may be clear or appear muddy and dim. As the lesion heals, only moderate pigment irregularities remain within the macular region.

Type 2

The entire subretinal serous exudate, located between the pigment epithelium and Bruch's membrane, shows diffuse fluorescent staining. When this type of lesion heals, more severe pigment irregularities remain within the macular region.

Type 3

This is a rare form of the disease and represents a combination of Types 1 and 2. One or several specific sites of origin for fluorescein leakage may be present, but there is also diffuse leakage over other areas.

Therapy. It is believed that light or xenon laser coagulation shortens the course of the disease. Depending on the location of the leakage source, such a treatment is indicated in the following: (*a*) prolonged course of more than 6-8 weeks duration, (*b*) if secondary retinal changes occur, and (*c*) in cases of recidivation (Wessing, 1973).

Drug Treatment. The author prefers to prescribe corticosteroids in different applications combined with radiation therapy.

Prognosis. The prognosis in terms of visual acuity is often good. Spontaneous remissions without functional losses are seen frequently. In only 5% of cases does the disease progress to disciform macular degeneration. Hemorrhages during the acute phase (chorioretinitis centralis serosa haemorrhagica) worsen the prognosis. Such hemorrhages may lead to scar formation and severe pigment irregularities within the macular region. The normal course of the disease is 8-10 weeks.

According to Sautter and Utermann (1964), quite often a transition to exudative macular degeneration is seen in patients with recurrent central serous chorioretinitis in their later years.

Circinate Retinopathy

Synonyms: Macular star figure, Fuchs' circinate retinitis.

Circinate retinopathy was first described in 1875 by Hutchinson, who termed it "symmetrical central chorido-retinal disease occurring in senile persons."

A true macular star figure does not represent the disease in and of itself. It is rather a symptom caused by local retinal hypoxia. A macular star figure may be associated with other ocular diseases, including arteriosclerosis (Fig. 120), Stage II of diabetic retinopathy (Fig. 98), branch or central vein occlusions, Coats' disease (external hemorrhagic retinopathy of Coats), and as an early or accompanying symptom of a disciform macular lesion (Figs. 119 and 120). Less frequently, it is seen in anemic or leukemic patients and may also be associated with glaucoma.

Circinate retinopathy most often becomes manifest between the 5th and 6th decade of life, but is sometimes seen in juvenile patients. Most frequently, the retinal lesions occur bilaterally; however, a unilateral star figure may persist for years. Women seem to be more prone to suffer from this disease (female: male, 3:2).

Histopathologically, this disease is characterized by degenerative foci and lipid deposits within the deeper retinal layers.

Ophthalmoscopical Appearance. Typical cases show sharply demarcated foci of lipid deposition at the posterior pole surrounding the fovea (Figs. 172–175). The deposited material may appear white or yellow and is often arranged in a horseshoe, circular, or garland pattern. The isolated lesions tend to accrue. Retinal vessels are not affected and may unimpededly pass the circinate figure. Less frequently, a similar star figure can be found in the retinal periphery immediately adjacent to hemorrhagic or proliferative areas (Fig. 174). The number of degenerative foci and hard exudates may vary. In most cases the macula shows some pathology (senile disciform or cystoid degeneration). This macular involvement is a determinant for the amount of functional loss (central visual loss, metamorphopsia, central scotoma). Spontaneous remissions are possible.

Therapy. The only known therapy is treatment of the underlying disease.

Septic Retinitis

A generalized sepsis often causes characteristic changes that can be observed ophthalmoscopically. These changes are precipitated partially by emboli from the causative organisms and partially by the toxic effects of the organisms. The severity of the disease depends on the virulence of the organisms, as well as on the number of organisms that have invaded the blood stream. The severity of the disease may also be modified by the patient's immunologic response.

Septic retinitis is associated most often with subacute bacterial endocarditis, phlebitis, puerperal infections, tuberculosis, and cachexia in tumor patients. *Staphylococci,* nonhemolytic *Streptococci, Meningococci,* and virus and fungal (*Candida albicans*) infections have been identified as most often causative. Despite the severe fundus involvement, patients normally have few subjective symptoms. A rare exception to this rule occurs with a septic embolic occlusion of the central retinal artery.

Hollwich (1982) differentiates between a simple septic retinitis and septic retinitis associated with metastatic ophthalmia.

Ophthalmoscopical Appearance. The bacterial or mycotic offender most often penetrates the vascular wall at the sites of vascular branching, causing retinal hemorrhages. In the classical form, these hemorrhages resemble Roth's spots (1872). A white or light-gray contrasting center is typical. Such lesions may also be found in areas apart from larger retinal vessels. The retinal or preretinal hemorrhages may be round, oval, or flame-shaped and may show a rapidly changing pattern.

A sympathetic ophthalmia is characterized by conjunctival chemosis, ciliary injunction, corneal and endothelial precipitates, a cellular reaction in the aqueous humor that can lead to a hypopyon, and a cellular reaction in the vitreous that may progress to a vitreous abscess. The optic disc becomes edematous, and the embolic lesions increase in size and show blurred margins.

Therapy. Therapy consists of antibiotic treatment for the causative infection.

Prophylaxis. If the patient's history reveals the presence of a congenital or acquired malformation of the heart valves, preoperative antibiotic therapy is indicated before dental, ear, nose, and throat, and urologic surgical interventions are performed (Heisig, 1981).

Choroiditis

Synonym: Posterior uveitis.

The extreme vascularity of the choroid (posterior uvea) seems to predispose it for occurrence of inflammatory processes that are transported into the vascular tissue via the blood stream. Such inflammation may result from tumor metastasis from other regions of the body, septic emboli, and microorganisms and their toxins.

Schreck (1977) defined a group of generalized diseases

that show a uveotropic character in that the most frequent manifestation sites are the anterior and posterior uvea. These diseases include tuberculosis, rheumatic diseases, and especially focal or localized infections. In the majority of cases, the etiology is unknown.

Ophthalmoscopical Appearance. One has to differentiate a central and peripheral choroiditis according to the localization of the inflammatory lesion, and a disseminated choroiditis from a localized or circumscribed choroiditis according to the inflammatory foci.

Subjective Symptoms. Peripheral inflammatory lesions usually do not cause any symptoms. Therefore, choroiditis is often diagnosed incidentally during a routine ophthalmoscopic examination. Sometimes patients report a light flicker in front of their eyes (photopsia) or report dark spots (scotoma). Lack of pain is characteristic, except for patients who suffer from Vogt-Koyanagi syndrome or Harada's syndrome in which encephalitis may be associated with the uveitis. The visual acuity is affected only in patients who have paracentral or central choroidal infiltrates. Micropsia or metamorphopsia may be present in these patients. Extensive scarring affects the mesopic vision and reduces the visual field.

Disseminated Choroiditis

The chronic course of disseminated choroiditis, which is characterized by intermittent inflammatory episodes, explains why an ophthalmoscopical examination may reveal fresh inflammatory infiltrates as well as old choroidal scars. Sometimes both types of lesions are seen immediately adjacent, indicating a perifocal spread from an earlier scarred choroidal area.

Fresh choroidal lesions located anywhere in the fundus measure between 0.25 and 1.5 optic disc diameters. The lesions are oval or round, light gray to yellow-green, and show blurred margins. The overlying retina may appear muddy because of exudates, and the usually unaffected retinal vessels may be partially masked. In other cases, the unaffected vessels course over the slightly elevated lesions.

A choroidal inflammation that is located close to the optic disc may cause the disc to appear blurred. In the advanced scar stage of this disease, irregularly configurated, partially confluxing choroidal scars may cover larger areas of the choroid. These lesions show a light yellow to white discoloration. Retinal exudates have disappeared by this stage and the white-yellow sclera is clearly visible through the atrophic choroid. Sometimes obliterated choroidal vessels are seen at the bottom of the scar. An initial fine granular pigmentation of the isolated foci is typical. In later stages the margins and centers of larger scars may show clumped dark pigmentations.

Complications. Choroidal or retinal hemorrhages, vascular ensheathing, perivascular nodules, and vitreous opacities may be associated with or complicate the course of disseminated choroiditis.

Central Localized Choroiditis

The hallmark of this entity is the presence of an isolated central group of lesions or a solitary large lesion. A causative protozoa infection (e.g., toxoplasmosis) must be ruled out.

Chorioretinitis

An inflammation that involves both the choroid and retina is defined as chorioretinitis (Figs. 176–188). Originally, the inflammation starts in the choroid, but the retina is often affected secondarily and permanently damaged. Isolated foci close to the optic disc are often referred to as juxtapapillary chorioretinitis (Fig. 185).

Jensen's Juxtapapillary Retinochoroiditis

This classic juxtapapillary retinochoroiditis is manifest by inflammatory chorioretinitis immediately adjacent to the optic disc, as the term indicates. The etiology of this disease is unknown. Several inflammatory and infectious processes are considered to be causative, e.g., tuberculosis or tuberculoallergenic reactions, syphilis, toxoplasmosis, and focal infections. Most often, patients of both sexes in the 3rd decade of life are affected.

Ophthalmoscopical Appearance. Early in the disease an oval elevated inflammatory lesion with blurred margins, which measures between 1 and 2 optic disc diameters, can be found immediately adjacent to the optic disc. The optic disc also shows blurred margins from the papilledema. The vessels close to the papillae are also distorted, and the arterioles overlying the inflammatory lesion are narrowed. The vitreous shows inflammatory involvement, and keratic precipitates can be seen on the corneal endothelium.

Diagnosis is confirmed if an irreversible arcuate visual field defect is present that resembles a comet's tail and originates from the blind spot. Within 3–4 months the inflammation subsides, and a chorioretinal scar with varying amounts of pigmentation is left. Recurrences located within the primary lesion, or adjacent to it, have been described.

Chorioretinitis of the Optic Disc

Schreck (1977) defines all inflammatory lesions of the Jensen's juxtapapillary type as chorioretinitis of the optic disc if the lesions are located some distance from the papilla rather than immediately adjacent to it.

Central Hemorrhagic Choroiditis

Synonyms: Juvenile exudative macular retinitis, juvenile disciform macular lesion, serous-hemorrhagic disciform macular detachment, focal macular choroiditis.

The appropriate term, focal (central) hemorrhagic chororiditis, is based on the suggestion of Schildberg and Wessing (1975). This entity represents localized or focal choroiditis and subretinal hemorrhages are present at an early stage. Fluorescein angiography reveals choroidal neovascularization that protrude into the subretinal space.

The etiology of this disease is unknown. Serologic screening for diseases associated commonly with uveitis is usually negative. A major characteristic of this disease is the acute onset with a mainly monocular severe visual loss. Other typical findings are a central scotoma and metamorphopsia. Central hemorrhagic choroiditis affects patients within the 3rd to 4th decade of life.

Ophthalmoscopical Appearance. Initially, a localized central retinal detachment may be observed. The serous fluid is soon replaced by recurrent subretinal hemorrhages. After these sickle-shaped or circular hemorrhages are resorbed, a pigmented scar remains. Frequently, isolated or multiple less pigmented chorioretinal scars of smaller diameter than the primary affected site can be found (see Fig. 189).

Differential Diagnosis. Early stages of central hemorrhagic choroiditis have to be differentiated from central serous retinopathy.

Therapy. The early phase may be treated with light coagulation of any localized choroidal neovascularization as verified by fluorescein angiography. Corticosteroids do not have any effect on the course of the disease.

Prognosis. The prognosis for full visual acuity is good.

Toxoplasmic Retinochoroiditis

Three different forms of choroiditis caused by toxoplasmosis have been identified: congenital form, acute acquired lesions, and late ocular recidivation (Huismans, 1979b).

Congenital Toxoplasmic Infection

The congenital form is characterized by the classic triad of hydrocephalus, intracranial calcification, and central retinochoroiditis (Janku, 1959). Other symptoms are jaundice, hepatosplenomegaly, and encephalitis.

Ophthalmoscopical Appearance. The majority of the cases show a monoocular involvement with prominent effects at the posterior pole. Morphologically, a macular rosette-shaped lesion can be observed in 40% of cases, a pseudocoloboma of the macula in 40% of cases, and an unspecific chorioretinitis in 20% of cases.

The macular rosette-shaped lesion, which is pathognomonic for congenital toxoplasmosis (François, 1963), has distinct central and peripheral zones. The central zone may appear as a vessel-free, homogeneous, unpigmented, gray-blue pseudotumor; as a pigmented, gray lesion; as an accumulation of black pigment; or simply as an atrophic area. Several partially excavated round chorioretinal scars separated by pigment accumulations fill the peripheral area. Extensions and projections of the central and/or peripheral pigmentations may create an arabesque-like picture (François, 1963).

A macular pseudocoloboma characteristically shows an oval, deeply excavated scar with irregular central and peripheral pigmentation. This scar is an important morphological hallmark for this disease (Hollwich, 1963b).

A less charactistic retinochoroiditis may be caused by a congenital toxoplasmic infection. This condition therefore has to be judged by the clinical situation, as well as by serological examinations (complement fixation test, Sabin-Feldman dye test, indirect fluorescein antibody test, indirect hemagglutination test, and a comparison analysis of blood and aqueous contents).

Late Ocular Recidivation

According to François (1963), late recidivations can be found in 70% of cases between the ages of 10 and 30, and are located mostly in the eye that was affected by the congenital lesion. In rare cases, a bilateral occurrence or a new manifestation in the previously healthy eye can be found. The late recidivation is caused by formation of cysts by the intracellular protozoan parasite. Rupture of these cysts then leads to the release of new parasites. The newly built inflammatory lesion is most often found in close proximity to the primary lesion.

Acquired Toxoplasmic Infection

Acquired toxoplasmosis is usually diagnosed between the ages of 10 and 40 and, unlike the congenital form, the central nervous system is rarely involved. Fundus abnormalities usually consist of a solitary inflammatory lesion that is initially yellow-gray. Over a period of months, the initially prominent lesion flattens. The degree of pigmentation may vary and retinal hemorrhages around the lesion margins are seen often over the years. A solitary lesion may be as large as 1 disc diameter, but satellite lesions are usually smaller. Rieger's central exudative retinitis is a special form of acquired toxoplasmic infection.

Therapy. Pyrimethamine (Daraprim) combined with sulfameth oxazole is a common treatment. Theodossiadis (1981) reported a successful treatment of active toxoplasmic chorioretinitis with argon laser coagulation. He suggested treatment of not only the entire area of acute inflammation, but also the adjacent scarred areas.

Chorioretinitis Associated with Listeriosis

Clinically, listeriosis represents a sporadically occurring, most often acute, and sometimes chronic, long-lasting infectious disease (Erdmann and Seeliger, 1968). It was first discovered in humans by von Nyfeldt in 1929. Seeliger and Potel (1969) differentiated five types according to their relative incidence: (*a*) acute septic type (newborn listeriosis or granulomatosis infantispectica); (*b*) listeriosis of the central nervous system (encephalitis, meningitis, meningoencephalitis); (*c*) glandular type (monocytic angina, lymphadenitis); (*d*) localized type (keratoconjunctivitis, skin listeriosis); and (*e*) chronic, septic type with isolated organ affection (abscess, endocarditis).

The involved organism (*Listeria monocytogenes*) is a Gram-positive bacteria that is rod-shaped and measures 0.3-3 μm in length and 0.5 μm in width. It belongs to the family of *Corynebacteriaceae*, is motile and peritrichous, and does not produce any spores. The organisms produce chains of 3-5 cells that are elongated and filamentous, which may be difficult to identify based on morphology alone.

L. monocytogenes contains antigens on the body (O-antigens) and on the lash (H-antigens). The term "*monocytogenes*" is based on the observation that this organism is quite often found in monocytic angina. It may be found in oral swabs, blood samples, or in tissue from glandular biopsies. For a long time this organism has been mistakenly identified as causative for infectious mononucleosis. The serotypes 1 and 4b seem to be the most offending forms of this organism in humans.

L. monocytogenes is a ubiquitous organism that lives in soil. Human infections may be caused exogenously by contact with infected animals and their feces (as with farmers), laboratory infections (as with veterinarians), by inhalation of listeria-containing dust, or by ingestion of contaminated food (milk, raw meat, fruit). Endogeneous infections are possible by hematogenous seeding organisms that are located in the intestine and/or male urethera of infected persons. A classic example of an endogenous infection is newborn listeriosis. Several different infectious modalities are possible. The placenta may become infected by bacteria from the mother, and the organisms may invade the fetus via the umbilical vein. Septicemia leads to hematogenous distribution of the organisms into all fetal organs. The fetus may also become infected secondarily when swallowing its own contaminated urine (Reiss et al., 1951). It is important that even when the mother is known to be the source of the fetal infection, she does not necessarily have to have any symptoms of the disease. Even after one child has been born with a listeriosis infection or has died because of this infection, the mother may completely recuperate without antibiotic treatment, and future children may be born healthy (Herrmann, 1961).

The newborn, if alive, is usually severely ill at the time of birth or will become so within a few days to 2 weeks thereafter. The clinical condition largely depends on the extent of hematogenous spread of the organism. Symptoms include a reduced general condition, malaise, diarrhea and vomiting, dysfunctions of the cardiovascular and pulmonary systems (dyspnea, cyanosis, apnea) caused by diffuse pneumonia and/or atelectasis of the lung, myocarditis, hepatosplenomegaly, and serous or purulent meningitis.

An adult infected with the organism seems to be more prone to develop encephalitis and may show symptoms of brainstem involvement. Disseminated ependymitis may cause an internal hydrocephalus. Histopathologically, foci of mononuclear cells that surround a necrotic area may be found within the tissue (listerioma).

Pink or blue skin lesions with yellow centers are indicative of this disease, but these lesions are not always present. Diagnosis is based on the patient's history and isolation of the organisms in the meconium or in the cerebrospinal fluid. Newborn listeriosis is found at an incidence of one case in 1500–2000 births.

The glandular type of listeriosis is characterized by a diffuse swelling of the lymph nodules. Clinically, influenza-like symptoms with angina and swelling of the throat and neck lymph nodules may be present. The lymph nodules may undergo necrosis and/or develop outer fistulas. The localized type of this disease shows purulent and pustulant skin lesions with accompanying lymphangitis. In rare cases, hematogenous meningitis has been described. Localized disease is frequently found in patients whose profession requires contact with infected animals or other sources of infection.

In addition to the search for bacteria in blood and other body secretions and tissues, a repeated serological analysis of the antibodies may help confirm the diagnosis. The two tests used for the antibody analysis are the Widal listeriosis test (Table 15) and the complement fixation test. A clinical example is shown in Figs. 193–195.

If the infection becomes clinically manifest, the O-titers show a positive agglutination at a dilution of 1:100 to 1:160 and higher. However, even in cases of a proven infection, the titers are often lower (Seeliger and Potel, 1969). The antibiotic of choice is ampicillin. Successful treatment has also been reported with tetracycline.

Listeriosis may affect the eye by causing conjunctivitis, and listeriosis associated with conjunctivitis in newborns has been reported (Burdin et al., 1965). Data from laboratory experiments show that listeria-containing specimens can cause keratoconjunctivitis in guinea pig and rabbit eyes. This conclusion may be extrapolated to clinical cases because human eyes can also suffer from keratoconjunctivitis after infection with this organism. However, this possibility is not often entertained clinically.

Table 15. Antibody Concentration[a]

	Listeriosis agglutination, concentration			
Antigen	24 May	14 June	28 June	19 July
Type 1, O-antigen	1:100	Negative	1:200	1:200
Type 1, H-antigen	1:50	1:100	1:50	1:50
Type 4, O-antigen	1:50	Negative	Negative	Negative
Type 4, H-antigen	1:50	Negative	1:50	Negative
	Therapy			
	Tetracycline Prednisolone	Tetracycline Prednisolone	Ampicillin	Ampicillin

[a]Widal's listeriosis test.

Goodner and Okumoto (1967) reported an acute anterior uveitis, and Cherednichenko (1962) described six cases of choroidal involvement in a series of 80 patients suffering from generalized listeriosis.

Toxocariasis

Beaver et al. (1952) described the childhood syndrome caused by infection by *Toxocara canis*, and they coined the term "visceral larva migrans syndrome." The secondary larvae of the canine roundworm are distributed to peripheral organs, especially to the liver, lungs, brain, and eyes, from the small intestine.

Intraocular toxocariasis was first described and emphasized by Wilder in 1950, who found larvae in histological sections of enucleated eyes that had been removed because of misdiagnoses. In most of these cases, the true diagnosis was pseudoglioma.

The characteristic finding of toxocariasis is an eosinophilic granulomatous response. The cellular infiltrates consist of eosinophils, plasma cells, lymphocytes, and foreign body giant cells. Sometimes, the center of the granulomatous foci contains complete or fragmented larvae.

The clinical symptoms are not specific and are often misinterpreted. Bronchopulmonary and gastrointestinal symptoms, as well as a lymphadenopathy, are the most prominent features. The blood count reveals an eosinophilia that may resemble eosinophilic leukemia. The invasion of the larvae into the central nervous system often leads to such misdiagnoses as epilepsy, encephalitis, acute menigomyelitis, stroke, brain tumor, and other diseases.

A toxocariasis infection may be proved serologically by a microprecipitation test using living *T. canis* larvae that have been developed in generations of mice, or by the enzyme-linked immunosorbent assay (ELISA). According to Schwarzhuber (1978), a titer of 1:320 is considered specific for a larvae invasion when the clinical history and laboratory diagnosis (complement fixation test) have ruled out filariasis.

Ophthalmoscopical Appearance. Eye lesions usually manifest themselves as a leukocoria. The fundus may show two different morphological types of infection depending on whether the larvae invasion is recent or long-standing. In a long-standing chronic larvae invasion a solitary, isolated ocular granuloma can be found. It is noteworthy that ocular involvement generally represents a late manifestation (3 months to several years after parasite invasion). Distribution of the larvae occurs via the arterial circulation (Figs. 190–203).

Acute Larvae Infection

It is exceptional to observe a *T. canis* larva during the initial invasion of the human eye. The diameter of the larva is between 0.018 and 0.020 mm, and the gray-white larva body is difficult to see during routine ophthalmoscopy. Therefore, direct proof of larvae invasion within the ocular circulation can be achieved only if a specific search for the organism is made by serial photography, based on a clinical suspicion for this disease.

Ophthalmoscopical Appearance. Some specific morphological features help to identify a larva within the fundus. The organism is most frequently found in the temporal fundus. Small retinal hemorrhages and localized retinal edema may be observed at the location of the parasite. Larvae can rapidly change position and morphological appearance, but ribbon-, band-, or ring-shaped lesions are seen most frequently. Once the accompanying retinal exudations increase, the larvae become even more difficult to locate. An inflammatory encapsulation ensues and punctate, hook-, or sickle-shaped pigmentations may be seen at the invasion site (Huismans, 1980c). At times, these pigmentations indicate the migration tract of the larvae along the fundus. The inflammation probably represents a local tissue reaction caused by complete or fragmented larvae or their metabolic products. Once the inflammatory encapsulation begins, the disease may be easily misdiagnosed since the encapsulations may resemble cotton wool exudates or the lesions in Jensen's juxtapapillary chorioretinitis (Figs. 198–203).

Chronic Larvae Infection

The most typical manifestation of a chronic infection is a solitary granuloma that is most often located near the posterior pole. Peripheral granulomas adjacent to the ora serrata are rare. The diameter of the lesion can exceed several optic disc diameters, and the center of the lesion contains the *T. canis* larva. The periphery of the lesion is characterized by pigment clumps of varying density and concentration, which sometimes imitate the concavity or outline of the larva body. According to long-term studies (Huismans, 1982c), a solitary granuloma does not necessarily represent an inactive scar, but it may be the source of recurrent chorioretinal inflammatory reactions that can occur within months or years after the initial invasion. The pigmentary irregularities in later stages increase the difficulty of an ophthalmoscopical-morphological diagnosis (Figs. 190–192).

Therapy. There is no absolute safe and efficient therapy. Anthelmintic drugs do not have any effect once the larvae are encapsulated. According to reports to date, a drug treatment seems to be efficacious only while the larvae are migrating through the host and are exposed to the drug. The most promising drug for treatment of this infection in humans is thiabendazole. This drug is also used in veterinary medicine (Seitz, 1984; Stoye, 1981).

In cases of early ocular involvement, a combination of systemic prednisolone, long-lasting sulfonamides, and tetracycline appears to have a positive effect (Huismans, 1977b). The rationale for this combination of drugs is to reduce the inflammatory activity and prevent secondary infections that develop because of the mechanical tissue damage caused by the larvae invasion and migration. A therapetic regimen should be started immediately because of the severity of the infection and even without the serological test results, which usually take some time to complete. Nolan (1968) recommend subconjunctival corticosteriod injections. Siam (1973) and Raistrick and Dean-Hart (1975) recommend the destruction of the larvae in situ by light coagulation.

Prophylaxis. Repeated anthelmintic drug treatment of pet dogs, especially young puppies up to 6 months, is recommended. At the age of 3 weeks, a puppy may already excrete embryonic eggs. These eggs mature in air at a temperature of 30°C within 30 days. After this period, *T. canis* larvae become capable of invading another organism. Puppy infection is usually prenatal (Stoye, 1981). The larvae are encapsulated within the muscles of the female dog, become activated by hormonal stimuli, and infect the dog fetus via the placenta. This cycle explains why a negative helminthic test in the female dog can not be considered conclusive that an infection with *T. canis* has not previously occurred. The most important postnatal infectious source for the puppies is the mother dog's milk (Stoye, 1981).

Hygienic Precautions. Puppies and young dogs should be kept away from children's playgrounds, parks, and beaches. If the clinical symptoms of a larva migrans-visceralis infection are present, especially after a person has spent some time in a tropical or Mediterranean area, repeated ophthalmoscopical examinations should be performed.

Echinococcus granulosus Infection

The hydatid of *Echinococcus granulosus* (canine tapeworm) is only rarely found in the human eye (vitreous, uvea, retina, and anterior chamber). In 1977, Huismans (1977e) reported only the 17th case in the literature in which the *Echinococcus* hydatid was located subretinally in a 2-year-old child (Fig. 204).

The diagnosis for this disease is based on characteristic ophthalmoscopical findings and serological diagnosis (complement fixation test, indirect hemogluttination test, precipitation test, and Casoni's skin test). The skin test must be performed at the end of the serological diagnosis. Because of the small size of the hydatids, such diagnostic methods as sonography, roentgenographic screening for calcification, or computed tomography are of limited value.

Ophthalmoscopical Appearance of Subretinal Hydatids. The posterior pole is most frequently affected. The infection most characteristically shows a large, smooth-surfaced tumor that measures up to several optic disc diameters, which may or may not be elevated. The tumor center appears umbilicated, and hemorrhages may be present around the tumor margins.

Therapy. Treatment of the lesion by laser coagulation was suggested by Bernsmeier in 1980. According to Minning (1969), scoleces may develop only after the hydatid cyst has exceeded a diameter of 20 mm. Anthelmintic drug treatment with mebendazole or flubendazole, combined with surgery when necessary, is used most often.

Cytomegalic Inclusion Disease

Synonyms: Cytomegalic inclusion retinitis, maladie des inclusions cytomégaliques, generalized cytomegalic inclusion disease, giant cell inclusion disease.

Cytomegalic inclusion disease is caused by a DNA virus of the same name. The virus was isolated by Smith and coworkers in 1970. The cytomegalic virus is a facultative pathogen that is closely related to herpes and varicella viruses. The exact incubation period is not known; however, it has been shown that the virus may survive for years in infected organs. Infected patients may excrete the virus for up to 30 months even with subclinical infections.

Affected humans are the source of infection, with an incubation period of approximately 2–10 weeks. The virus is transmitted via dust, smears, droplets, blood transfusions, and bone marrow transplantation. Individuals undergoing immunosuppressive and cytostatic therapy for leukemia or malignant lymphomas, patients on dialysis treatment, or organ transplant patients are at increased risk for this infection.

Primary infection must be differentiated from a reinfection or a reactivation of a latent infection.

The virus is a ubiquitous organism found worldwide. In western Europe, a positive complement fixation test for cytomegalic virus is found in 20–30% of 1-year-old children, and in 40–60% of persons older than 30 years.

Clinical Appearance. Two types of cytomegalic inclusion disease must be differentiated, a congenital form and an acquired, adult form. Congenital cytomegalic inclusion disease is a diaplacental infection caused by transfer of viremia from the mother. The severity with which the embryo or fetus is affected may vary markedly. Embryopathic, generalized, and localized types of infection can be found. Most often congenital cytomegalic inclusion disease results in gross malformation or death of the newborn infant.

The cerebral form of infection is characterized by hydrocephalus, microcephalus, congenital encephalopathy, and intracranial calcifications. Symptoms identifying ocular involvement include microphthalmia, optic nerve coloboma, and optic nerve hyperplasia. If the embryo was infected before the 3rd month of gestation, complete aplasia of the retinal vessels may occur. Decreased growth of the body is another general symptom. The generalized form of this disease often leads to premature birth.

Organ manifestations that may occur include:

Brain	Encephalitis with postinflammatory loss of brain substance, cerebral convulsions, paresis, cerebral hemorrhages, mental retardation
Eye	Chorioretinitis, optic nerve atrophy, cataract
Heart	Valve malformations, myocarditis
Lung	Acute interstitial pneumonia, bronchopneumonia
Liver	Hepatomegaly, hepatitis, cirrhosis
Spleen	Splenomegaly
Gastrointestinal	Ulcers, enteritis
Hematopoietic system	Hemolytic anemia, thrombocytopenia
Skeletal system	Metaphysical irregularities
Salivary glands	Enlargement of parotid glands
Endocrine glands	Pancreas, thyroid, and suprarenal glands may be affected

The generalized form of cytomegalic inclusion disease can be found with or without associated embryopathy. The localized form is considered an incomplete form of a generalized infection.

Acquired Postnatal Form of Cytomegalic Inclusion Retinitis. The acquired form observed in newborns or infants resembles a generalized septicemia that is resistant to most antibiotics. The adult form is characterized by recurrent fever or there may be few clinical symptoms. Lymphadenopathy resembling infectious mononucleosis may be present, but tests for mononucleosis are negative. The respiratory system may be affected by influenza-like symptoms. Bronchopneumonia, atypical pneumonia, or influenza-like illness are other manifestations of this disease. The gastrointestinal system may be affected by gastric ulcers, enteritis, and ulcerative colitis. Other signs are hepatosplenomegaly, myocarditis, generalized vasculitis, and/or an infection of the hematopoietic system. The salivary glands and kidneys may be affected but infection in these organs can remain latent. Polyneuropathy, arthritis, and labyrinthitis also have been observed.

Ocular involvement may be manifest as a severe bilateral conjunctivitis with lid edema, dacryoadenitis, scleritis, corneal lesions, keratomalacia, chorioretinitis, necrotizing retinitis, necrotic panuveitis, and/or moderately pigmented, isolated retinochoroidal scars.

Differential Diagnosis. Conjunctival toxoplasmosis, optic nerve atrophy, pscudorctinitis pigmentosa, cataract.

Confirmation of the Diagnosis. It may be extremely difficult to culture the virus since the organism loses its infectious qualities once it is frozen. In addition, the virus grows only in diploid cells.

Serologic Diagnosis. Increasing titers in the complement fixation test, especially during pregnancy, are indicative. Low titers in a newborn's serum do not rule out an infection because there may be a delay in the production of antibodies. A high titer represents an active and relatively recent infection by the cytomegalic virus. An ELISA allows for the following conclusions: if anticytomegalic antibodies are IgM positive, the infection is most likely acute; if the antibodies are IgG positive, it is most likely that the infection took place earlier. However, virus reactivation can not be ruled out completely.

Cytologic Findings. Cytomegalic virus-containing cells are acidophiles, which are mononuclear with an eccentric nucleus and typical inclusions. These inclusions reveal a dense center with a lighter periphery ("owl eye cells"). The diameter of infected cells may measure up to 30 mm. The inclusions can be intranuclear and intracytoplasmic. Laboratory tests of fresh urine (without any stablizing agents), sputum, cerebrospinal fluid, blood (leukocytes), aqueous humor, vitreous humor, and cervical mucosa may be used to identify the virus. However, virus identification can be difficult.

Histological Diagnosis. A tissue biopsy, e.g., a liver biopsy, can confirm the histological diagnosis.

Ocular Differential Diagnosis. The ophthalmoscopical differental diagnosis for this disease includes retinitis of different etiologies: herpes simplex, sporotrichosis or Schenck's disease, toxoplasmosis, leukemic retinopathy, Behçet's syndrome, sympathetic ophthalmia, necrotic melanoma, necrotic retinoblastoma, primary reticulum cell sarcoma of the retina, uveal and retinal metastases, multiple retinal infarctions, vascular occlusions of the retina and choroid, hyperlipidemia, Coats' disease and secondary Coats' disease, Harada's disease, or acute multifocal placoid pigment epitheliopathy (Figs. 205–207).

Therapy. Treatment with vidarabine (Vira-A) infusion therapy and other drugs may be effective.

Subacute Sclerosing Panencephalitis

Synonyms: Dawson's subacute sclerosing leukoencephalitis, Van Bogaert's disease, Pette-Döring disease (nodular panencephalitis).

The etiology of this disease is unknown. For a long time it had been considered a degenerative disease, but it is now recognized as a late manifestation of a slow virus infection (measles virus). The latter assumption is based on elevated measle-antibody titers found in the serum and cerebrospinal fluid of affected persons. Antigens to the measles virus are found by immunohistological evaluation of biopsy and autopsy material of the central nervous system. The patient's history usually reveals that an uncomplicated measles infection occurred years before onset of the neurological symptoms.

Histopathologically, the disease is characterized by a panencephalitis that shows perivascular cellular infiltrates, consisting mostly of lymphocytes and plasma cells. Disseminated glial nodular calcification may be found in the cerebral cortex (particularly in the parietooccipital cortex), the nuclei of the telencephalon, and in the brainstem. In addition, inclusion bodies may be found in central nervous system cells.

This disease occurs in children of school age. Boys are most often affected. Initial symptoms are psychic alterations that may develop over months. According to Mumenthaler (1976) and Soyka (1975), such symptoms are irritation, energy loss, fatigue, alterations in motivation and intellectual skills, and aphasia. As the disease becomes progressively more severe, extrapyramidal, hyperkinetic symptoms, such as chorea and athetosis, may ensue. Other possible symptoms include myoclonic disorders that may be induced by noise or other external stimuli, cerebral convulsions, cranial nerve palsies, and/or delirium. The patient eventually reaches a severe vegetative state that progesses to cerebral coma and death.

Diagnosis. In the initial stage, bilateral, periodically occurring groups of slow, high peaks, which are considered pathognomonic, appear in the electroencephalogram (EEG). Analysis of the cerebrospinal fluid reveals a moderate pleocytosis and a markedly increased gamma globulin fraction. Both the cerebrospinal fluid and serum show an increased concentration of antibodies to the measles virus.

Ocular Effects. Since the parietooccipital region of the brain is most often affected, cortical symptoms such as central agnosia, cortical blindness, hallucinations, nystagmus, and dysfunctions of the III and VI cranial nerves are frequently present. Therefore, the eye may show a severe visual loss without any direct involvement of the retina. In the literature, such a combination of symptoms was found in 30% of cases.

Ophthalmoscopical Appearance. If the retina is directly involved, the typical ophthalmoscopical findings are bilateral macular lesions in the form of an acute central chorioretinitis. Peripheral chorioretinal scars without signs of an acute inflammation also have been described. In later stages, papilledema and optic nerve atrophy may be present. Pülhorn (1976) reported an acute necrotizing retinitis associated with a subacute sclerosing panencephalitis. The visual field may be affected, showing a central scotoma and severe concentric constrictions of the outer borders.

Therapy. No effective ocular treatment is known. Any therapeutic regimen must be symptomatic. Lund et al. (1983) reported some success with ribavirin (Virazole) or vidarabine (Vira-A). This treatment did not restore the patient to health (restituo ad integrum), but did prevent the otherwise lethal outcome of this disease.

Tapetoretinal and Tapetochoroidal Degenerations

Retinitis Pigmentosa

Synonyms: Retinopathy pigmentosa, pigmentary retinopathy, pigmentary retinal dystrophy, peripheral tapetoretinal degeneration, peripheral tapetoretinal dystrophy. The term "retinopathy" is the more accurate one since this entity does not represent an inflammatory disease and the suffix "itis," although entrenched in clinical usage, is inaccurate. This disease can be better described as a hereditary, progressive dystrophy of the outer retinal layers (rods and cones) and, in later stages, of the bipolar and ganglion cell layers (Figs. 208–219).

Retinitis pigmentosa is the classic example of the large variety of tapetoretinal degenerations. This latter term describes degenerative and heredity diseases of the retinal pigment and neuroepithelium.

Isolated retinitis pigmentosa may occur sporadically or be transmitted as an autosomal recessive trait, but it also may be inherited in an autosomal dominant trait and, rarely, in an X-linked recessive manner.

Ophthalmoscopical Appearance. The optic nerve head has a pale yellow waxy appearance with blurred margins, indicative of an ascendent retinal optic nerve atrophy. The central retinal artery and the central retinal vein and their major branches are narrowed. The arterioles may appear extremely thin and may even be obliterated peripherally (Figs. 211–215). A characteristic finding is a star-shaped or bone spicule-shaped dark-brown to black pigmentation. Occasionally, the pigmented areas appear dusty or granulated rather than having the classic bone spicule shape. The pigmented areas also have processes and projections connecting adjacent lesions in a net-like fashion. The total number of lesions may vary markedly, but as the disease progresses, the number of lesions increases. Initially, these lesions are found in the midperiphery of the retina and progress centrally, usually without involving the macula and periphery. As the pigment epithelium becomes atrophic, obliterated sclerotic choriodal vessels become visible. In later stages, the macula is affected and may show a cystic macular degeneration or, rarely, a macular hole.

In addition to the typical isolated form of retinitis pigmentosa, atypical forms occur that include the inverse or central type of retinitis pigmentosa, in which pigmentation within the macular area is an initial finding. When the changes are confined to a single sector of the fundus, the disease is called sector retinitis pigmentosa. In the unilateral form of the disease, pigmentation is seen in only one eye.

Pigmentary retinopathy is sometimes associated with systemic disorders, some of which are summarized in Table 16.

Diagnosis (Figs. 208–219). Objective symptoms are based on the typical ophthalmoscopical findings. The electroretinogram (ERG) response is extinguished, and the B-wave is absent. An electrooculogram (EOG) may show pathological findings. These signs can be identified before clinical symptoms are evident. Subjective symp-

Table 16. Syndromes with a Retinitis Pigmentosa-like Pigmentary Degeneration

Pigmentary degeneration may be a partial symptom in patients with:
Cockayne's syndrome
Bassen-Kornzweig's syndrome
Sjögren-Larsson syndrome
Laurence-Moon-Bardet-Biedl syndrome
Refsum's syndrome
Spielmeyer-Stock disease

toms include hemeralopia, which may be noted early in the patient's school-age years (Figs. 216 and 217).

Visual Fields. Early on, sickle-shaped or ring-shaped scotomas in the midperiphery of the visual field are noted. As the disease progresses, the visual field becomes more and more constricted, and finally, only a small (10°) central visual field remains. Such tubular vision prevents normal three-dimensional orientation.

Visual Acuity. In many cases, visual acuity remains intact and provides sufficient vision for normal function over the years. However, an associated component of this disease is development of a posterior polar cataract (cataracta complicata). Such a cataract causes an exaggerated loss of vision because of its central location in the already compromised visual field. In addition, if the macula becomes involved as the disease progesses, severe visual loss ensues.

Therapy. No therapy is known. According to recent findings, retinitis pigmentosa may be caused by an abetalipoproteinemia. Some patients lack the abetalipoprotein B responsible for the transportation of cholesterol in the blood. The lipid-soluble vitamins A, D, E, and K are absorbed at a reduced rate because of this alteration of lipid metabolism. Therefore, vitamin substitutes and a fat-reduced diet may possibly slow the progress of the disease.

Atypical Pigment Degenerations of the Retina

Synonyms: Retinitis punctata albescens, progressive albipunctate dystrophy.

The fundus shows multiple wide dots, which are diffusely scattered, and abnormal fundus reflexes. These round or oval lesions are not usually found in the macular region. In advanced stages, peripheral bone spicule-shaped pigmentations may be found in some cases. Retinal vessels may be narrowed, and the optic disc may appear pale. This disease always occurs bilaterally and symmetrically, and the lesions are primarily found in the peripheral retina. Functional abnormalities of the retina are similar to those seen with retinitis pigmentosa. Hemeralopia is an early symptom, although it does not develop in all patients. The visual fields are concentrically constricted. Normally, alterations in color vision (achromotopsia) do not occur, but this symptom has been reported.

Central visual acuity may remain intact over a period of several years, but the general course of the disease is slowly progressive. Atypical pigment retinal degeneration is inherited as an autosomal recessive (rarely dominant) trait.

Several cases have been described in which typical retinitis pigmentosa was observed with retinitis punctata albescens within the same family.

Retinitis Pigmentosa without Pigment

Retinitis pigmentosa without pigment (sine pigmento) is similar to the more typical form of the disease except for the absence of pigmented bone spicules. The optic disc shows varying degrees of atrophy and has a waxy yellow appearance. The retinal vessels appear narrow. Pigmentations are absent or, in cases of retinitis pigmentosa with reduced pigment (paucipigmentosa), are extremely rare. This latter form of the disease is rare before the age of 30 years. This entity is transmitted as an autosomal dominant or recessive trait.

Hereditary Diseases Mimicking Retinitis Pigmentosa

Fundus Albipunctatus

A harmless variation, fundus albipunctatus has to be differentiated from retinitis punctate albescens. Numerous small, round or disciform, white lesions are visible in the extreme retinal periphery. These small dots may partially overlap or line up like pearls on a necklace. Occurrence is generally bilateral. The optic disc and retinal vessels appear normal. Neither an ERG nor EOG show any pathological signs. The only functional loss is night blindness. The disease is transmitted as an autosomal recessive trait that does not progress. Familial occurrence is typical.

Fundus Flavimaculatus

The term "fundus flavimaculatus" denotes a bilateral, symmetrical, slowly progressive fundus condition with yellow or yellow-white, round or linear, pisiform flecks that vary in size, shape, and density. Histopathological examination reveals that the lesions are located at the level of the pigment epithelium. The ERG remains unchanged; the EOG is often subnormal (in 50% of cases associated with Stargardt's syndrome or macular degeneration). Visual acuity is good if no macular degeneration is present. The disease may remain stationary or show a very slow progression. It is transmitted as an autosomal recessive trait.

Fundus Pulverulentus

Fundus pulverulentus can be identified by central posterior (around the posterior pole and optic disc) and midperipheral or peripheral spotty and/or granular pigmentations. The optic disc and retinal vessels remain unchanged. The lesions are symmetrical and are situated within the level of the retinal pigment epithelium. An ERG is normal, and visual acuity is affected only by a moderate decrease throughout life. This entity is not associated with other abnormalities and represents a heredofamilial disease.

Reticular Dystrophy of the Retinal Pigment Epithelium

In this entity, small granulated, round, black pigment spots that resemble a halo are present in the macula. Fishnet-like pigmentations are found around the posterior pole. These bilateral, symmetrical lesions are most often located in the retinal pigment epithelium. Results from an ERG and from an EOG are normal, and the visual acuity is not affected. This anomaly is inherited as an autosomal recessive trait. Familial occurrence is typical.

Pseudoretinitis Pigmentosa

Synonyms: Retinopathy pseudopigmentosa, secondary pigmentary degenerations of the retina.

Several nonhereditary acquired diseases may produce a unilateral or bilateral pigmentinopathy with fundus changes resembling those of retinitis pigmentosa. Pseudoretinitis pigmentosa may develop following trauma (retinitis sclopetaria or late stage commotio retinae), in cases of siderosis retinae, after successful repositioning of a detached retina (peripheral reattachment lines), following inflammation or virus infection (measles, mumps, polymyelitis, rubella, varicella), stage III congenital syphilis, toxoplasmosis, and as an age-related degeneration in an otherwise normal eye (Fig. 220).

In cases of pseudoretinitis pigmentosa, a normal ERG helps to rule out a primary pigmentary degeneration. An ERG has only limited value because a subnormal ERG does not allow for a differentiation and is only an indication for the degree of retinal damage. Depending on the underlying disease, monocular or binocular involvement is possible, but occurrence is most often monocular.

Choroideremia

Synonym: Central progressive choroidal atrophy.

Choroideremia, first described by von Mauthner in 1871, can be classified as a tapetochoroidal degeneration. This progressive disease first becomes manifest in juvenile patients. The sclerosis of choroidal vessels progresses and the disease ends with complete choroidal atrophy. Amaurosis can be expected within the 3rd to 4th decade of life. Since the macula usually remains intact until the final stage, macular visual acuity may remain good. Early in the disease, an alteration in dark adaptation (hemeralopia) can be found. Visual field defects are initially difficult to prove. In the final stage, visual fields are markedly constricted ("gun barrel" vision). The EOG shows a reduced basic potential. The ERG sometimes has a B-wave that later diminishes. Fluorescein angiography reveals large areas of pigment epithelial defects that can be seen in the first stages. In advanced cases, the choroidal vessels are almost entirely destroyed and the white sclera is bared. Choroideremia is a sex chromosome transmitted condition that affects men and is usually carried without symptoms by women.

Ophthalmoscopical Appearance. Initially, the optic nerve head, retinal vessels, and posterior pole are unchanged. At an early stage, the choriocapillaris and pigment epithelium become atrophic. Also, the pigment of the intervascular choroidal spaces disappears and then a depigmented zone develops, surrounding the optic nerve head. These changes cause easy visibility of large choroidal vessels that continue to rarify and obliterate over large areas. Atrophic areas conflux, and such depigmented areas continue to spread peripherally. Irregularly disseminated bone spicule-like pigmentations supplement the opthalmoscopical appearance. In the final stage, the bare sclera becomes visible, and the fundus loses all structure. In this stage, the retinal vessels may become constricted, and the optic nerve develops a waxy ascendent optic nerve atrophy.

Female carriers of the disease may show minor fundus changes, including minimal midperipheral pigmentary changes. If there is a suspicion that a child is carrying the disease, evaluation of other family members may be useful because characteristic findings often can be seen in other family members.

Therapy. No therapy is known.

Prophylaxis. When a genetic expression of choroideremia is known, prenatal identification of the embryo's sex during the first 3 months of pregnancy may be useful.

Gyrate Atrophy

The first description of this disease was by Jacobsohn in 1888, who termed his findings "retinitis pigmentosa atypica." Today's commonly used term for this slowly progressive disease, "gyrate atrophy," was coined by Fuchs in 1896. This condition shares some similarities with choroideremia, and both diseases are classified as tapetochoroidal degenerations. Typically, gyrate atrophy is associated with hyperornithinemia and has a hereditary, metabolic etiology. When this disease is combined with myopia and cataract (star-shaped posterior polar cataract, scutiform anterior or posterior cataract, or total cataract), the refractive error averages −7 diopters (Franceschetti, 1963). In most cases the myopia is related to defects in the crystalline lens.

This disease is transmitted as an autosomal recessive trait. Consanguinity of the parents has been described. The clinical course is characterized by hemeralopia that becomes manifest during childhood. Visual field changes result in a concentric constriction. At times a ring scotoma (but never a central scotoma) can be found. The characteristic, slowly progressive decrease in visual acuity is most pronounced during the 2nd and 3rd decades of life. In extreme cases, visual acuity may be decreased to light perception. Initially, the ERG is normal; in later stages, it becomes subnormal or is extinguished. Distortions in color vision (blue-yellow perception) have been described. No characteristic fluorescein angiographic findings have been reported in the literature. Schäfer and Tenner (1970) reported an irregular background hyperfluorescence that begins in the early arterial phase and ends with the efflux of fluorescein dye from the fundus. This phenomenon probably occurs because choroidal fluorescence becomes visible in areas where the retinal pigment epithelium is defective.

Ophthalmoscopical Appearance. Sharply demarcated atrophic choroidal lesions can be found (Figs. 221 and 222). These lesions subsequently accrue and may assume garland-shaped formations that extend centrally and peripherally. Sometimes quite large, irregularly disseminated pigmentations resembling bone spicules can be seen in the atrophic margins. The large choroidal vessels become visible due to the loss of pigment epithelium and intervascular melanocytes, and the choroidal vessels are obliterated. Initially, the retinal vessels are unchanged, but in later stages of the disease the vessels may decrease in thickness. The optic disc is not affected at first, although it may become surrounded by an atrophic peripapillary choroidal zone. As the disease advances, the optic disc becomes pale yellow, indicating an ascendent optic nerve atrophy. The macular region remains intact until the final stage of the disease. Rarely, atrophy may begin at the posterior pole (Komoto, 1914).

Therapy. If the finding of hyperornithinemia is verified, an adequate dietetic regimen should be stressed. *Note:* In cases of choroidal vascular occlusion, gyrate atrophy-like lesions may be found (Neubauer, 1955). However, in these cases, retinal vessels and the optic nerve head remain unchanged and there is no hemeralopia.

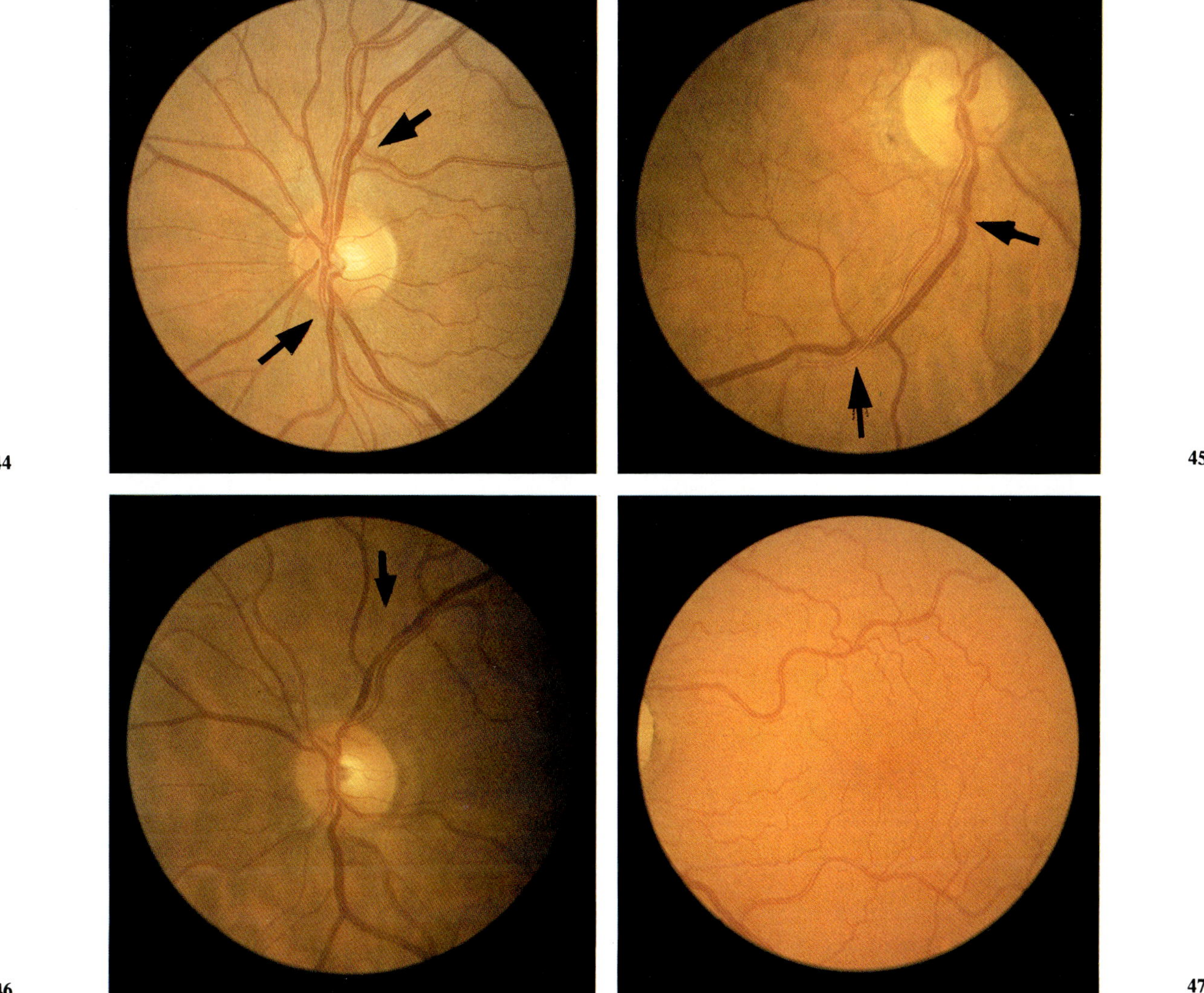

Figure 44. Left eye of a 27-year-old male patient with early stage hypertension.

Clinical Findings

The patient had a history of arterial hypertension for 5 years. Blood pressure, with antihypertensive therapy, was 160/95 mm Hg measured on both arms. Both eyes were ametropic. Visual acuity was 20/20, the refractive media were unremarkable, and visual fields were normal. The fundus examination revealed an AV crossing (*arrows*) that appeared thickened where it passed over the arteriole (*upper arrow*).

Figure 45. Right eye of a 73-year-old male patient with early stage hypertension. The findings in this eye are consistent with fundus scleroticus D, according to Sautter's classification (Table 13). A combination of arteriosclerotic and hypertensive vascular abnormalities can be seen.

Clinical Findings

The patient had a clinical history of arterial hypertension for 10 years. Despite antihypertensive therapy, blood pressure was still 190/110 mm Hg (measured on both arms). The eye was slightly hyperopic (+1 diopter sphere) with a beginning cataract. Visual fields were normal. There are AV crossings present in the posterior pole (*arrows*). Note the very pronounced arterial reflex (wire reflex).

Figure 46. Left eye of a 48-year-old female patient with early stage hypertension.

Clinical Findings

The patient had a 2-year history of arterial hypertension. Blood pressure was still elevated despite antihypertensive therapy (140/100 mm Hg measured on both arms). A refraction of +0.25 sphere, −0.5 cylinder, axis 0° was corrected for a visual acuity of 20/20 in both eyes. The refractive media and visual fields were normal. This fundus is an example of a parallel Gunn's sign (*arrow*). A segmental narrowing of some vessels, mainly venules, was evident at the site where the vessels are parallel and in close proximity to each other.

Figure 47. Left eye of a 49-year-old female patient with early stage hypertension.

Clinical Findings

The patient had a 2-year history of known arterial hypertension. Despite antihypertensive therapy, blood pressure measured on the right arm was 220/115 mm Hg and 170/105 mm Hg on the left arm. Visual acuity was 20/20 in both ametropic eyes. The refractive media and visual fields were normal. Note the corkscrew-like appearance of the perimacular venules.

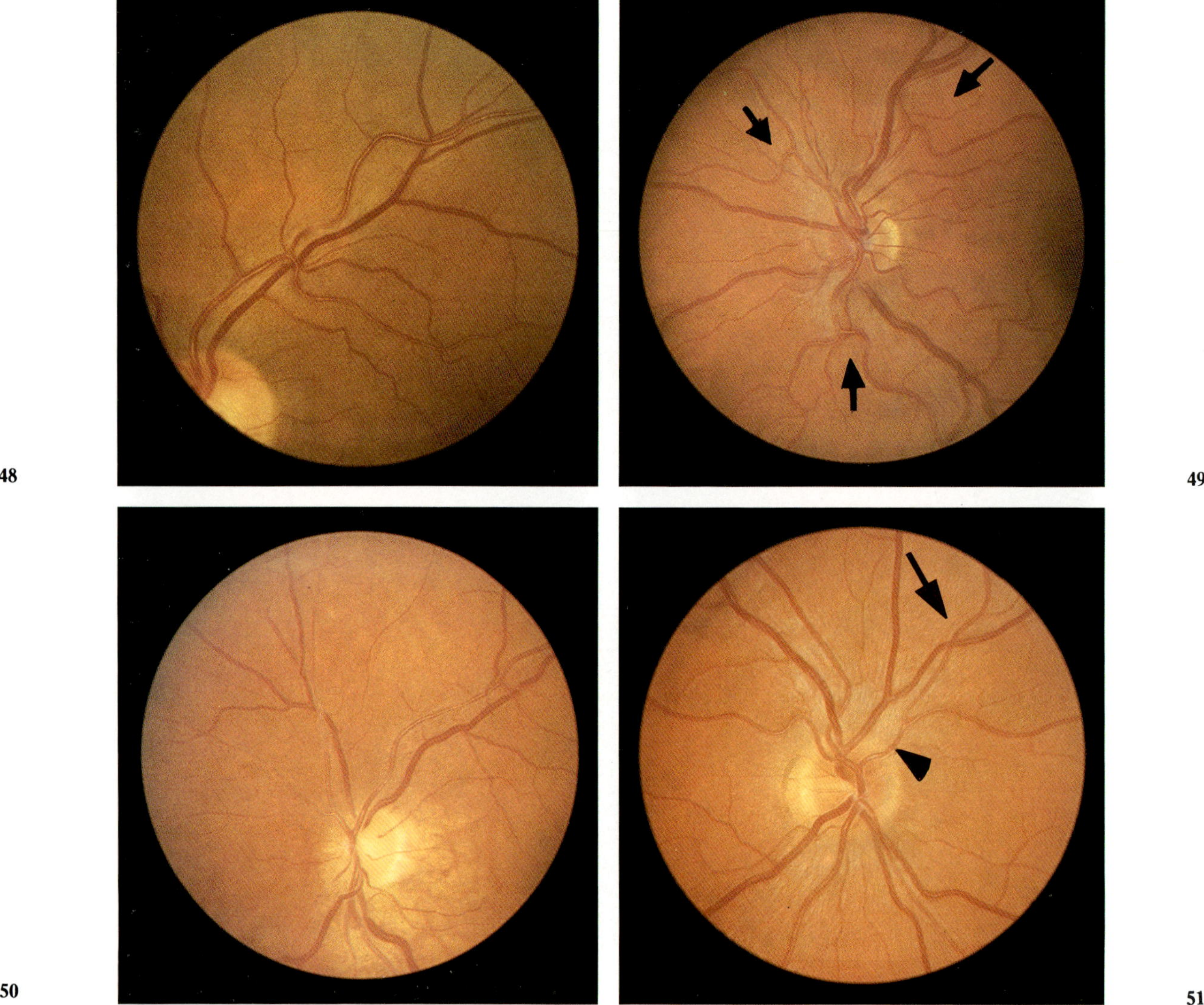

Figure 48. Left eye of a 57-year-old female patient with early stage hypertension.

Clinical Findings

There was a history of known arterial hypertension for 8 years. Under therapy, blood pressure was 165/95 mm Hg (measured on both arms). With a correction of +1.5 sphere, −1.0 cylinder, axis 0°, visual acuity could be corrected to 20/30. The refractive media and visual fields were normal. Fundus examination revealed AV crossings and the classical copper wire arteriolar appearance seen with hypertension.

Figure 49. Left eye of a 44-year-old female patient with advanced stage hypertension.

Clinical Findings

The patient had a 10-year history of arterial hypertension. Even with antihypertensive therapy, blood pressure was 190/105 mm Hg (measured on both arms). The left eye was slightly hyperopic with a refraction of +1 diopter sphere, but visual acuity in both eyes was 20/20. The refractive media and visual fields were normal. This fundus clearly shows omega branching (*arrows*) with widely spread arterioles, a type of branching that indicates high blood pressure.

Figure 50. Left eye of a 46-year-old female patient with advanced stage hypertension.

Clinical Findings

The patient had known arterial hypertension for 20 years. Despite treatment, blood pressure was 230/150 mm Hg (measured on both arms). Refraction was −0.75 diopters sphere and visual acuity was 20/25. Endocrine, renal, and drug-induced hypertension were ruled out by an extensive clinical workup. This most likely represents a case of primary hypertension. Very bright arterial reflexes (silver wire reflexes) were noted in a fundus examination.

Figure 51. Left eye of a 40-year-old female patient with early stage hypertension.

Clinical Findings

The patient had a 3-year history of arterial hypertension. Blood pressure was 150/95 mm Hg with antihypertensive treatment. Visual acuity was 20/20 in both eyes. The refractive media and visual fields were normal. A salus sign can be seen at the AV crossing supratemporally (*arrow*). The arterioles show caliber irregularities (*arrowhead*).

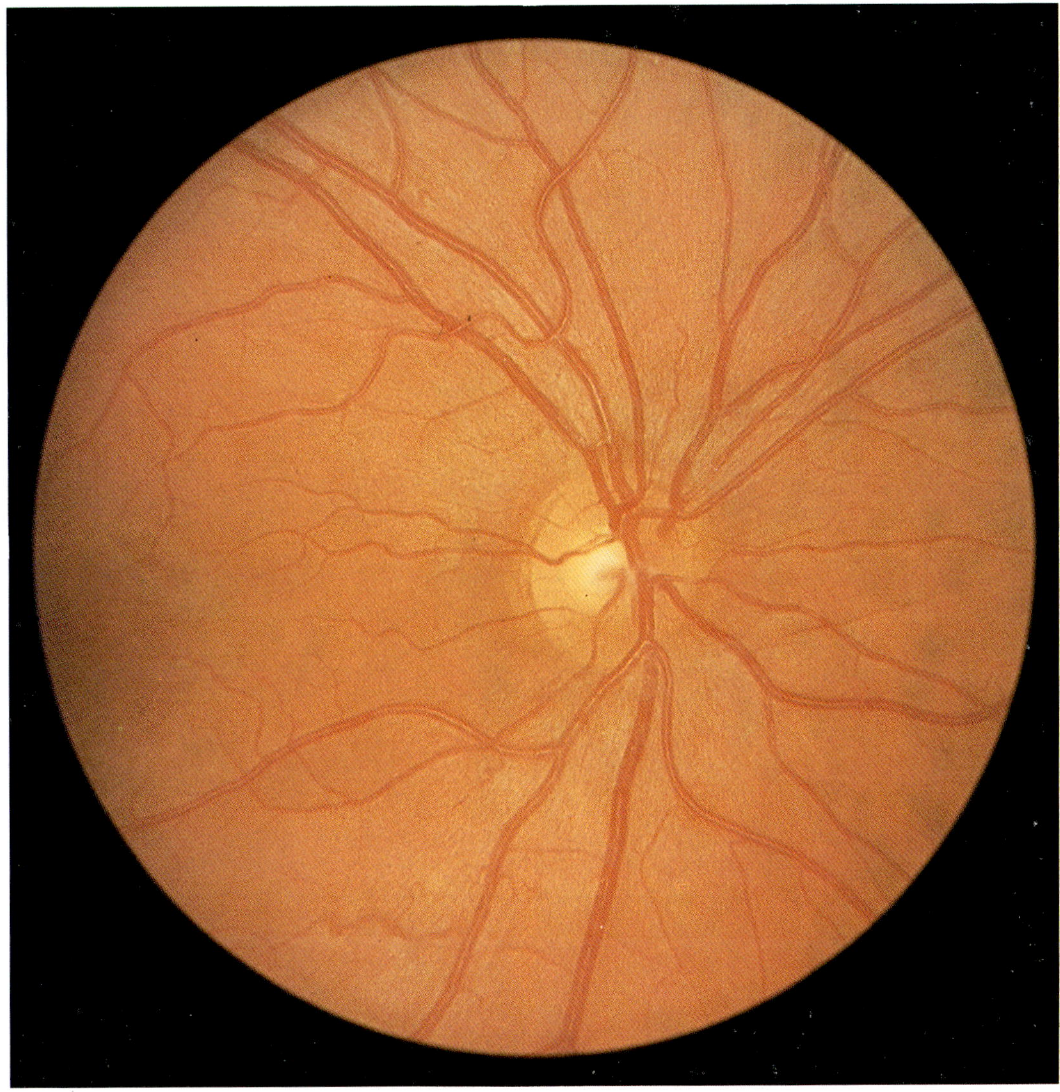

52

Figure 52. Right eye of a 19-year-old male patient with early stage arterial hypertension (primary hypertension).

Clinical Findings

There was a known history of arterial hypertension for 3 years. Blood pressure, despite antihypertensive therapy, was 210/110 mm Hg (measured on both arms). Visual acuity in both ametropic eyes was 20/20. The retractive media were clear and the visual fields were normal. Causes for the hypertension, including renal (chronic glomerulonephritis, chronic interstitial nephritis, cystic kidneys, obstructive pyelonephritis, renal artery stenosis), endocrine (Cushing's disease, hyperaldosteronism, pheochromocytoma, adrenocortical hypertonia), and drug-induced etiologies, were ruled out by an extensive workup. The fundus shows caliber irregularities of the arterioles and copper wire reflexes. A trifurcation rather than the normal bifurcation of the temporal superior arteriole is an interesting vascular variation in this fundus. At this site, the arteriole branches show moderately increased tortuosity.

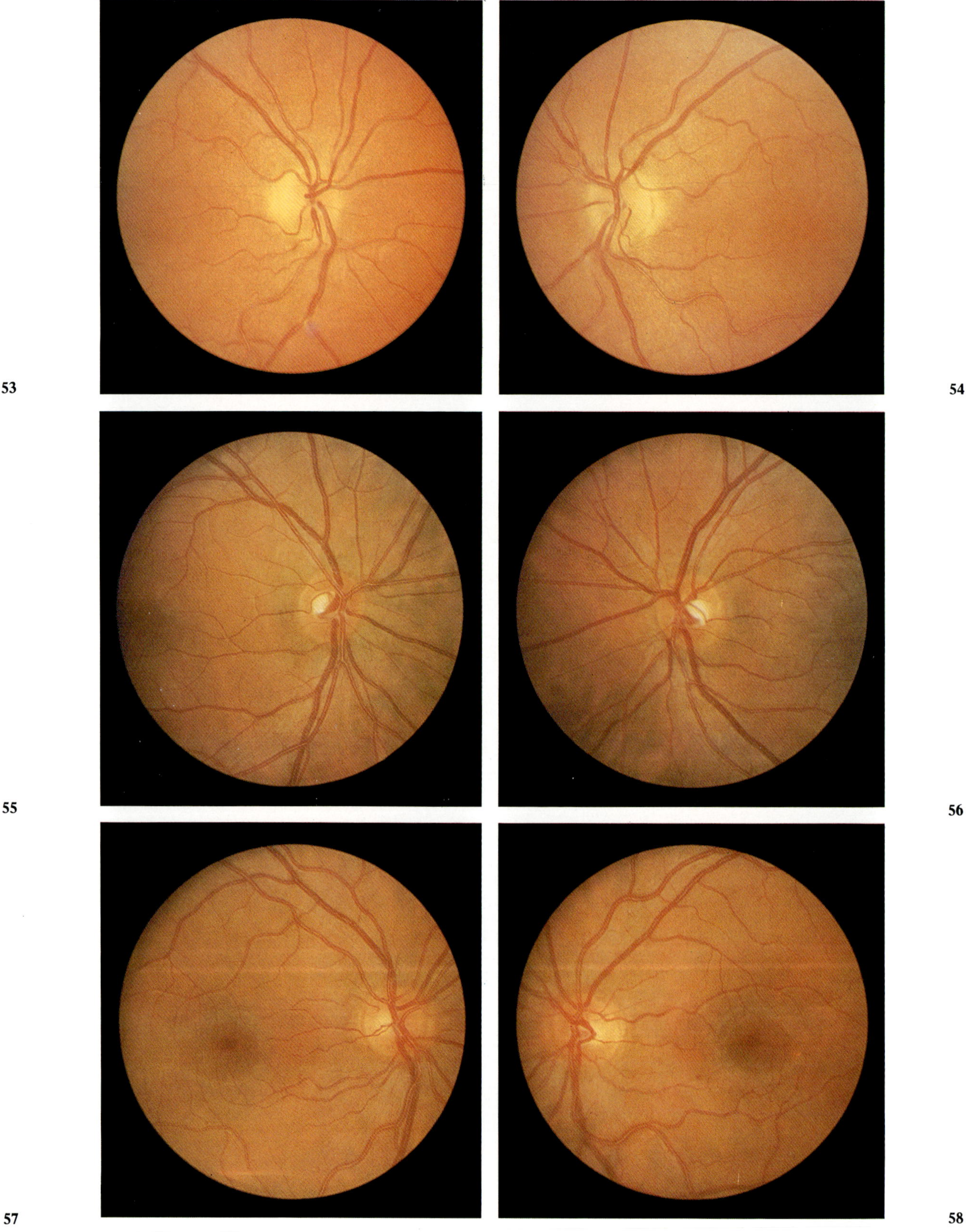

53

54

55

56

57

58

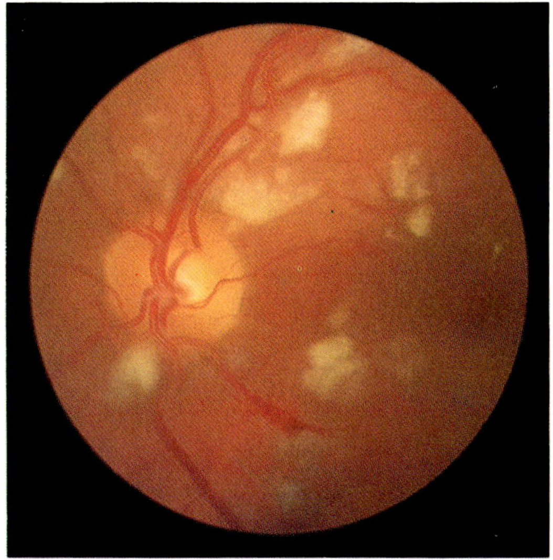
59

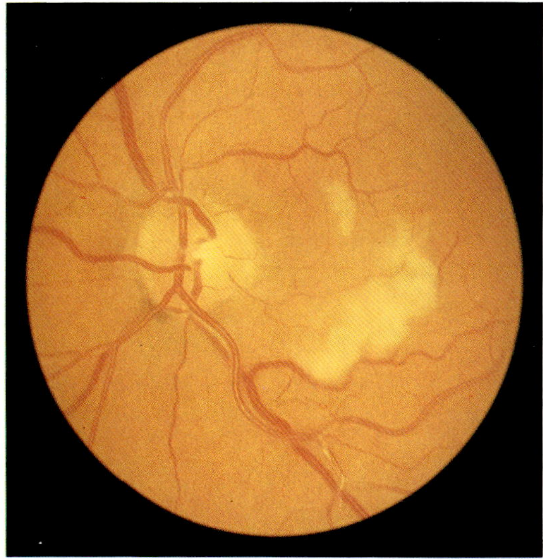
60

Figures 53 and 54. Right and left eyes of a 36-year-old female patient with late stage hypertension caused by chronic pyelonephritis.

Clinical Findings

There was a history of known arterial hypertension for 4 years. Despite therapy, blood pressure was 220/120 mm Hg (measured on both arms). Both eyes were ametropic and visual acuity was 20/20. The refractive media were clear and visual fields were normal. The posterior pole shows an increased tortuosity of the arterioles and caliber irregularities. Isolated punctate hemorrhages are present. The arteriovenous ratio was 1 : 3.

Figures 55 and 56. Right and left eyes of a 20-year-old male patient with early stage hypertension (primary essential hypertension).

Clinical Findings

The patient has a 4-year history of arterial hypertension. Even with antihypertensive therapy, blood pressure was 200/115 mm Hg on the right arm, and 190/110 mm Hg on the left arm. Visual acuity in both ametropic eyes was 20/20. The refractive media were clear and visual fields were normal. The patient's mother also suffered from hypertension (see Fig. 50).

Ophthalmoscopical Examination

Caliber irregularities of the arterioles and engorgement of the retinal veins were seen. The arteriovenous ratio was 1 : 3.

Figures 57 and 58. Right and left eyes of a 24-year-old male patient with early stage hypertension (primary essential hypertension).

Clinical Findings

The patient had a history of known arterial hypertension for 3 years. Despite therapy, blood pressure was 190/110 mm Hg (measured on both arms). Visual acuity of both ametropic eyes was 20/20. The refractive media were clear and visual fields were unchanged. The fundus shows increased tortuosity of the arterioles and caliber irregularities. At some sites, the diameter of the arterioles and venules is identical. Isolated punctate hemorrhages can be seen surrounding the macular region.

Figure 59. Left eye of a 29-year-old male patient with early stage hypertension.

Clinical Findings

Blood pressure readings were extremely varied and periodically spiked as high as 250/140 mm Hg. Visual acuity in both eyes was 20/30. Visual field testing showed a mild constriction of the peripheral borders. There were multiple cotton wool exudates. An early stage macular star figure is present (hard exudates). The retinal vessels have caliber irregularities. The ratio between arteries and veins was 1:3. The arterioles are partially masked. Band- or flame-shaped hemorrhages are present. Based on repeated laboratory analyses, a visual fields chromocytoma or any other endogenous cause of hypertension could be ruled out. A renal vascular etiology was also ruled out based on x-ray examination and serum renin analysis. There was also no indication for any parenchymatous renal disease. Therefore, this condition had to be considered a primary essential hypertension.

Figure 60. Left eye of a 68-year-old patient with early stage renal hypertension caused by chronic pyelonephritis.

Clinical Findings

The patient had a history of arterial hypertension for 20 years. Blood pressure, despite antihypertensive therapy, measured on the right arm was 240/110 mm Hg, and on the left arm was 180/100 mm Hg. With a correction of +1.0 sphere, −0.75 cylinder, axis 90°, the best visual acuity was 20/100. There was a beginning cataract in both eyes. Visual field testing revealed a central scotoma with a concentric constriction of the peripheral margins. The fundus shows increased arteriolar tortuosity, caliber irregularities, and patchy arteriole ensheathing (see branches of inferotemporal artery). Several AV crossings are present, particularly in the papillary and peripapillary regions. The retinal veins are engorged. There are large yellow-white ischemic areas at the posterior pole.

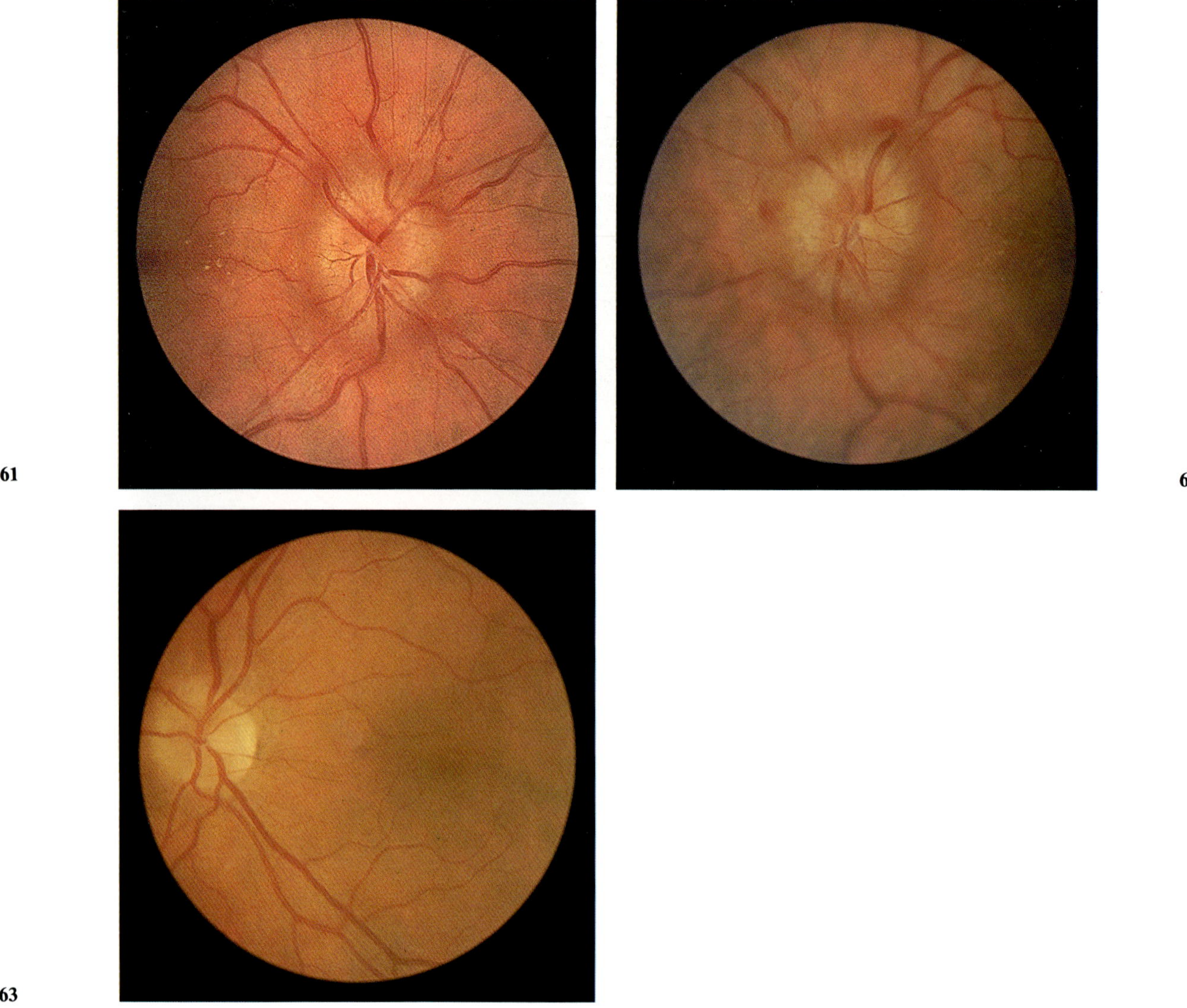

Figures 61 and 62. Right eye (Fig. 61) and left eye (Fig. 62) of a 30-year-old female patient with early stage hypertension.

Clinical Findings

Both eyes were slightly myopic (−0.75 diopters sphere) with visual acuity of 20/20. Testing of the visual fields revealed an enlargement of the blind spot with normal peripheral margins. Intraocular pressure in both eyes was 16 mm Hg. Exophthalmometry measurements were 14-92-14 mm. Pupillary reaction and corneal sensitivities were normal in both eyes and the patient did not complain of double images. Blood pressure measured on the right arm was 200/130 mm Hg. A fundus examination revealed an edematous, elevated optic disc in both eyes (2 diopters, right eye, and 2.5 diopters, left eye). The optic disc capillaries are hyperemic and no central excavation is discernible. Isolated punctate and small dot-and-blot hemorrhages are seen in the peripapillary area. The retinal veins are engorged and tortuous and the arteries appear narrow with caliber irregularities. At some sites, neither arteries or veins are visible (especially in Fig. 62). The arteriovenous ratio was 1:3. Drusen are present between the optic disc and the macula (Fig. 61). Renal, endocrine, drug-induced, and cerebral causes for the papilledema were ruled out. The condition spontaneously slowly resolved, and therefore, the bilateral papilledema was most likely caused by the hypertension.

Figure 63. Fundus of the left eye of the same patient as in Figures 61 and 62, 1 year after the first examination. Blood pressure was then controlled at 130/90 mm Hg (measured on both arms).

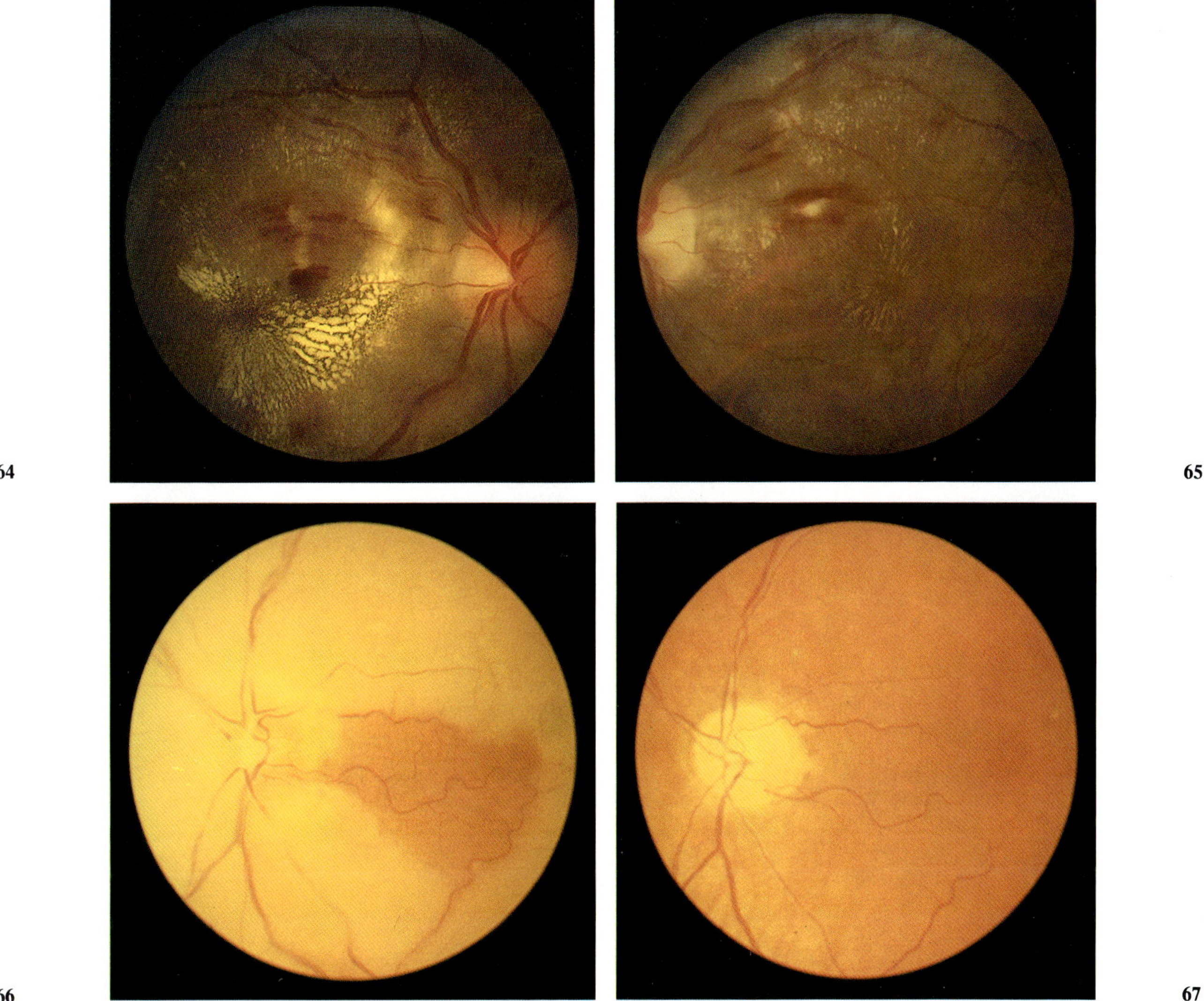

Figures 64 and 65. Right eye (Fig. 64) and left eye (Fig. 65) of a 17-year-old male patient with late stage hypertensive retinopathy, chronic glomerular nephritis, and terminal renal insufficiency.

Clinical Findings

With a refractive correction of −0.5 diopters sphere, visual acuity in the right eye was 20/400, and 20/200 in the left eye. The refractive media were clear. Visual field examination revealed a central scotoma and a concentric constriction of the visual field margins, leaving a residual field of 40°. Intraocular pressure in both eyes was 14 mm Hg. The patient had undergone dialysis therapy for 2 years. Blood pressure was 180/120 mm Hg. The fundi in both eyes show the characteristic changes of late stage hypertensive retinopathy. The optic discs are hyperemic with discrete margins but are not elevated. The retinal venules show only moderate changes. The retinal arterioles reveal severe caliber irregularities. Some arterial segments are not discernible. There are cotton wool exudates on both posterior poles, but these are more evident in the right eye. Hard exudates have formed an incomplete macular star figure in the right eye. Multiple hemorrhages are present.

Figures 66 and 67. Left eye of a 65-year-old male patient with central retinal artery occlusion with residual perfusion by a cilioretinal artery.

Clinical Findings

The eye was slightly hyperopic (+1.5 diopters sphere) and visual acuity in the right eye was 20/20, and 20/30 in the left eye. The refractive media were clear. A visual field remnant is present that corresponds to the area supplied by the cilioretinal artery and resembles a horizontally oriented keyhole. Intraocular pressure in both eyes was 14 mm Hg. Blood pressure was 160/85 mm Hg, and the blood sedimentation rate was 20/46 mm. Doppler sonography did not reveal any abnormalities of the internal carotid artery.

Clinical Course

The ischemic retinopathy caused a vascular optic atrophy, but visual acuity remained 20/20. An internal examination revealed cardiac insufficiency. Note in Figure 66 how the normal color of the retinal area that receives its blood supply from the central retinal artery contrasts with the ischemic, edematous retinal areas.

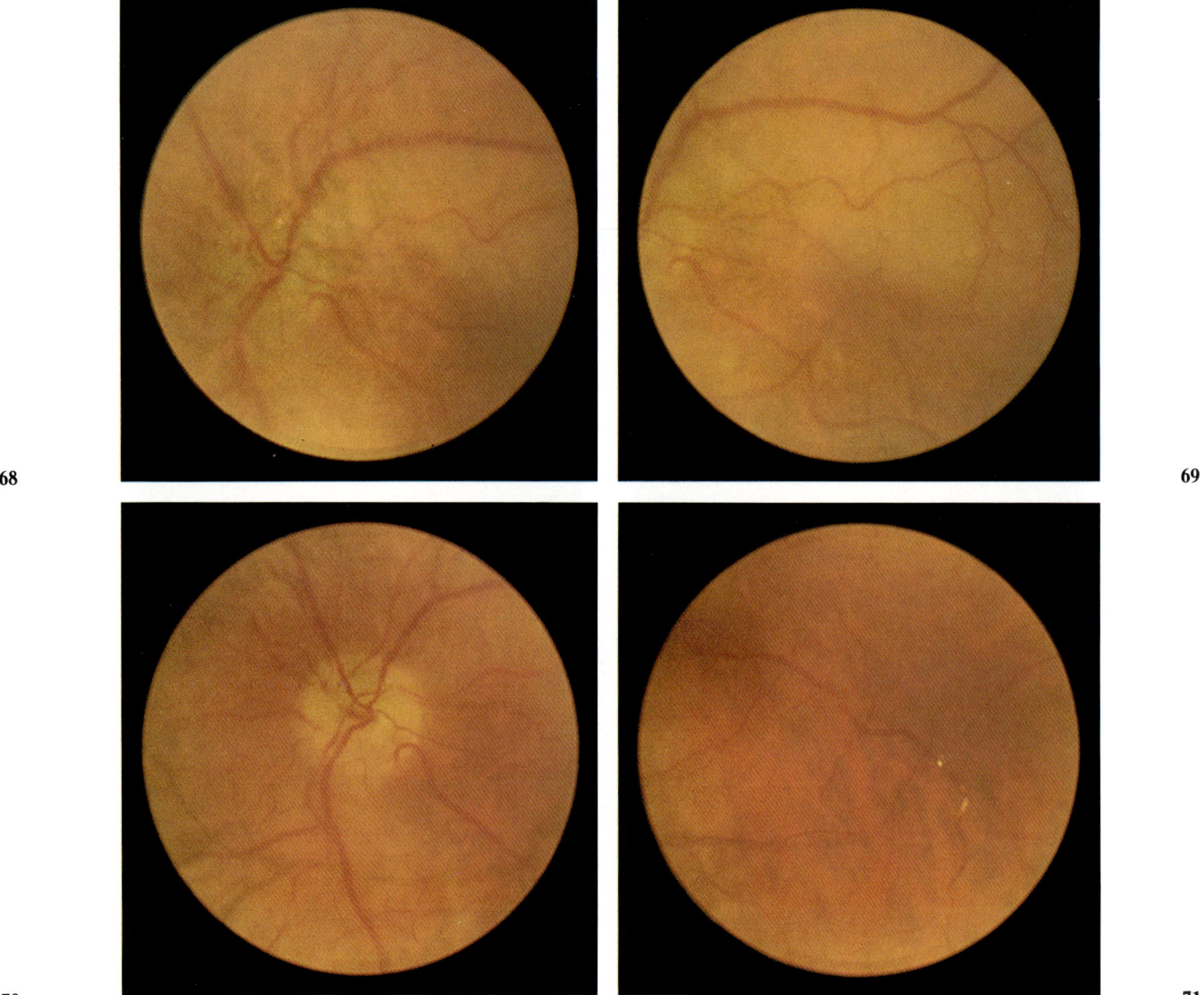

Figures 68–71. Left eye of a 78-year-old male patient with central artery occlusion and a cilioretinal artery.

Clinical Findings

Examination revealed stenosis of the left carotid artery and arterial hypertension. The refraction in both eyes was +0.75 sphere, and visual acuity in the right eye was 20/400 that could be improved to 20/30 when the patient turned his head toward the right. There was a visual field remnant in the left eye consistent with the retinal area supplied by the cilioretinal artery. Intraocular pressure in the right eye was 14 mm Hg, and 16 mm Hg in the left eye. A beginning cataract was seen by slitlamp examination. Blood pressure was 190/140 mm Hg, and the blood sedimentation rate was 15/35 mm. Doppler sonography showed a distortion of the blood flow within the internal carotid artery (see Fig. 7).

Clinical Course

The disease progressed and a vascular optic atrophy developed. Note in Figure 71 the presence of two cholesterol emboli in the cilioretinal artery.

Figures 72 and 73. Right eye of a 59-year-old male patient with central retinal occlusion associated with arterial hypertension.

Clinical Findings

The patient's history revealed that visual acuity abruptly decreased the night following extensive consumption of alcohol. Eighteen hours after the first symptoms occurred, examination revealed that the right eye was amaurotic with an amaurotic pupil reaction. Intraocular pressure was 16 mm Hg. Blood pressure was 180/120 mm Hg measured on both arms, and the blood sedimentation rate was 16/44 mm. The retina is extensively edematous and pale with a classic cherry-red spot in the macula. Doppler sonography did not reveal any vascular abnormalities of the internal carotid artery. Retinal doppler sonography (Huismans, 1983b) revealed only irregularly deformed complexes along the x axis of the hemotachometer printout. A physical examination revealed no abnormalities, and an ECG showed no irregularities a physical examination revealed no abnormalities, and an ECG showed no irregularities.

Laboratory Findings

Normal blood cell count, serum protein of 7.7%, albumin 41.4%, α_1-globulin 6.9%, α_2-globulin 6.9%, β-globulin 12%, gamma globulin 16.2%, creatinine 1.1 mg/100 ml, Quick test 78%, partial throm-

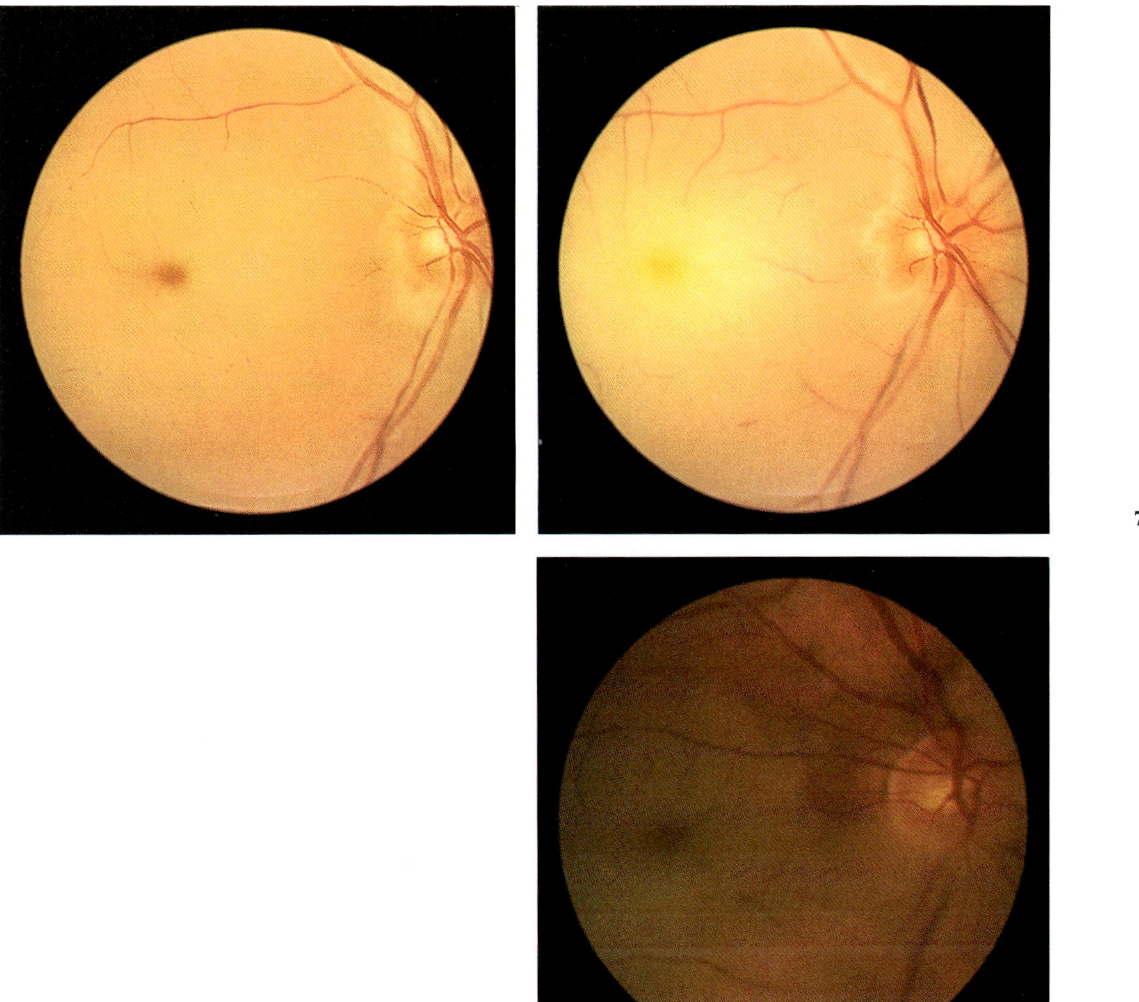

boplastin time 25.8 seconds, prothrombin time 17.4 seconds, fibinogen 410 mg/100 ml, platelets 300,000. The urine contents were unremarkable. Blood pressure taken in a supine position was 210/125 mm Hg on the right arm, and 220/125 mm Hg on the left arm. In an erect position, blood pressure was 230/130 mm Hg on the right arm, and 250/140 mm Hg on the left arm. Blood glucose concentration was 120 mg/100 ml.

Clinical Course

Despite extensive treatment (paracentesis, lowering of the blood pressure, infusion therapy, Diamox therapy, and radiation therapy) visual acuity could not be improved. Only a small visual field remnant remained superotemporally. The patient's fundus 3 days after the first examination is shown in Figure 73. The cherry-red spot has already been replaced by a xanthochromatic fovea and retinal edema has decreased. The eye later developed a vascular optic atrophy.

Figure 74. Right eye of a 70-year-old male patient with occlusion of branch arterioles associated with arterial hyptertension.

Clinical Findings

The eye was hyperopic with a refractive error of +2.0 diopters sphere. Visual acuity in the right eye was hand movements, and 20/25 in the left eye. Intraocular pressure in both eyes was 16 mm Hg. There was a sector-shaped visual field remnant in the right eye with a central scotoma. A beginning cataract was present. Blood pressure measured on both arms was 190/110 mm Hg. Blood sedimentation rate was 30/54 mm. Doppler sonography revealed no abnormalities of the blood flow in the internal carotid artery. A temporal artery biopsy did not show temporal arteritis.

Clinical Course

Visual acuity did not improve and a vascular optic atrophy developed.

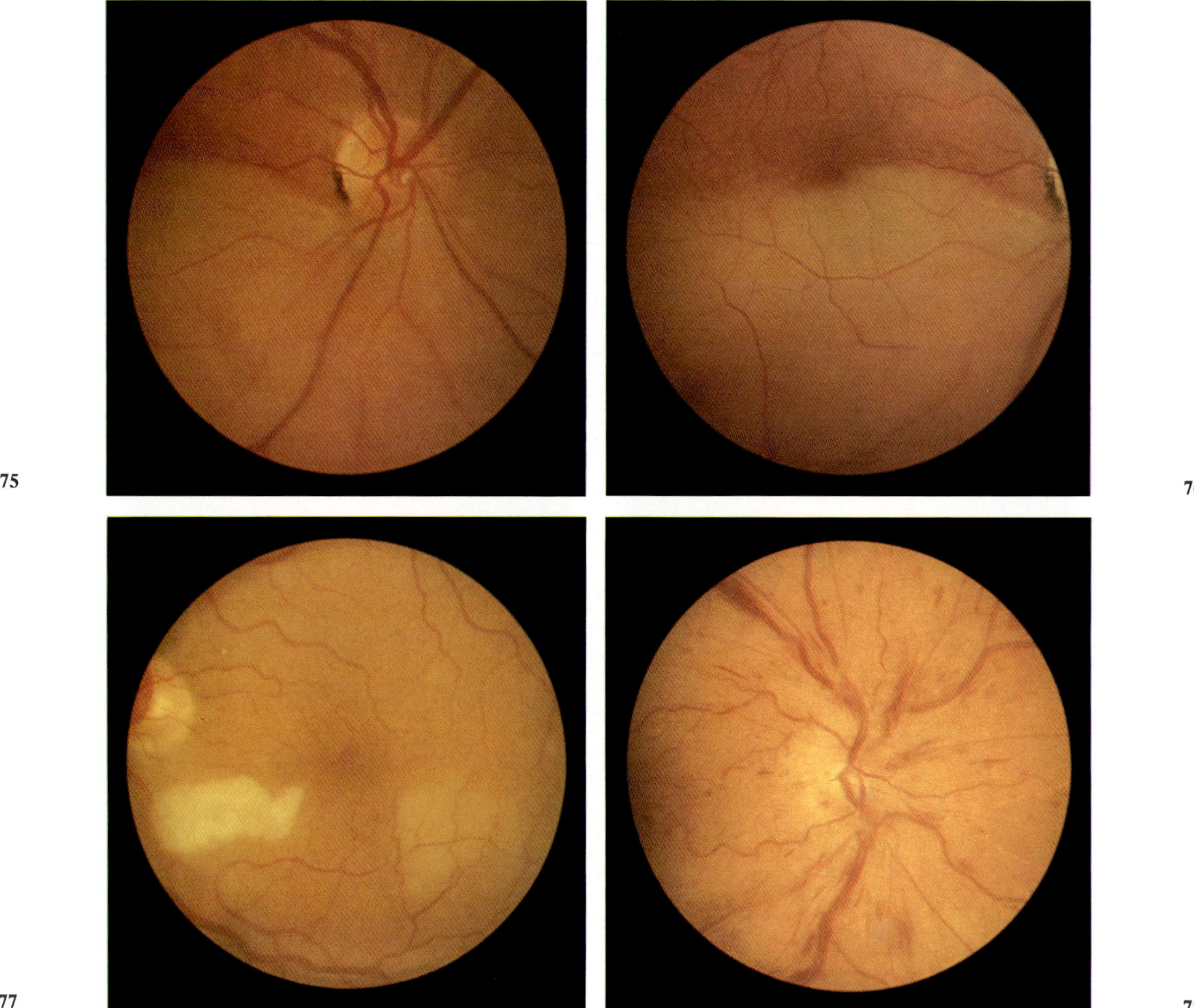

Figures 75 and 76. Right eye of a 60-year-old female patient with occlusion of branch arterioles associated with arterial hypertension following a myocardial infarction.

Clinical Findings

The refractive error in the right eye was +1.25 sphere, −0.75 cylinder, axis 90° with visual acuity of 20/100. The error in the left eye was +0.75 diopters sphere and visual acuity was 20/25. Examination of the refractive media revealed the presence of a beginning cortical and nuclear cataract. Intraocular pressure was 12 mm Hg. There was a visual field defect in the right eye involving the entire superior half. Blood pressure was 170/110 mm Hg, and the blood sedimentation rate was 28/40 mm. Doppler sonography revealed no abnormalities in the internal carotid artery.

Clinical Course

Final visual acuity was to 20/30.

Figure 77. Left eye of a 65-year-old patient with occlusions of branch arterioles associated with arterial hypertension and diabetes mellitus.

Clinical Findings

Blood glucose concentration was 160 mg/100 ml. With a correction of −0.5 diopters sphere, visual acuity in the left eye was 20/100, and 20/50 in the right eye. Intraocular pressure was 14 mm Hg in both eyes. Both eyes showed the presence of a beginning cataract. Blood pressure measured on the right arm was 180/100 mm Hg, and 180/95 mm Hg on the left arm. Blood sedimentation rate was 20/48 mm. Doppler sonography showed no internal carotid artery abnormalities.

Clinical Course

This patient died from a myocardical infarction on the same day of the ocular examination.

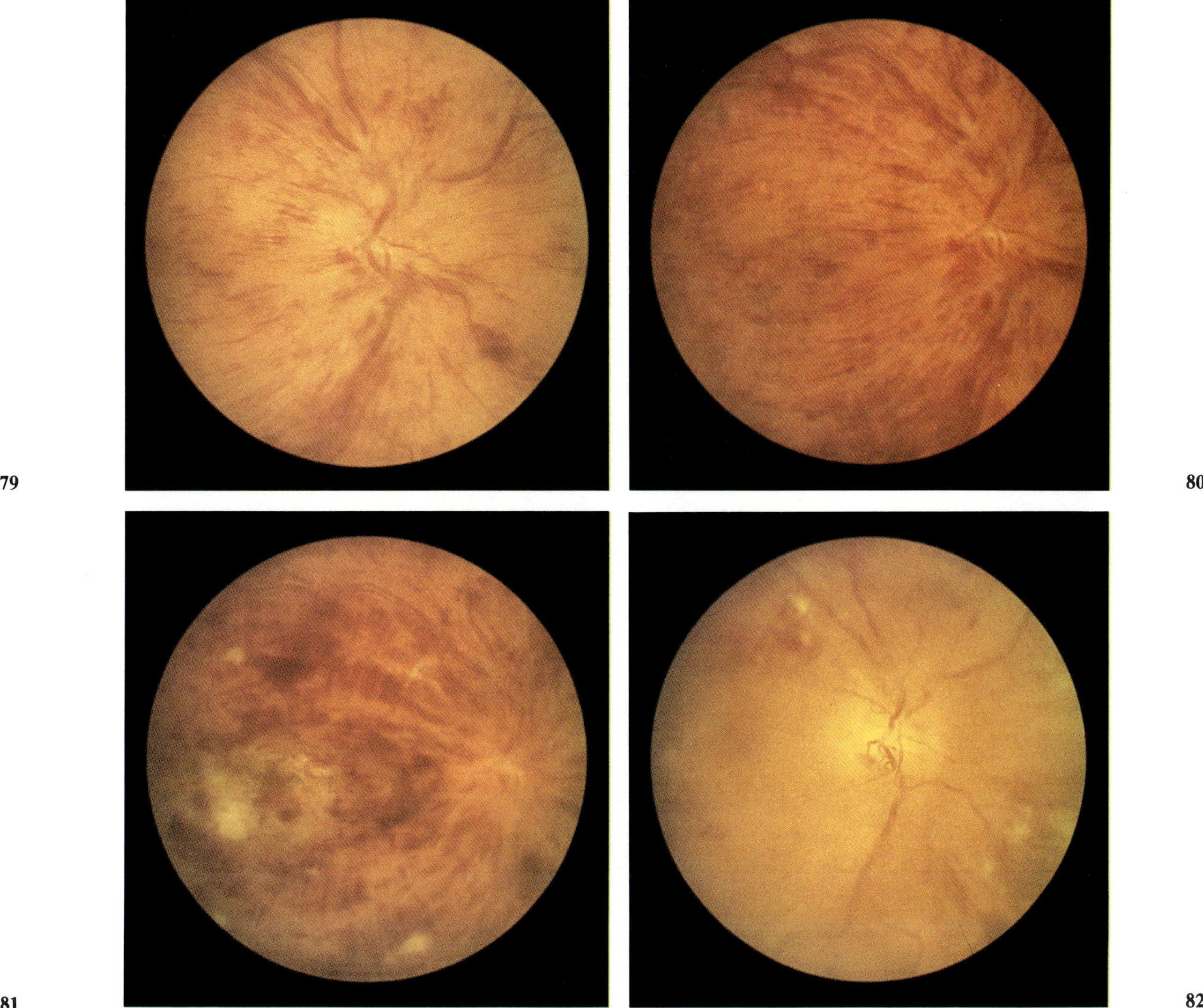

79 80

81 82

Figures 78–82. Right eye of a 53-year-old male patient with central retinal vein occlusion associated with arterial hypertension.

Clinical Findings

The patient had complained of blurred, hazy vision for 1 week and markedly decreased visual acuity 2 days prior to the examination. The right eye was emmetropic. Visual acuity was 20/700 in the right eye and 20/20 in the left eye. Intraocular pressure was 14 mm Hg in both eyes. The anterior segment showed no abnormalities. Figure 78 shows the posterior pole as it appeared during the first ophthalmic examination. The optic disc has blurred margins, particularly in the nasal quadrant, but there is no exudation in the central excavation. All retinal veins are engorged and tortuous. The arteries appear narrow, and isolated segments are masked by the peripapillary edema. Flame- or band-shaped hemorrhages can be seen, especially at AV crossings. Punctate and linear hemorrhages extend into the periphery and the macula is edematous. The left visual field was normal, but the right visual field had a central scotoma and a concentric constriction. Blood pressure was 220/120 mm Hg, and blood sedimentation rate was 20/36 mm. Doppler sonography did not show any abnormalities of the internal carotid artery. The hypertension was treated with propranolol hydrochloride and bendroflumethiazide. The patient also received prednisolone and a rheologic agent.

Clinical Course

The fundus appearance worsened until full-blown hemorrhagic retinopathy developed. The last fundus photograph (Fig. 82) was taken 6 months after the occlusion. The entire retina is edematous, the veins are still engorged, and hemorrhagic exudates are present in the midperiphery. AV shunts have developed on the optic disc. Visual acuity at this time was 20/1000 with an eccentric fixation. Intraocular pressure was 16 mm Hg. There was a centrocecal scotoma and a concentric constriction of the outer margins.

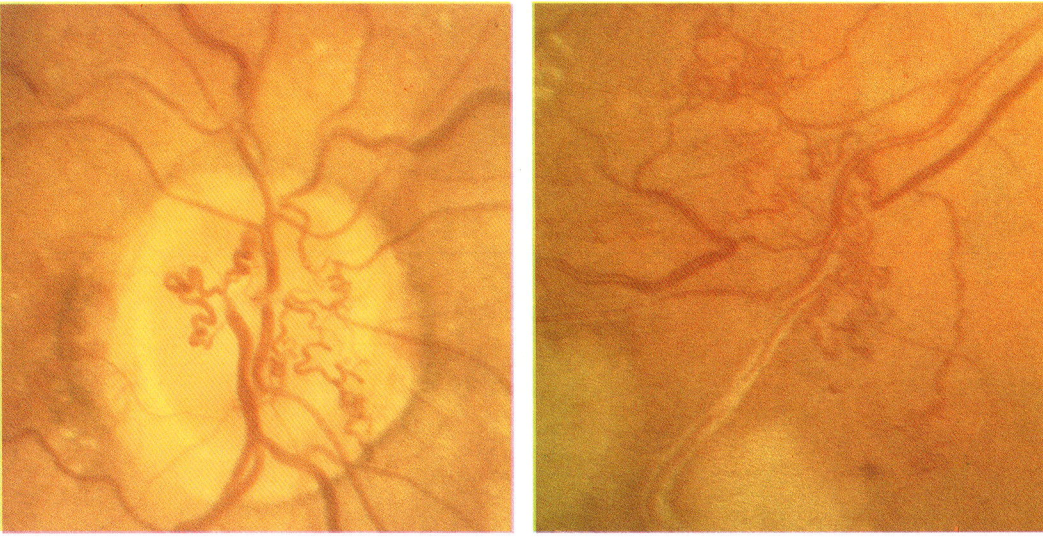

Figures 83 and 84. These figures of the same eye as in Figs. 78–82 show arteriovenous shunts that arose following the central retinal vein occlusion (Fig. 83) and a branch vein occlusion (Fig. 84). These two figures represent the status of the fundus after light coagulation of the peripheral neovascularizations that had caused recurrent vitreal hemorrhages.

85

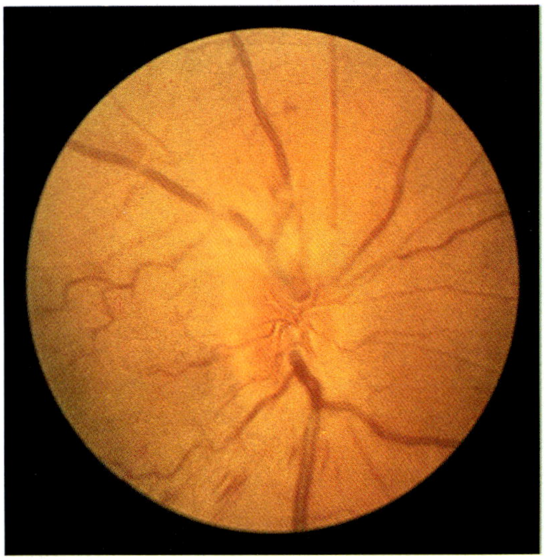

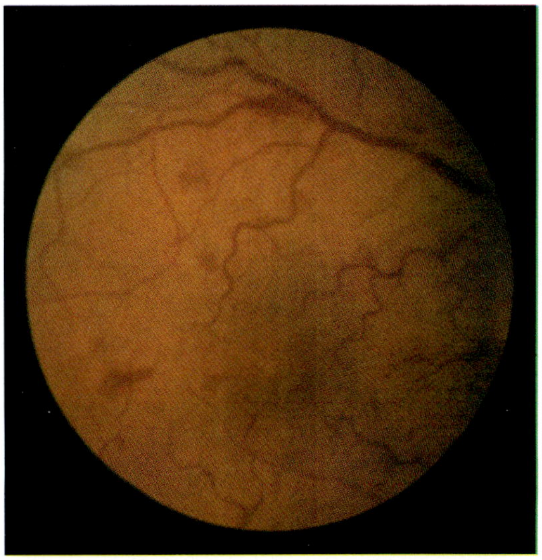

86

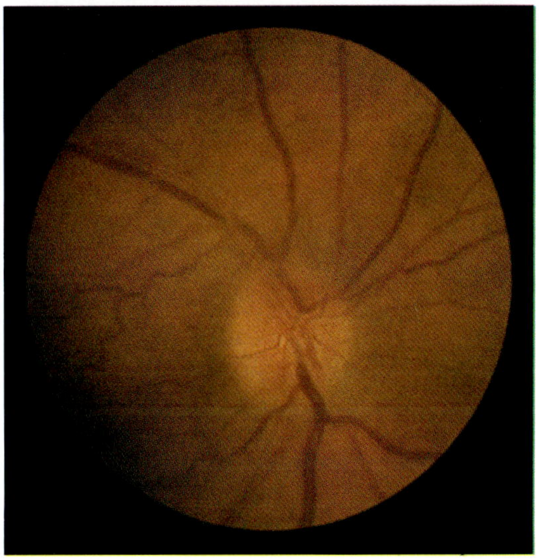

87

Figures 85-87. Right eye of a 46-year-old male patient with prethrombosis of the central retinal vein. (Differential diagnosis: venous stasis retinopathy.)

Clinical Findings

The patient noticed visual disturbances 8 hours prior to the ocular examination. He was able to view only contours of certain objects. Both eyes were emmetropic. Visual acuity in the right eye was 20/50 and in the left eye was 20/20. Intraocular pressure was 14 mm Hg in both eyes. Visual field testing showed a relative central scotoma (test mark: I/3, Goldmann perimeter). The outer margins of the visual field were slightly constricted. Blood pressure measured on the right arm was 120/80 mm Hg, and on the left arm was 100/80 mm Hg. Blood sedimentation rate was 22/45 mm. The optic disc in the right fundus was hyperemic with blurred margins and engorged and dilated veins. Arteries can not be seen in the peripapillary area because of the retinal edema, but visible arteries in other parts of the retina appear to be normal. The macula is also edematous. Dot and blot and flame-shaped hemorrhages extend into the retinal periphery. Slitlamp examination of the anterior segment was normal, and doppler sonography of the internal carotid artery was also normal.

Laboratory Findings

Normal differential blood cell counts, and normal red blood cell counts. The Quick test was 80%; the prothrombin time, the partial thromboplastin time, fibrinogen, platelets, and leading time were all normal. The serum fat, liver enzymes, and electrolytes were not elevated. The urine status was unremarkable. An ECG showed a partial blockage of the right ventricular bundle sinus rhythm.

Therapy

Osmotic therapy with Dextran and sorbitrate was performed. A regimen of prednisolone was introduced in addition to radiation therapy.

Clinical Course

Full visual rehabilitation was achieved with a visual acuity of 20/20.

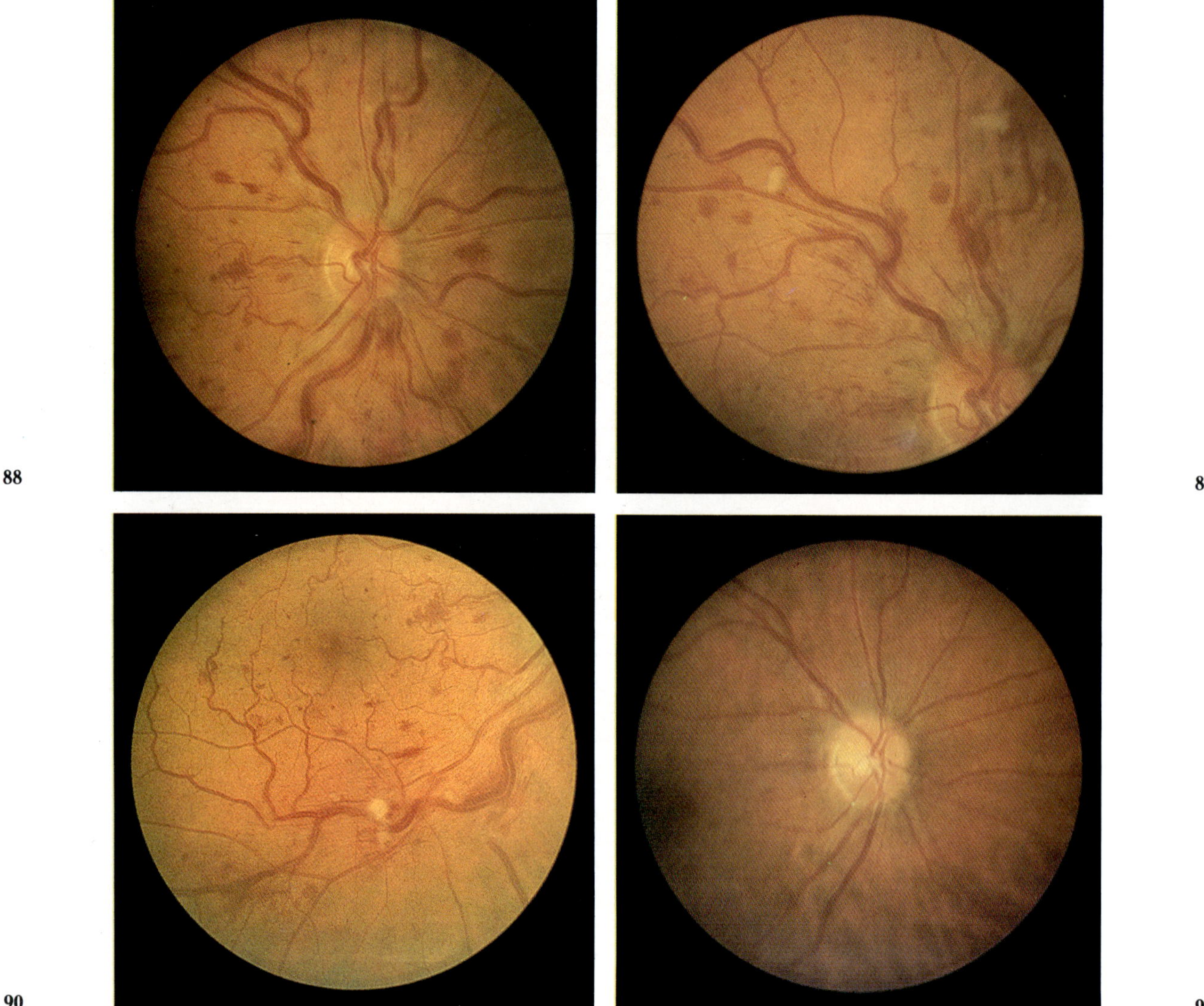

Figures 88–91. Right eye of a 40-year-old male patient with syphilitic retinal angiopathy. Ten years prior to the ophthalmic examination, the patient had suffered from a balanic syphilitic lesion while spending some time in a tropical region. At that time the infection was treated with penicillin. After the patient returned home, he was treated by a dermatologist for herpetic superinfected balanitis with associated inguinal lymph nodular swelling.

Clinical Findings

The patient presented with a prethrombosis of the central retinal vein. Both eyes were emmetropic with visual acuity of 20/20, and the visual fields were normal. Blood pressure was 140/80 mm Hg, and blood sedimentation rate was 40/86 mm. The fundus shows an optic disc with blurred margins and a hyperemia. The retinal veins are engorged and the arteries appear narrow. The arteriovenous ratio was 0.5 : 3. Peripherally, AV crossings are present. Cotton wool exudates are present, and dot and blot or flame-shaped radial retinal hemorrhages extend into the retinal periphery. As seen in Figure 88, the posterior pole is also affected. The anterior segment did not show any abnormalities. Doppler sonography revealed no abnormalities of the internal carotid artery. The laboratory diagnosis revealed a Quick's test of 83%, and a prothrombin time of 20.7 seconds. The white and red blood cell counts were normal. The *Treponema pallidum* hemagglutination test was positive (1:80). Cerebrospinal fluid showed a markedly elevated protein concentration (1.0 gm/100 ml). Neurologic and neuroradiologic examinations, as well as an orbital computed tomography, were unremarkable.

Therapy

The patient was treated with 60 million units of penicillin and vitamin C injections.

Clinical Course

The therapy was stopped after 2 months. Visual acuity at that time was 20/25 to 20/30. It is noteworthy that the patient did not suffer from any subjective symptoms during the entire observation period. The fundus changes were found during a routine examination.

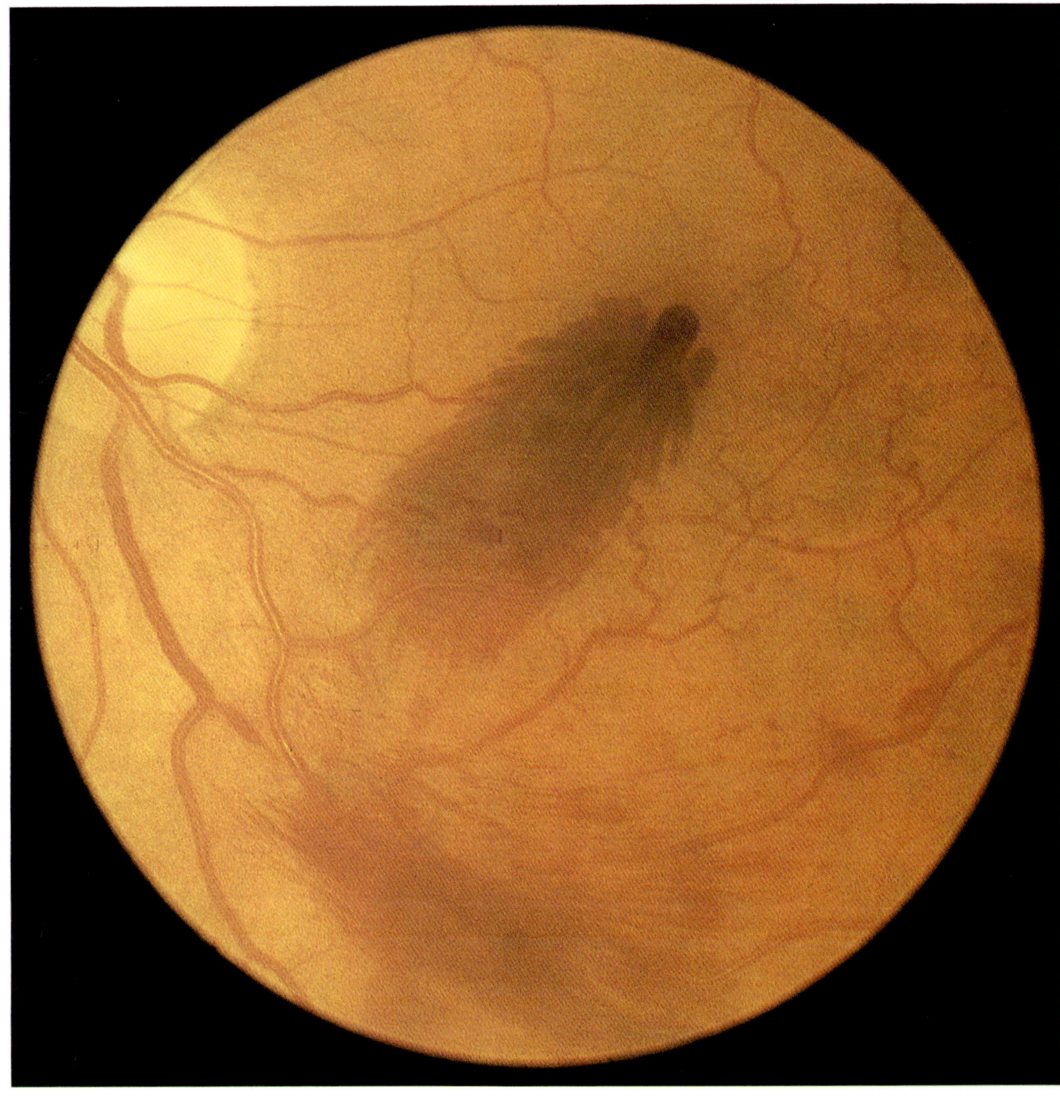

92

Figure 92. Left eye of a 61-year-old male patient with retinal branch vein occlusion and macular hemorrhage associated with arterial hypertension.

Clinical Findings

Visual acuity in the right eye was 20/20 and in the left eye 20/200. Intraocular pressure in the right eye was 12 mm Hg and in the left eye 14 mm Hg. Blood pressure was 165/100 mm Hg measured on both arms. The fundus showed a fan-shaped retinal hemorrhage overlying major branches of the inferior temporal artery and vein. The arteries showed omega-like branching. Wand reflexes were enhanced. The veins appeared engorged, but only the macular venules showed increased tortuosity. There was a large central hemorrhage extending into the macular region. The anterior segment was normal. Doppler sonography showed a normal blood flow in the internal carotid artery and coagulation tests were normal. An ECG revealed a sinus tachycardia. The patient was treated with oral anticoagulants, acetylsalicylic acid (aspirin), and radiation therapy.

Clinical Course

Full visual rehabilitation was achieved with visual acuity of 20/20.

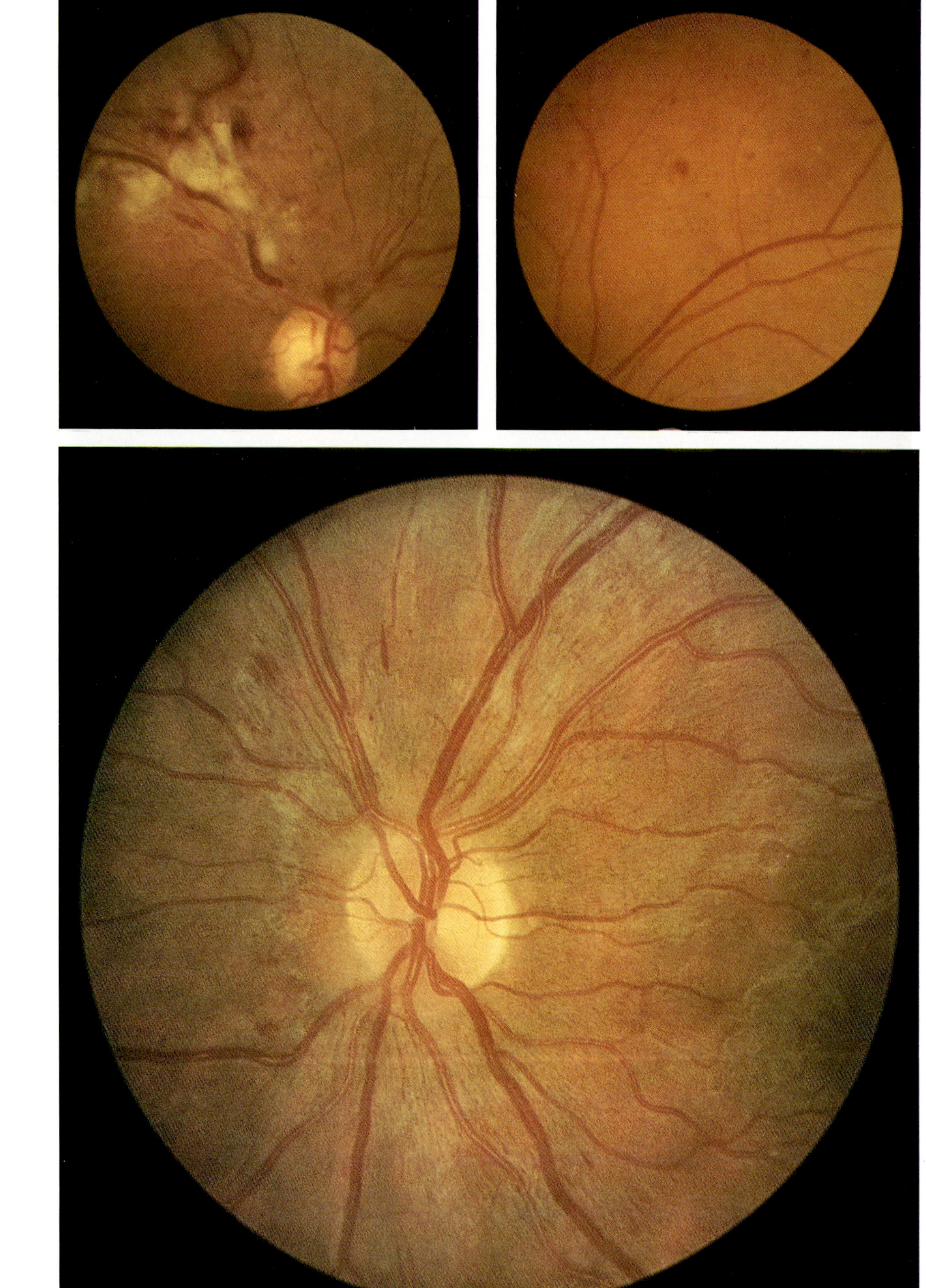

93

94

95

96 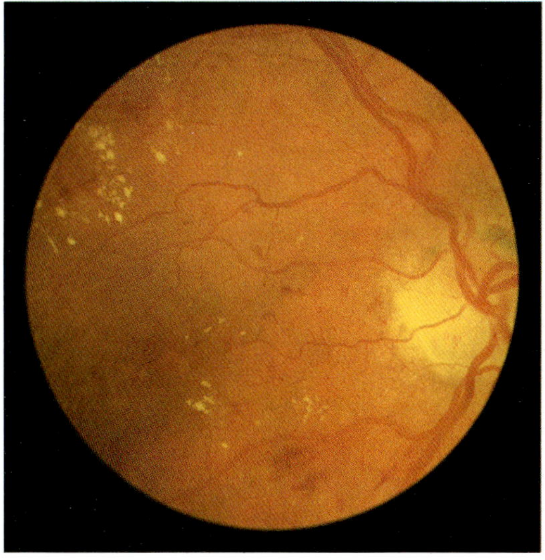

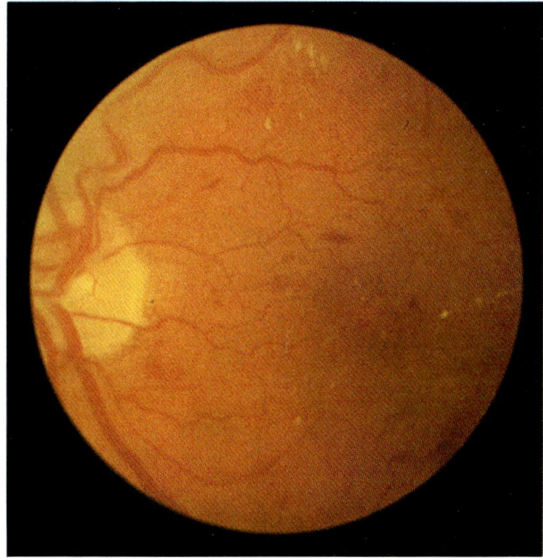 97

Figure 93. Right eye of a 63-year-old female patient with branch vein occlusion.

Clinical Findings

Both eyes showed a refractive error of +0.5 sphere, −1.0 cylinder, axis 90°. Visual acuity in the right eye was 20/200 and 20/25 in the left eye. Intraocular pressure in both eyes was 14 mm Hg. Visual field testing in the right eye showed a sector-shaped defect that extended from the blind spot inferonasally. Blood pressure was 220/110 mm Hg measured on the right arm and 230/115 mm Hg measured on the left arm. Fundus examination showed a normal optic disc. The superotemporal vein appears interrupted at several sites, caused by masking of the vessel by retinal edema and cotton wool exudates. The superotemporal vein and its branches are connected by retinal hemorrhages extending into the peripheral retina. The arteries appear narrow. The arteriovenous ratio was 0.5:3. The anterior segment was normal and doppler sonography showed a normal perfusion of the internal carotid artery. Coagulation tests were normal.

Therapy

Treatment consisted of oral anticoagulants and acetylsalicylic acid.

Clinical Course

The eye developed AV shunts and retinal neovascularizations (retia mirabila). These newly formed vessels caused recurrent vitreous hemorrhages. Subsequently, the superotemporal retinal quadrant was treated with xenon light coagulation. Following this therapy no other complications were observed.

Figure 94. Left eye of a 56-year-old female patient with Stage 1 diabetic retinopathy.

Clinical Findings

The patient had an 11-year history of diabetes. Visual acuity in both eyes was 20/60. Bilateral complicated cataracts (permeability cataracts) were present (Pau and Graeber, 1969). Blood pressure was 140/80 mm Hg.

Therapy

After a therapeutic trial with oral antidiabetic drugs failed, the patient was treated with insulin (400 international units in the morning, 22 units at night).

Figure 95. Left eye of a 12-year-old male patient with Stage 1 diabetic retinopathy and arterial hypertension.

Clinical Findings

The patient had a 6-year history of diabetes. The blood glucose concentration at the time of the examination was 160 mg/100 ml. Both eyes were slightly myopic (−1.0 diopter sphere), but visual acuity in both eyes was 20/20 and the refractive media were clear. Blood pressure was 145/95 mm Hg.

Therapy

The patient was treated with 24 units of insulin in the morning and 10 units at night. The number of microaneurysms was reduced markedly within a few weeks.

Figure 96. Right eye of a 50-year-old female patient with Stage 2 diabetic retinopathy.

Clinical Findings

The patient had an 8-year history of diabetes. Blood glucose concentration varied between 140 and 250 mg/100 ml. Visual acuity was 20/50. Blood pressure was 170/110 mm Hg. Note the presence of several hard exudates and retinal hemorrhages.

Therapy

The patient was treated with an oral antidiabetic drug.

Figure 97. Left eye of the same patient seen in Figure 96 with Stage 1 to 2 diabetic retinopathy.

Clinical Findings

This photograph shows that diabetic retinal changes are not always synchronous in both eyes. Visual acuity in this eye was 20/50.

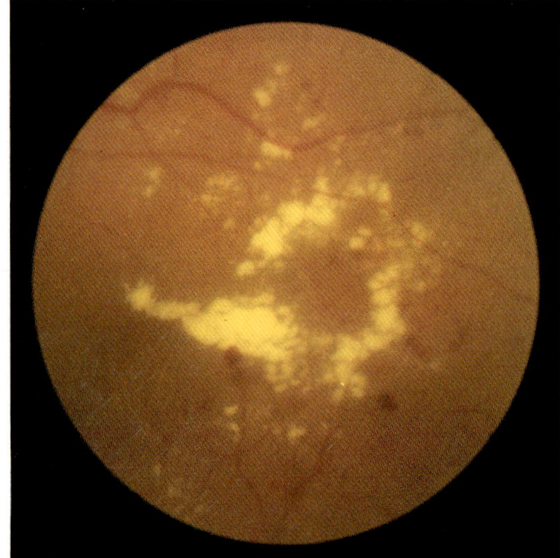

98

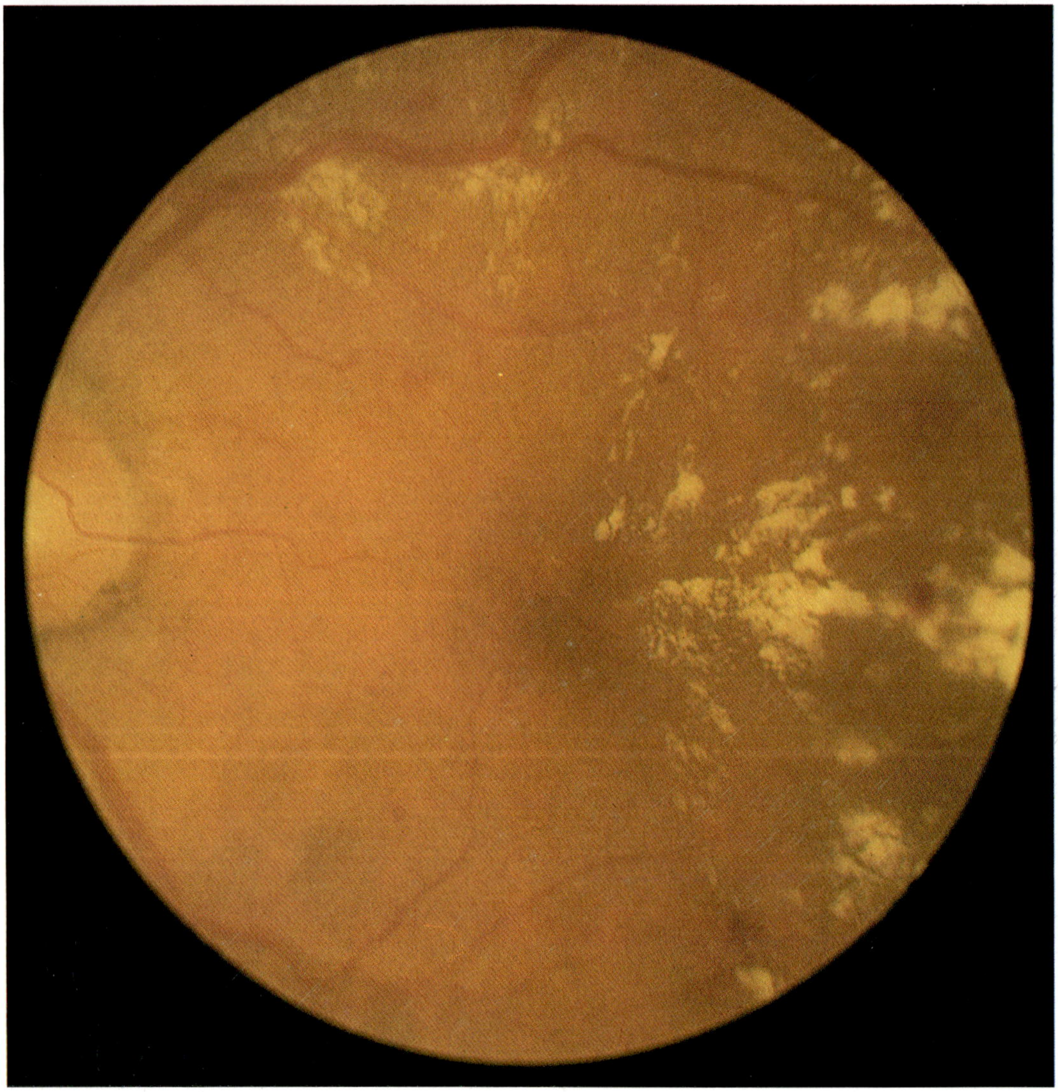

99

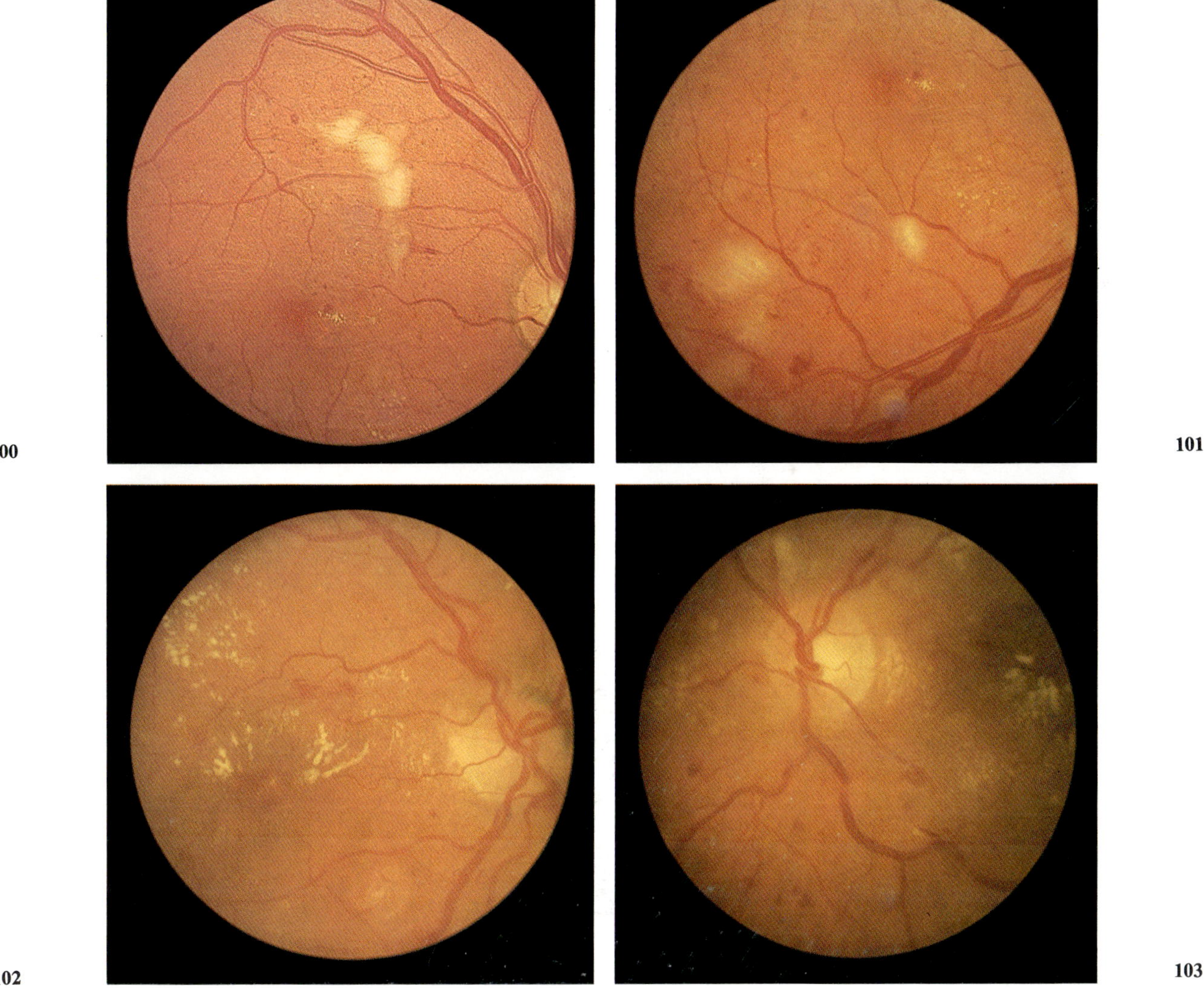

Figure 98. Left eye of a 77-year-old female patient with Stage 2 diabetic retinopathy.

Clinical Findings

The patient had a 20-year history of diabetes. Blood glucose concentration was approximately 200 mg/100 ml. Visual acuity was 20/200, and a nuclear cataract was present. Blood pressure was 150/90 mm Hg. Note the extensive retinal exudates, small hemorrhages, and microaneurysms.

Therapy

The patient was treated with an oral antidiabetic drug.

Figure 99. Left eye of a 67-year-old female patient with Stage 2 diabetic retinopathy.

Clinical Findings

The patient had a 27-year history of diabetes mellitus. Blood glucose concentration was 145 mg/100 ml. Visual acuity was 20/50. Blood pressure was 160/90 mm Hg, and blood sedimentation rate was 50/75 mm. Serum cholesterol was 335 mg/100 ml. Triglycerides were 207 mg/100 ml, and the β-lipoproteins were 927 mg/100 ml.

Therapy

The patient was treated with 20 units of insulin daily.

Figures 100 and 101. Right eye of a 22-year-old female patient with Stage 2 diabetic retinopathy and Kimmelstiel-Wilson disease.

Clinical Findings

The patient had a 2-year history of diabetes. Blood glucose concentration was 240 mg/100 ml. Visual acuity was 20/30. Blood pressure was 125/85 mm Hg. Note the hard and soft exudates and the presence of punctate hemorrhages and microaneurysms.

Therapy

The patient was treated with 32 units of insulin in the morning and 60 units at night.

Figures 102 and 103. Right and left eyes of a 49-year-old female patient with Stage 2 diabetic retinopathy and Kimmelstiel-Wilson disease.

Clinical Findings

The patient suffered from arterial hypertension and had a 7-year history of diabetes. Visual acuity in both eyes was 20/1000. Blood pressure was 240/140 mm Hg. Note the presence of extensive hard exudates, retinal hemorrhages, and microaneurysms.

Laboratory Findings

Blood glucose concentration 532 mg/100 ml, cholesterol 406 mg/100 ml, serum urine concentration 85 mg/100 ml, creatinine level 1.4 mg/100 ml. Urine protein level was 5%.

Therapy

The patient was treated with 24 units of insulin in the morning and 12 units at night.

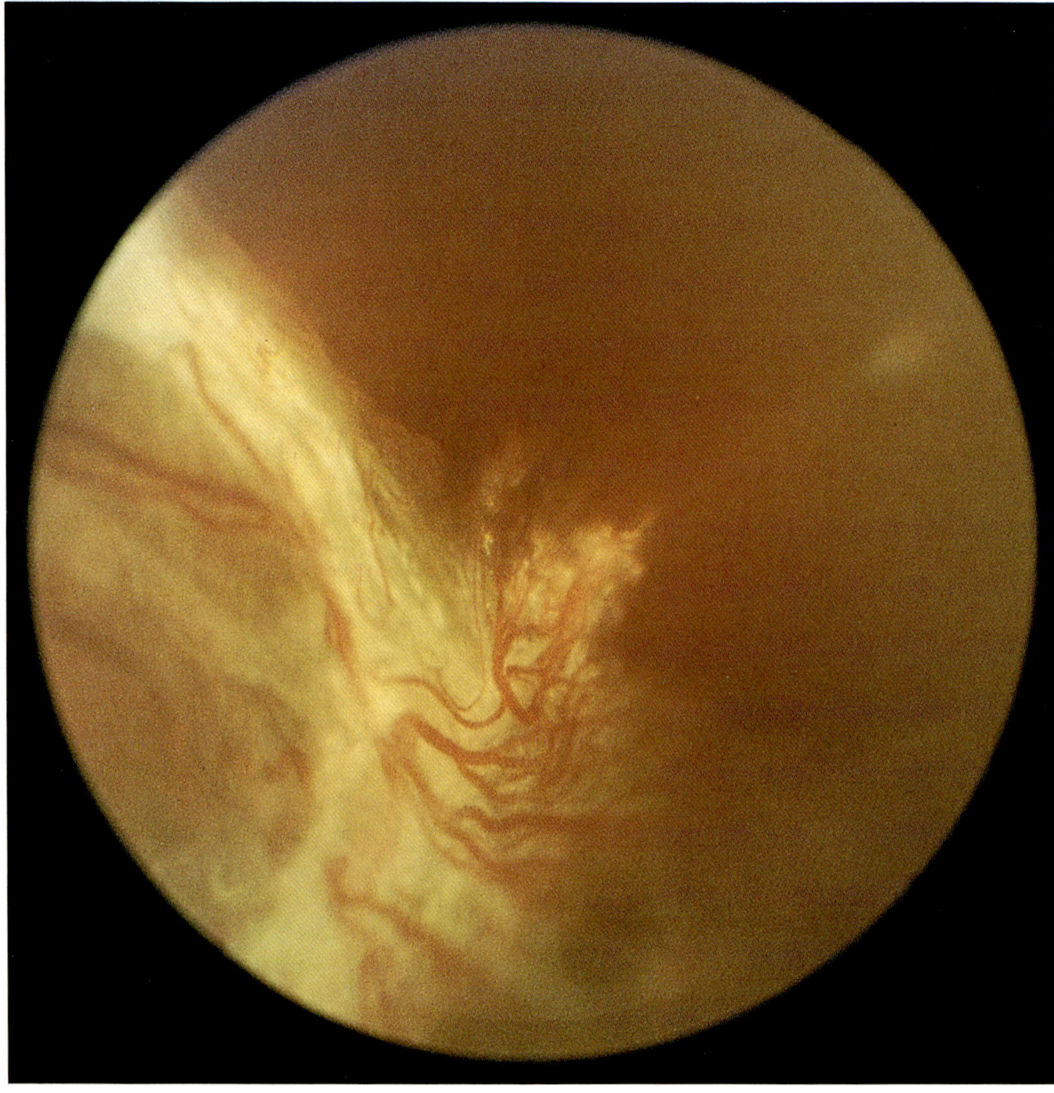

104

Figure 104. Left eye of a 27-year-old male patient with Stage 3 diabetic retinopathy.

Clinical Findings

The patient had a history of diabetes for 4 years. Blood pressure was 120/80 mm Hg. The eye was amaurotic. Extensive neovascularization had developed despite repeated laser and xenon light coagulations.

Therapy

The patient was treated with 20 to 24 units of insulin three times daily. With this treatment the blood glucose concentration during the day varied between 149–252 and 144–254 mg/100 ml. Other laboratory parameters were unremarkable.

Figure 105. Left eye of a 42-year-old male patient with Stage 2 diabetic retinopathy.

Clinical Findings

The patient was seen 3 days after a laser coagulation treatment. Blood glucose concentration was 290 mg/100 ml. Visual acuity was 20/200, and the visual field showed a relative central scotoma. Blood pressure was 145/90 mm Hg. The anterior segment showed no abnormalities. There are extensive hard exudates surrounding the posterior pole, as well as the flame-shaped and dot and blot hemorrhages. The edematous retina overlying the laser lesions appears white around the macular area.

Therapy

The patient was treated with 36 units of insulin in the morning and 16 units at night.

Clinical Course

After 2 weeks, visual acuity recovered to 20/30.

Figures 106 and 107. Right and left eyes of a 60-year-old female patient with Stage 2 diabetic retinopathy.

Clinical Findings

Both fundi had been treated with retinal laser coagulation 3 years earlier. With a refractive correction in both eyes of +1.5 sphere, −0.75 cylinder, axis 90°, visual acuity in the right eye was 20/40, and 20/1000 in the left eye. A partial macular hole was present in the left eye. Both eyes had a nuclear cataract combined with a beginning cortical cataract. The visual field in the right eye was tunneled, and the visual field in the left eye showed a central scotoma. Blood pressure was 150/95 mm Hg. Blood glucose concentration was 190 mg/100 ml.

Therapy

The patient was treated with 28 units of insulin in the morning and 12 units at night.

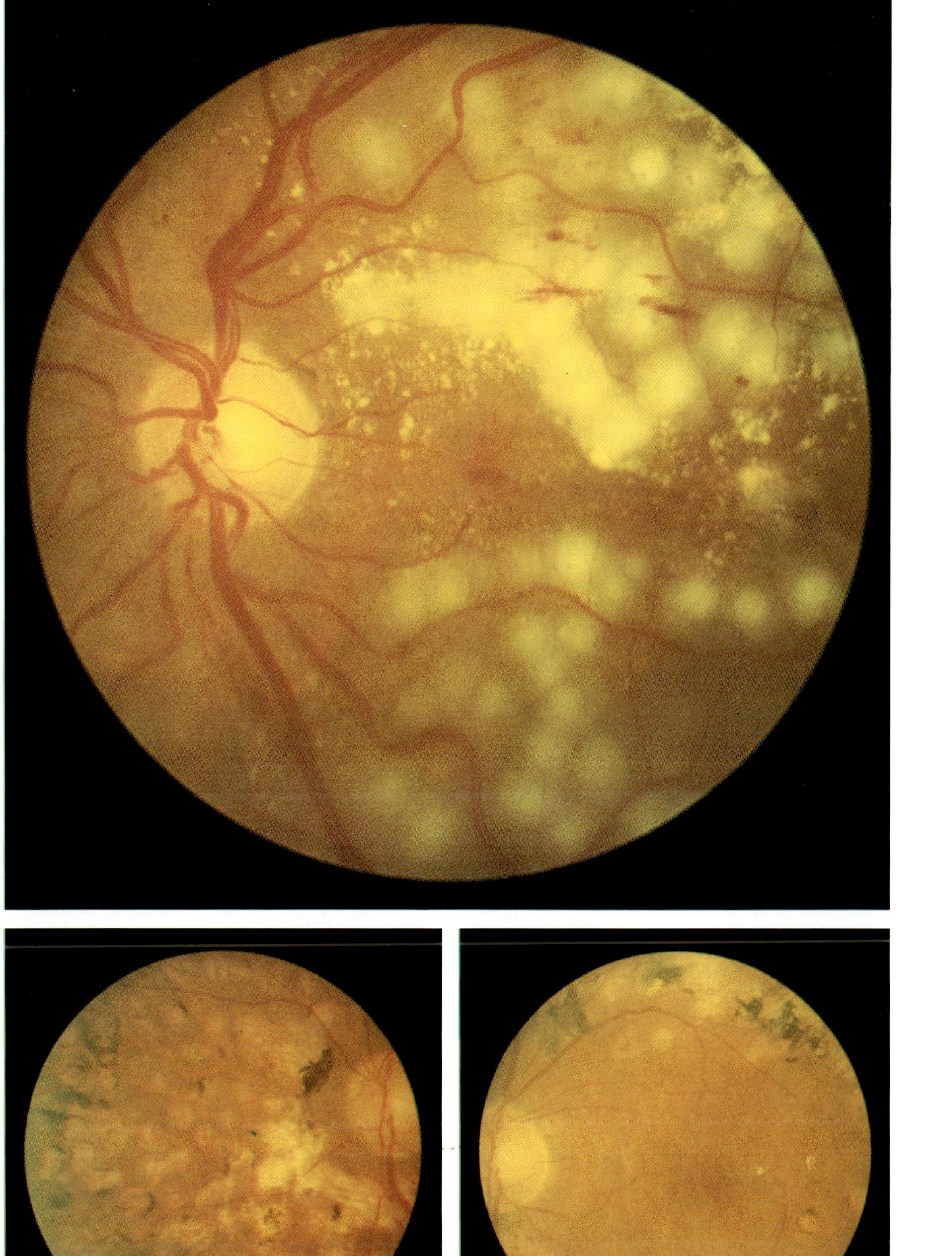

105

106

107

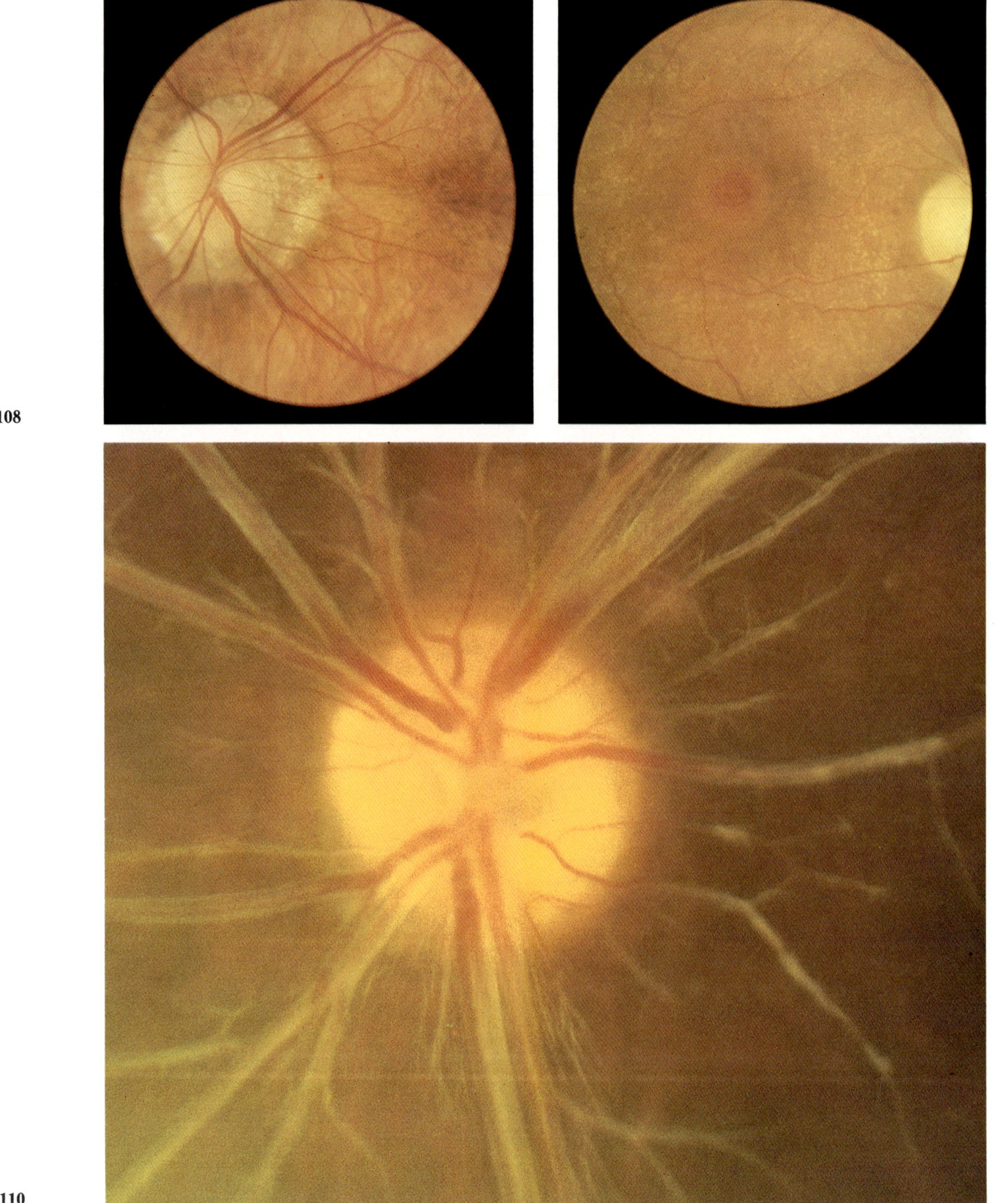

108

109

110

Figure 108. Left eye of a 63-year-old male patient with an arteriosclerotic fundus (fundus scleroticus A; Table 13, Sautter).

Clinical Findings

The refraction in both eyes was +1.5 sphere, −0.5 cylinder, axis 90°. Visual acuity in the right eye was 20/25, and in the left eye was 20/30. A beginning cataract was present in both eyes. Intraocular pressure was 14 mm Hg in both eyes. Visual fields were normal. Doppler sonography did not reveal any alteration in blood perfusion in the internal carotid artery. Ophthalmodynomography showed a difference in the blood pressure between the brachial and ophthalmic artery and a reduced pulsation volume. The pressure in the brachial artery was 160/90 mm Hg, and in the ophthalmic artery, 140/75 mm Hg. The pulsation volume was 35 μl. Examination of the fundus revealed an extensive inferotemporal crescent. The choroid is atrophic, and atrophy of the choriocapillaris caused the larger choroidal vessels to become visible. There are pigment irregularities in the macular region.

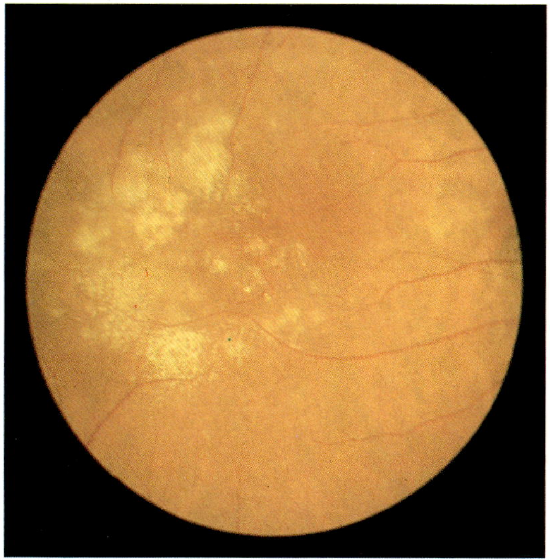

111

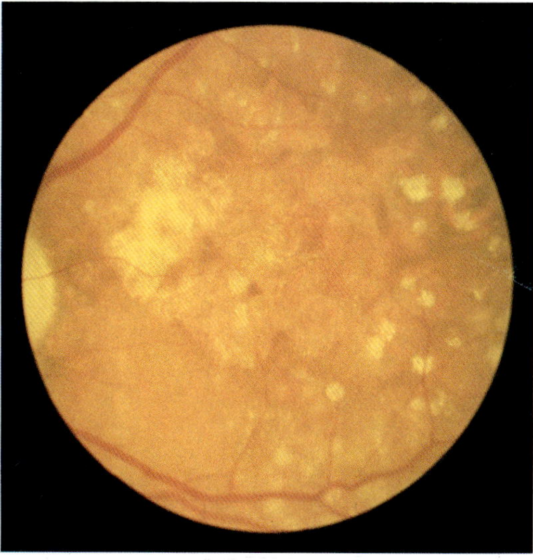

112

Figure 109. Right eye of a 72-year-old female patient with arteriosclerotic fundus (fundus scleroticus A; Table 13, Sautter), with an age-related (senile) partial macular hole.

Clinical Findings

Refraction in both eyes was −0.75 sphere, −1.0 cylinder, axis 90°. Visual acuity in the right eye was 20/700, and in the left eye 20/50. There was a beginning cataract. Intraocular pressure in the right eye was 14 mm Hg, and in the left eye, 16 mm Hg. There was a central scotoma in the visual field of the right eye. Blood pressure was 155/90 mm Hg. There are numerous age-related drusen at the posterior pole, and the optic disc shows a typical age-related pallor. A central, red macular hole is present.

Figure 110. Left eye of a 69-year-old female patient with optic atrophy and generalized vascular ensheathing.

Clinical Findings

The patient had cerebral convulsions following meningoencephalitis. This disease also caused amaurosis in the left eye. Refraction in the right eye was −0.5 cylinder, axis 160°, and visual acuity was 20/20. In the left eye the refraction was −1.0 sphere, but the eye was amaurotic with a secondary divergent strabismus. Both corneas showed a pronounced arcus senilis. A beginning cataract was also present. Intraocular pressure was 16 mm Hg. The visual fields and fundus in the right eye were normal. Visual fields in the left eye could not be evaluated. The optic disc of the left eye appears pale, the margins are well demarcated, and the disc is not elevated. All retinal vessels show a white ensheathing. The normal vascular reflex was only visible at a small portion of the vessels underlying the optic disc. The posterior pole shows pigmentary irregularities, but the peripheral retina was unremarkable. Blood sedimentation rate was 10/31 mm.

Laboratory Findings

Red blood cell count was 4.3 million erythrocytes and 7800 leukocytes. The differential white cell count showed 11 band neutrophils, 49 segmented neutrophils, 32 lymphocytes, and 1 basophil. Electrolytes, alkaline phosphatase, creatinine, and blood glucose concentrations were all normal. Serum cholesterol was 263 mm/100 ml. High-density lipoprotein (HDL) fraction was 77 mg/100 ml; low-density lioprotein (LDL) fraction was 161 mg/100 ml. The triglycerides were 122 mg/100 ml. Cerebrospinal fluid was clear and showed a glucose concentration of 60 mg/100 ml, cells 5/3. Screening for protein in the spinal fluid was negative (Pandy's reaction).

Internal Examination

Vertigo similar to that seen in Ménière's disease was caused by distortions of the cerebral blood supply with aortal sclerosis.

Ear, Nose, and Throat Examination

Ménière's disease-like symptoms of cerebral etiology were found. An EEG was unremarkable. Blood pressure was 170/110 mm Hg.

Therapy

The patient was treated with anticonvulsants and rheologic drugs.

Figure 111. Right eye of a 75-year-old female patient with arteriosclerosis (fundus scleroticus B; Table 13, Sautter).

Clinical Findings

Both eyes were hyperopic (+2.75 sphere). Visual acuity in the right eye was 20/60, and in the left eye, 20/50. Bilateral cortical and nuclear cataracts were present. Intraocular pressure was normal. Both visual fields showed relative central scotomas; a nonspecific constriction of the visual field was limited to 45°. The mesopic vision was distorted. Blood pressure was 160/85 mm Hg. Age-related drusen that had accrued to form larger plaques were present at the posterior pole. The macular region shows pigment irregularities.

Figure 112. Left eye of a 74-year-old female patient with arteriosclerosis (fundus scleroticus B; Table 13, Sautter).

Clinical Findings

The refractive error in the right eye was +1.0 sphere, and in the left eye was +1.0 sphere, −0.5 cylinder, axis 75°. Visual acuity in the right eye was 20/60 and in the left 20/200. Intraocular pressure in both eyes was 14 mm Hg. There was nonspecific constriction of the outer margins of the central 40° of both visual fields, and there was a relative central scotoma in both eyes. Blood pressure was 160/90 mm Hg. The fundus shows a central depigmented area. The underlying choriocapillaris is atrophic, and the lesion resembles a central macular dystrophy.

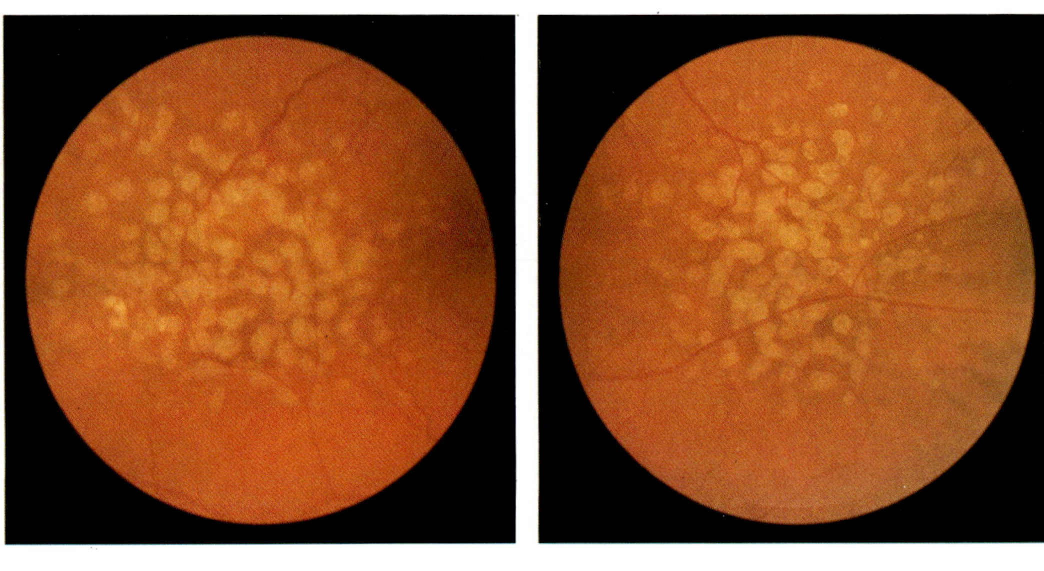

Figures 113 and 114. Right and left eyes of a 49-year-old female patient with arteriosclerosis (fundus scleroticus B; Table 13, Sautter).

Clinical Findings

Visual acuity in both eyes was 20/20 and both eyes were emmetropic. The refractive media were clear. Intraocular pressure in the right eye was 14 mm Hg and in the left eye, 16 mm Hg. The visual fields were normal. Blood pressure was 140/80 mm Hg measured on both arms. Both fundi show large age-related drusen that extend from the posterior pole toward the equator.

Figures 115–117. Left eye of a 65-year-old female patient with arteriosclerosis (fundus scleroticus C; Table 13, Sautter).

Clinical Findings

Refraction in both eyes was +0.5 sphere. Visual acuity was 20/20 in the right eye and hand movements in the left eye. A beginning cataract was present. Intraocular pressure in both eyes was 14 mm Hg. The right visual field was normal, but the left visual field showed a large central scotoma. Doppler sonography showed no abnormalities of the internal carotid arteries. Ophthalmodynomography showed a difference in pressure between the brachial and ophthalmic arteries. The blood pressure in the brachial artery was 150/85 mm Hg and the pressure in the ophthalmic artery was 140/63 mm Hg. Pulsation volume was 65 μl. Figures 115 and 116 illustrate an extensive choroidal hemorrhage that frames the optic disc superiorly and inferiorly and extends toward the macular region in an arcuate pattern. The retina, especially the papillomacular bundle, is edematous.

Clinical Course

As shown in Figure 117, the posterior pole underwent extensive scarring and glial proliferation. Kuhnt-Junius disease (disciform macular degeneration) was diagnosed.

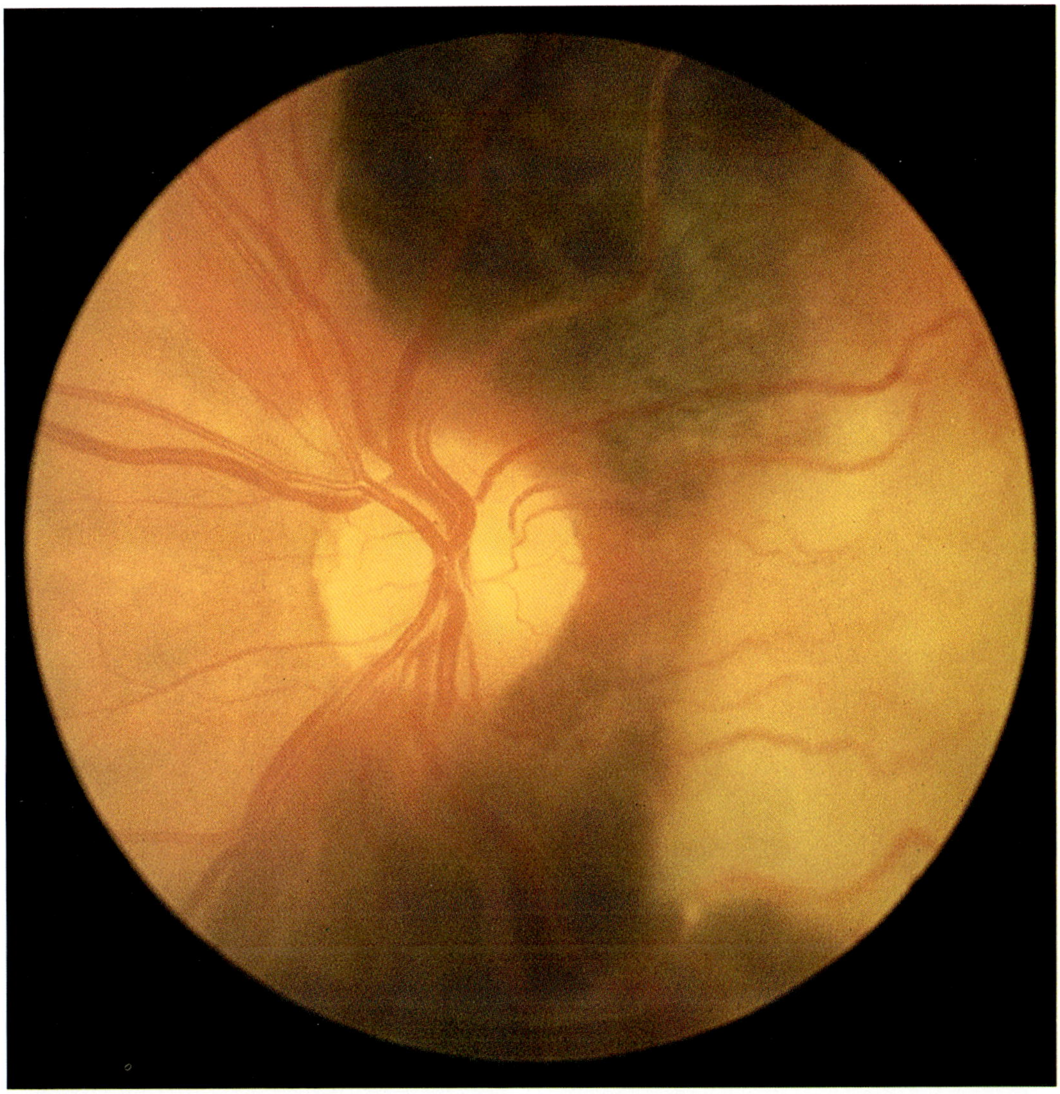

115

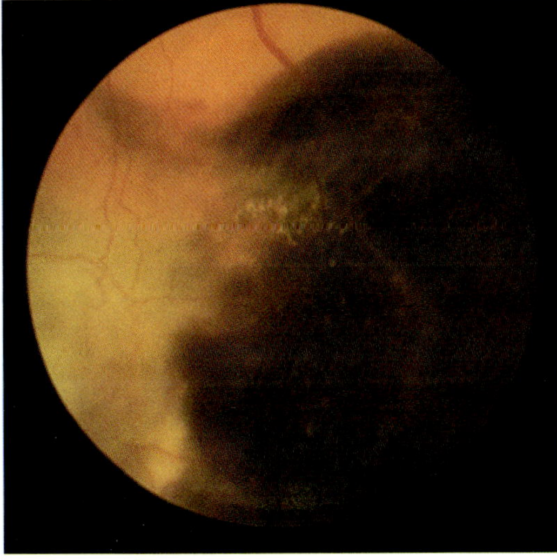

116

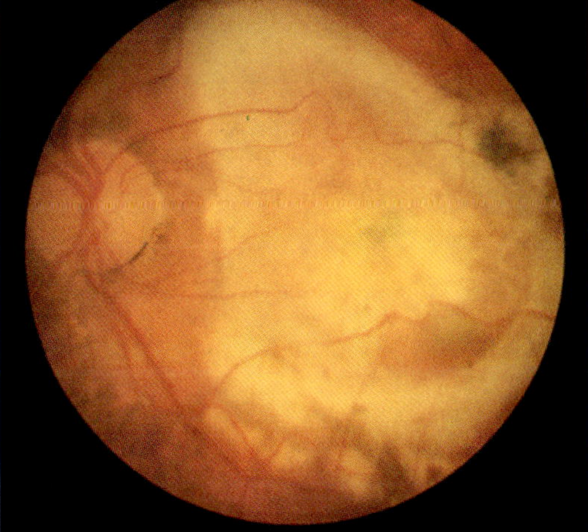

117

118

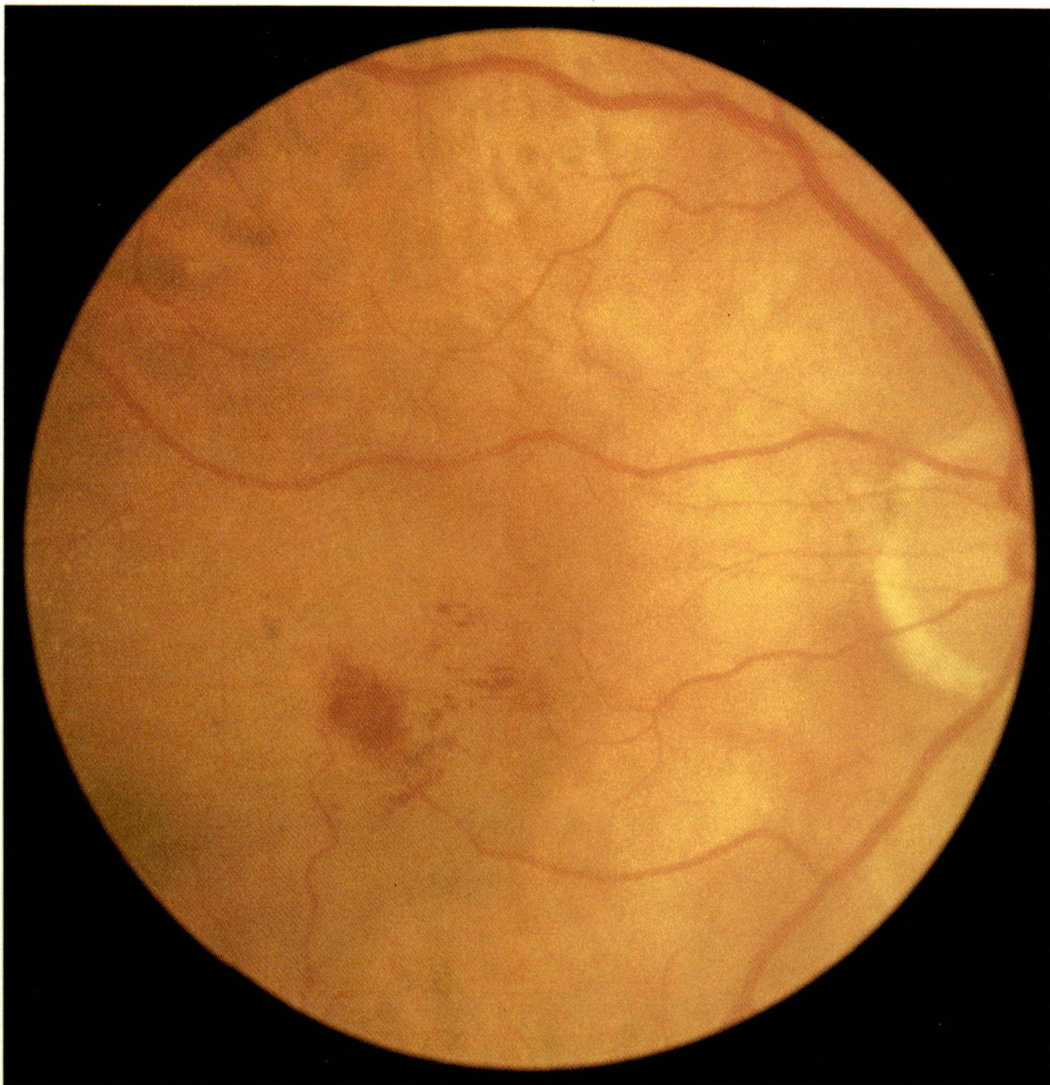

Figure 118. Right eye of a 70-year-old female patient with arteriosclerosis (fundus scleroticus C; Table 13, Sautter).

Clinical Findings

The eye was hyperopic, +1.25 sphere; visual acuity was 20/1000. Intraocular pressure in both eyes was 14 mm Hg. There was a central scotoma in the visual field of the right eye and concentric constrictions of the outer margins. Doppler sonography showed normal blood flow. Ophthalmodynomography showed cerebral hypotension. The blood pressure in the brachial artery was 130/85 mm Hg and in the ophthalmic artery was 115/65 mm Hg. Pulsation volume in the right eye was 68.1 μl and in the left eye was 81.3 μl. A macular edema (macular insudation) is present (Sautter, 1961). There are retinal hemorrhages in the elevated part of the retina.

119 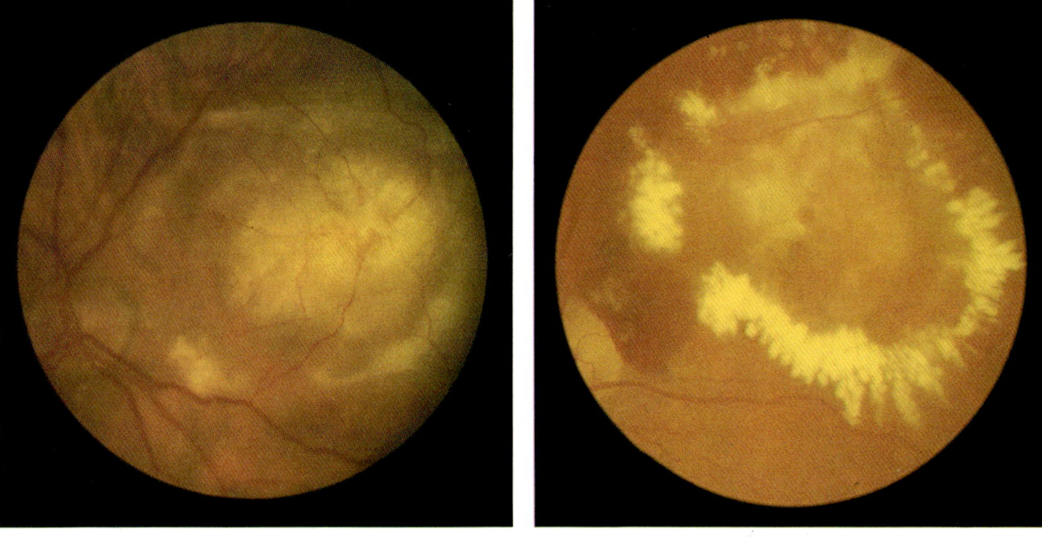 120

Figure 119. Left eye of a 76-year-old female patient with arteriosclerosis (fundus scleroticus C; Table 13, Sautter).

Clinical Findings

Visual acuity was 20/1000. The entire macular area shows an extensive disciform lesion with glial proliferation, indicative of disciform macular degeneration (Kuhnt-Junius disease).

Figure 120. Left eye of a 60-year-old female patient with arteriosclerosis (fundus scleroticus C; Table 13, Sautter).

Clinical Findings

Visual acuity was 20/1000. The posterior pole shows a developing disciform lesion (Kuhnt-Junius disease).

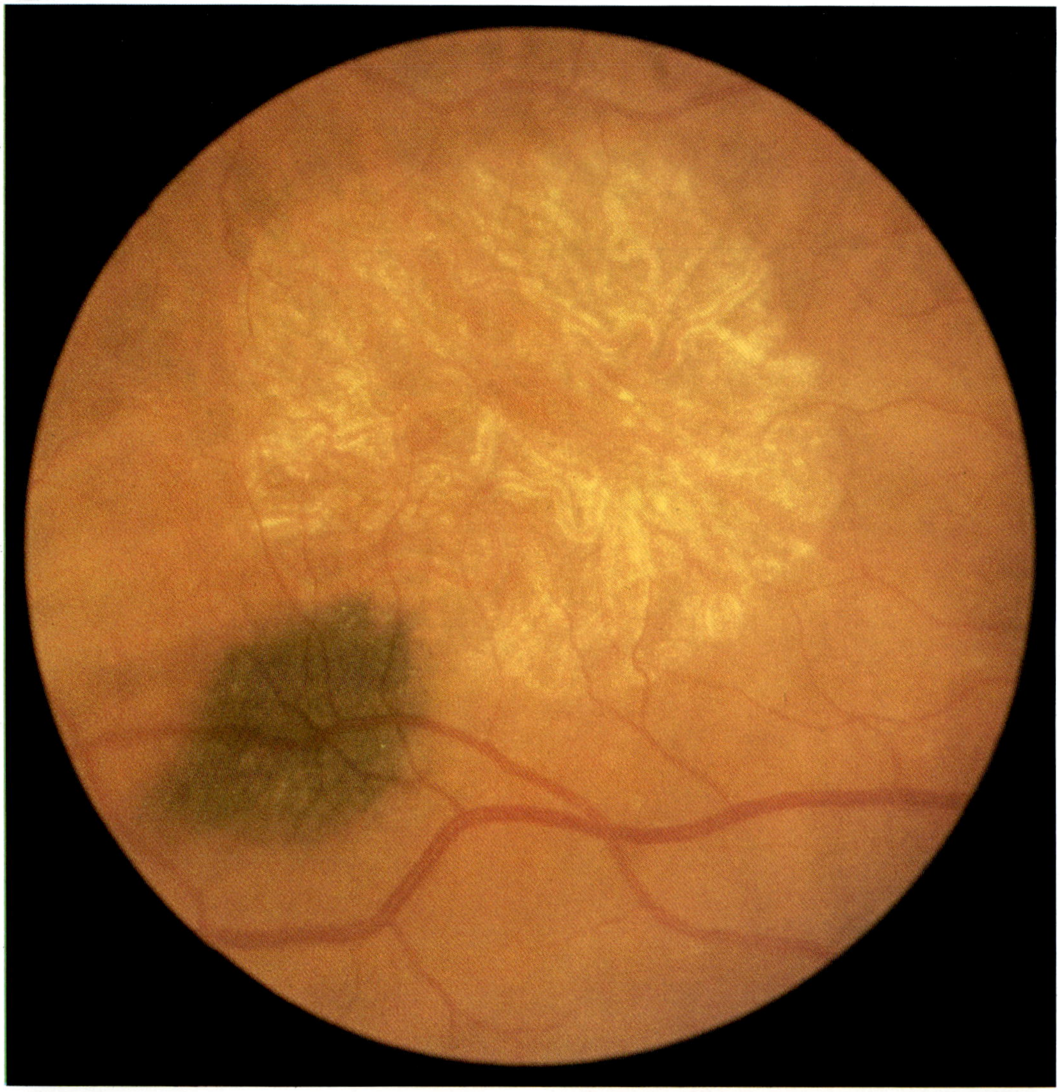

121

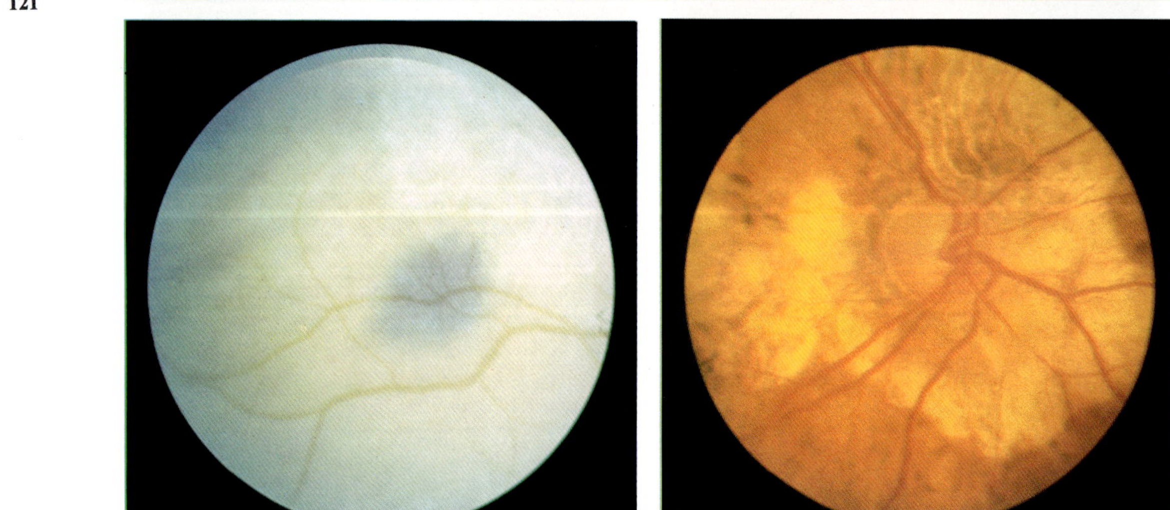

122

123

124

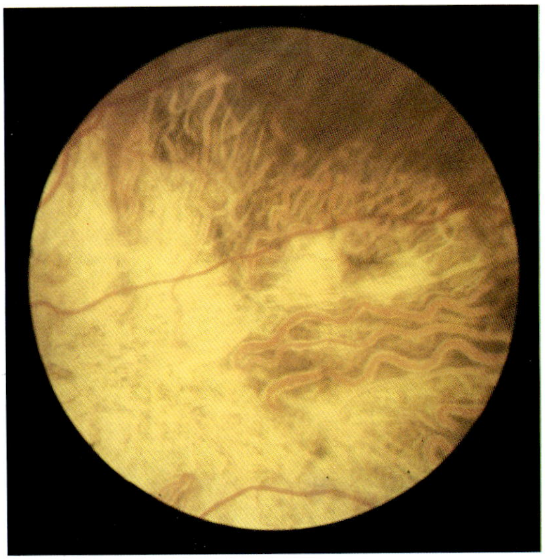

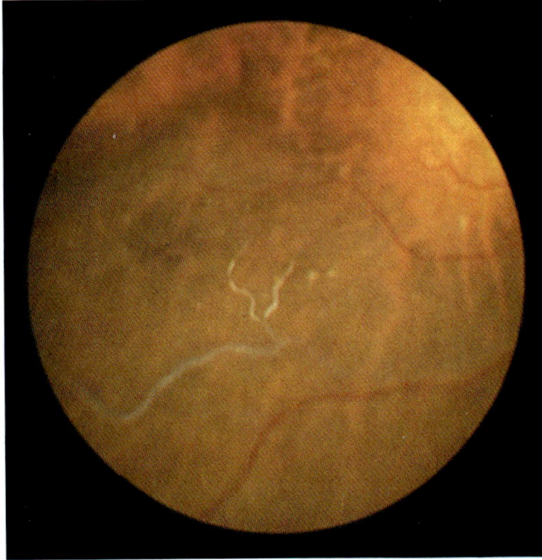

125

Figures 121 and 122. Left eye of a 72-year-old female patient with exudative macular degeneration following x-ray therapy and central retinal choroidal scarring.

Clinical Findings

Refraction in both eyes was +1.0 sphere. Visual acuity in the right eye was 20/1000 and there was a beginning cataract. Intraocular pressure in both eyes was 14 mm Hg. There was a central scotoma and a concentric constriction of the peripheral margins leaving a 15° visual field. Note the presence of a small choroidal nevus. The eye underwent a retrobulbar irradiation with 0.5 Ci in several fractions: the surface irradation dose was 150 rad, a single dose was 50 rad.

Figure 123. Right eye of an 86-year-old male patient with arteriosclerosis (fundus scleroticus D; Table 13, Sautter).

Clinical Findings

The refraction in both eyes was +2.25 sphere. Visual acuity in the right eye was 20/25, and in the left eye was 20/30. A nuclear cataract was present. Intraocular pressure was 16 mm Hg in both eyes. Visual field testing showed a mild concentric constriction of the outer margins but no scotomas were present. Blood pressure was 160/90 mm Hg. Doppler sonography revealed normal perfusion of blood in the internal carotid artery. The fundus showed a choroidal atrophy. The choriocapillaris atrophy revealed obstructed larger choroidal vessels. Intervascular spaces show varying degrees of pigmentation, which give the appearance of a tigroid senile fundus. The optic disc is excavated. The superotemporal vein shows nicking at the site where it crosses over the optic disc margin. Intraocular pressure was not elevated.

Figure 124. Left eye of a 70-year-old male patient with arteriosclerosis (fundus scleroticus D; Table 13, Sautter).

Clinical Findings

Both eyes were hyperopic with a refractive error of +2.0 sphere. Visual acuity in the left eye was 20/1000, and a nuclear cataract was present. Intraocular pressure in both eyes was 14 mm Hg. There was a central scotoma in the visual field with normal outer margins, and a distortion in the mesopic vision. Doppler sonography was normal. The fundus shows areas of choroidal atrophy with depigmentation and larger choroidal vessels are visible. Blood sedimentation rate was 30/56 mm. Serum cholesterol was 292 mm/100 ml (normal is between 150 and 250 mg/100 ml). Triglycerides were 297 mg/100 ml (normal is 50 to 200 mg/100 ml).

Figure 125. Right eye of a 90-year-old female patient with arteriosclerosis (fundus scleroticus D; Table 13, Sautter).

Clinical Findings

A refractive error of +12.0 sphere combined with 0.75 cylinder, axis 90° was corrected to a visual acuity of 20/25 in this aphakic eye. An arcus senilis was present. Intraocular pressure was 15 mm Hg. Visual fields were normal. Some fundus vessels are completely obliterated and occluded. The choroid shows an atropic sclerosis with a beginning senile tigroid fundus.

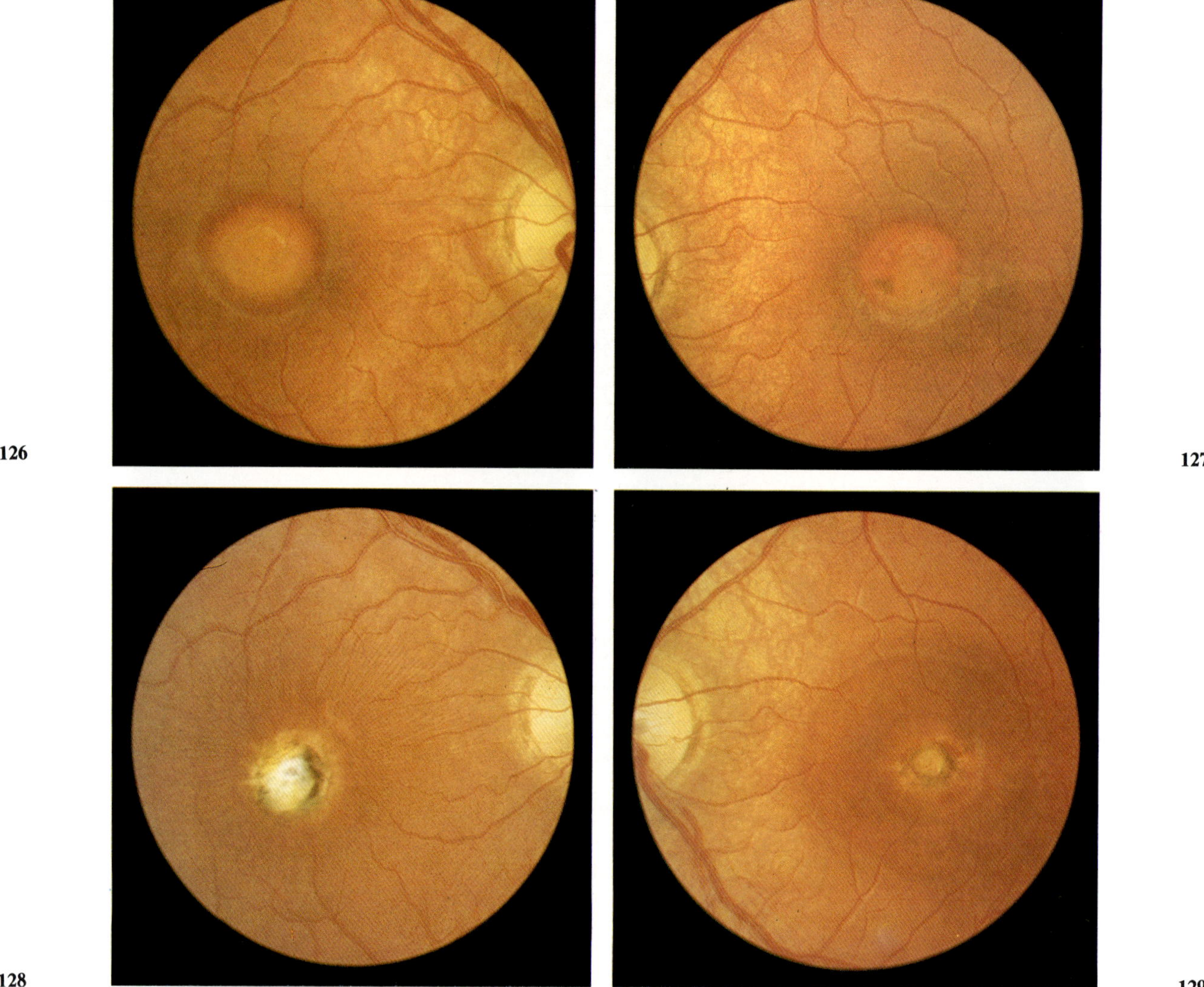

Figures 126–129. Right and left eyes of a 3-year-old male patient with Best's vitelliform dystrophy.

Clinical Findings

Refraction in both eyes was +1.75 sphere. Visual acuity in the right eye was 20/60 and in the left eye, 20/50, tested with the illiterate E chart. The patient showed an intermittent, turning divergent strabismus. The refractive media were clear and color vision was not affected. The anterior segment was normal. This disease did not appear in the family history of this patient. The father was emmetropic and the mother was myopic (−12.5 sphere). Figures 126 and 127 illustrate the characteristic "egg yolk" appearance of this normally hereditary disease. The disease progresses as these cysts rupture and scar to the end stage of pigmented chorioretinal atrophy, as illustrated in Figures 128 and 129.

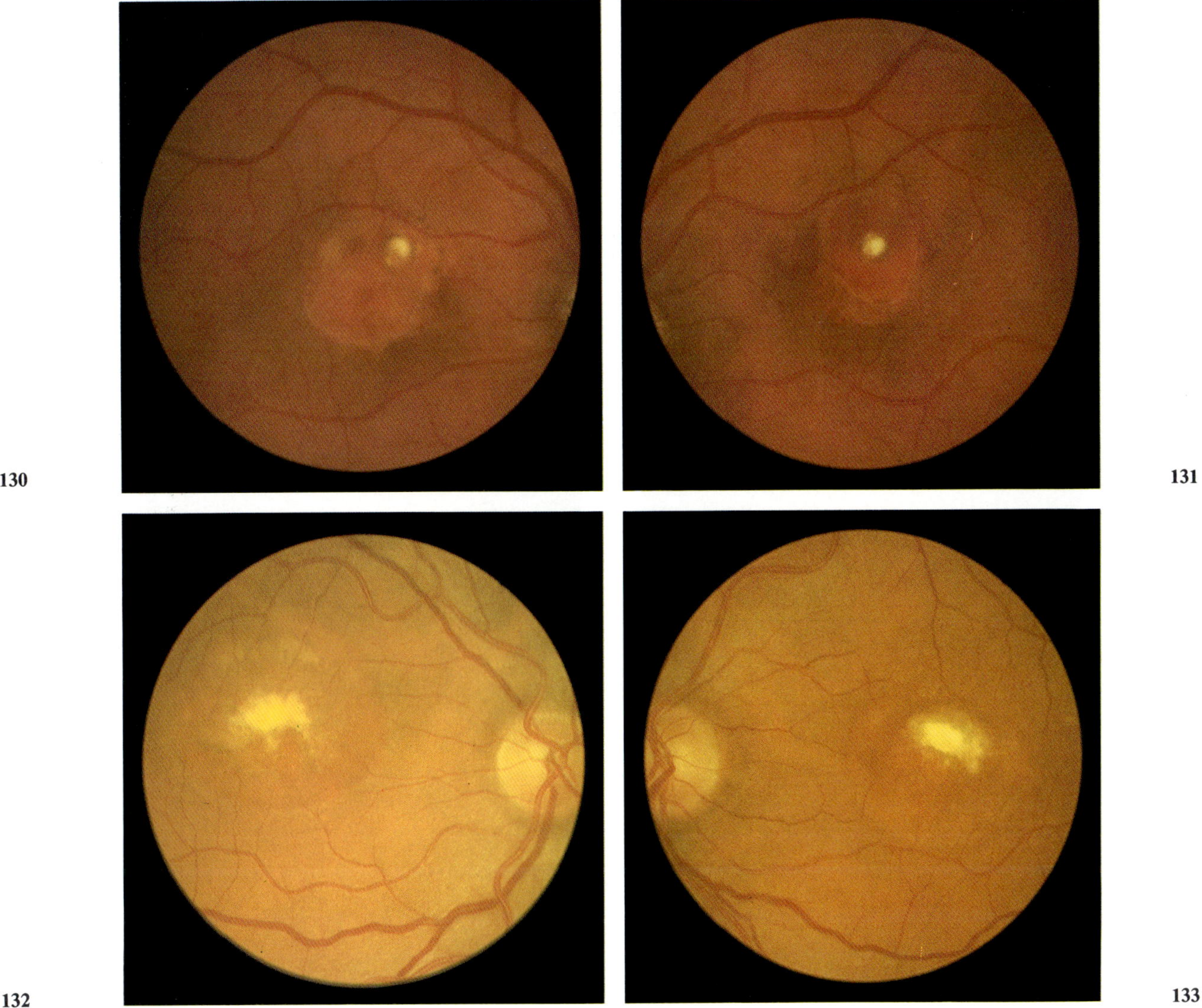

130 131

132 133

Figures 130 and 131. Right and left eye of a 16-year-old male patient with Best's vitelliform dystrophy.

Clinical Findings

Both eyes were emmetropic with visual acuity of 20/20. The refractive media and visual fields were normal and mesopic vision was intact. No distortion in dark adaptation and color vision were noted. Both maculas show the typical lesion of the disease. The patient's mother also had this disease. She presented with a bilateral disciform lesion (Huismann, 1977a).

Figures 132 and 133. Right and left eye of a 42-year-old male patient with Best's vitelliform dystrophy.

Clinical Findings

Refraction in both eyes was +0.25 diopters sphere. Visual acuity in the right eye was 20/100 and in the left eye 20/200. The refractive media were clear. The visual fields showed a central 5° scotoma in both eyes. The mesopic vision was distorted, but color vision was normal. The fundi showed a symmetric lesion resembling the "scrambled egg" stage of Best's vitelliform dystrophy. Prior to this examination, the lesions had been misdiagnosed as tuberculosis.

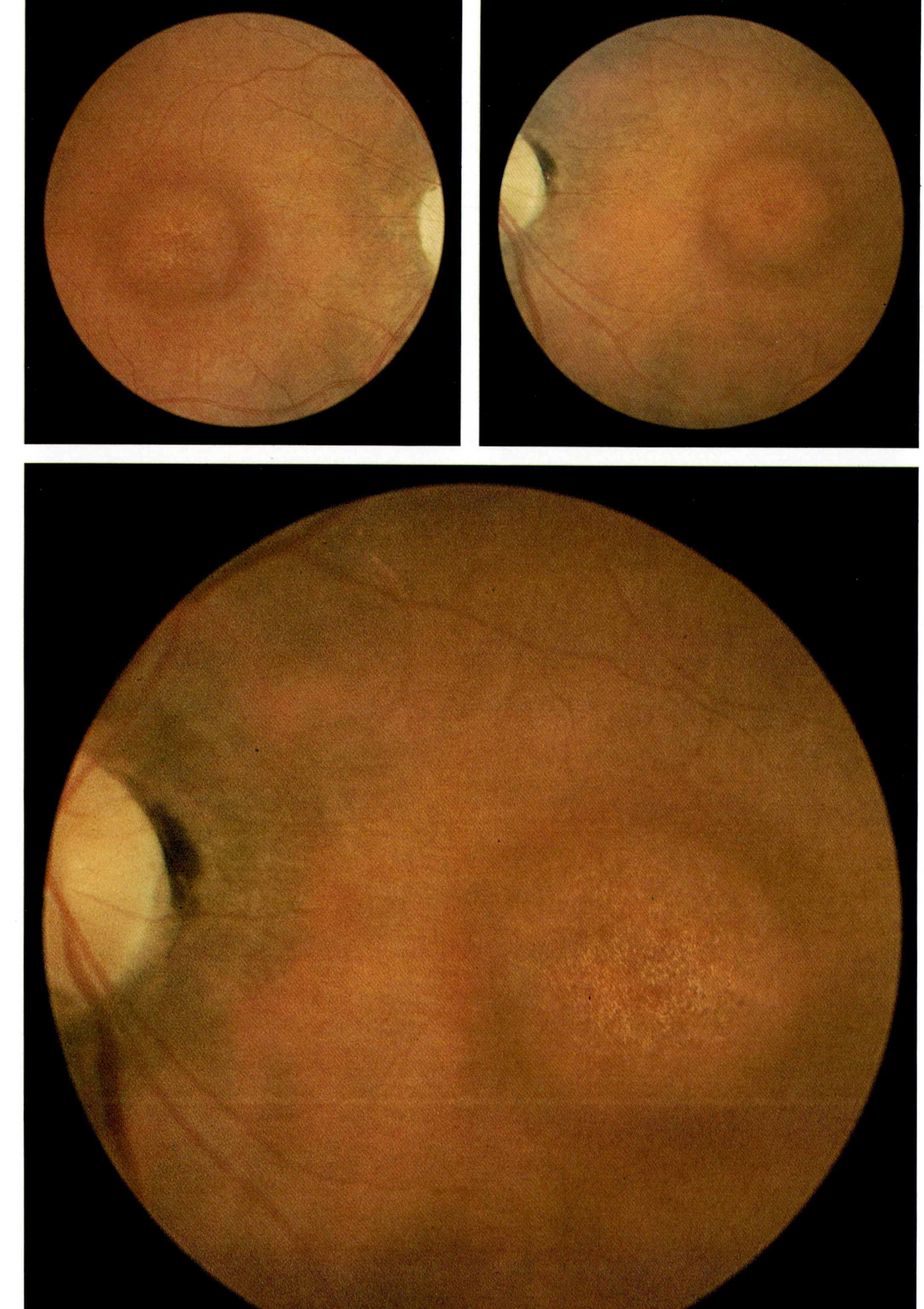

134

135

136

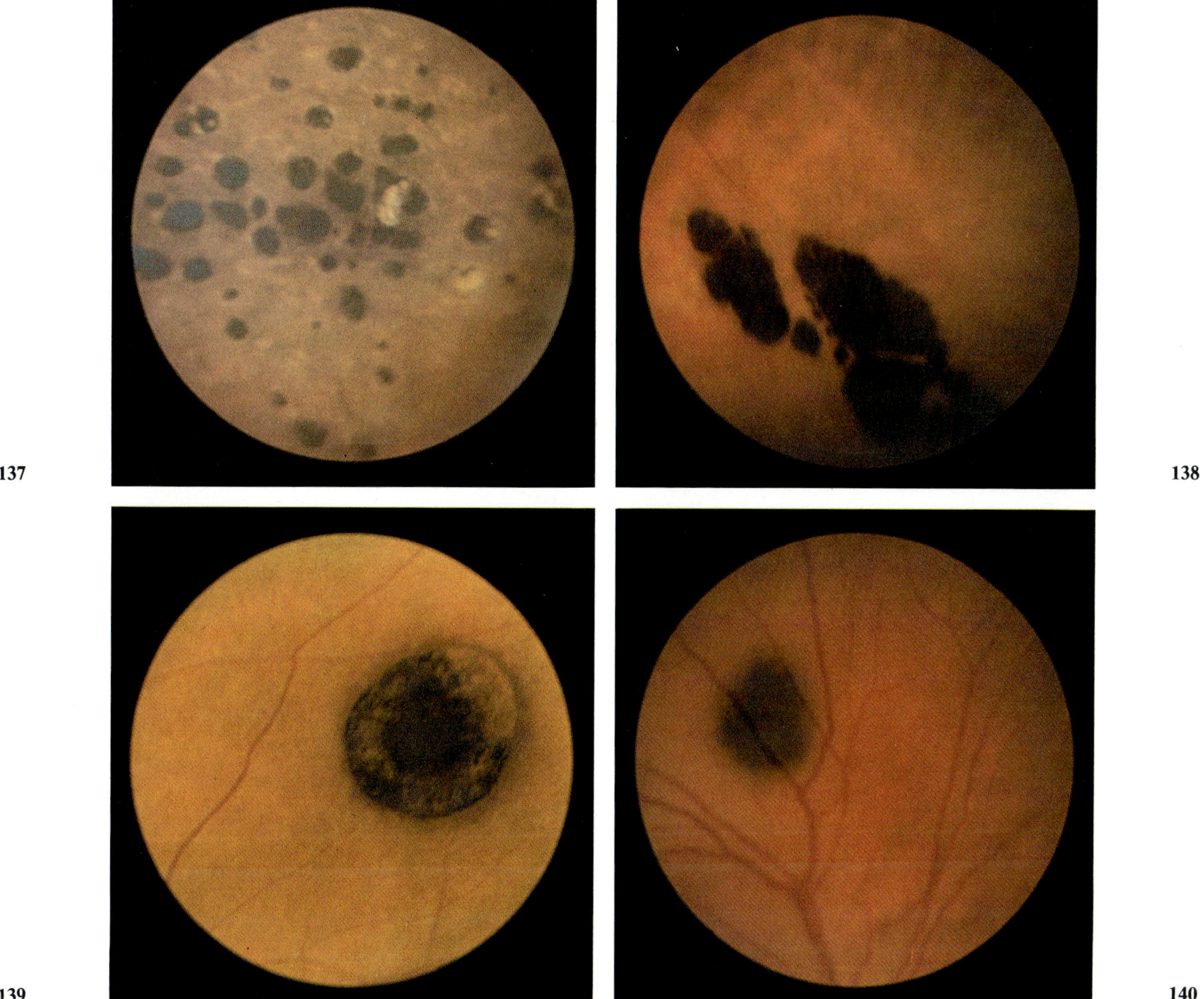

Figures 134–136. Right and left eyes of a 14-year-old female patient with Stargardt's disease.

Clinical Findings

With a correction of +1.5 sphere, −1.0 cylinder, axis 70°, visual acuity in the right eye was 20/200. With a correction of +1.0 sphere, −0.75 cylinder, axis 155°, visual acuity in the left eye was 20/100. There was a bilateral central scotoma with normal visual field margins, and mesopic vision was affected. There was a deuter anomaly. The family history could not be explored. Intoxications that could cause the macular changes were ruled out. Figure 136 shows the left eye 2 years later.

Figure 137. Left eye of an 18-year-old male patient with nevi and grouped nevoid pigmentation of the retina. The patient also suffered from a debilitating disease.

Clinical Findings

The refraction in this eye was −2.0 sphere, −2.25 cylinder, axis 0°. The refractive media were clear.

Figure 138. Left eye of a 20-year-old male patient with nevi and grouped nevoid pigmentation of the retina.

Clinical Findings

The eye was emmetropic. Visual acuity was 20/20 and the refractive media were clear.

Figure 139. Left eye of a 40-year-old male patient with hyperplasia of the retinal pigment epithelium.

Clinical Findings

The eye was hyperopic (+1.0 diopters sphere). With correction, visual acuity of 20/20 could be achieved. The refractive media were clear.

Figure 140. Right eye of a 52-year-old male patient with a choroidal nevus.

Clinical Findings

The refraction was +0.75 sphere. Visual acuity in both eyes was 20/20 and the refractive media were clear.

Clinical Course

The lesion did not show any changes over a period of 8 years.

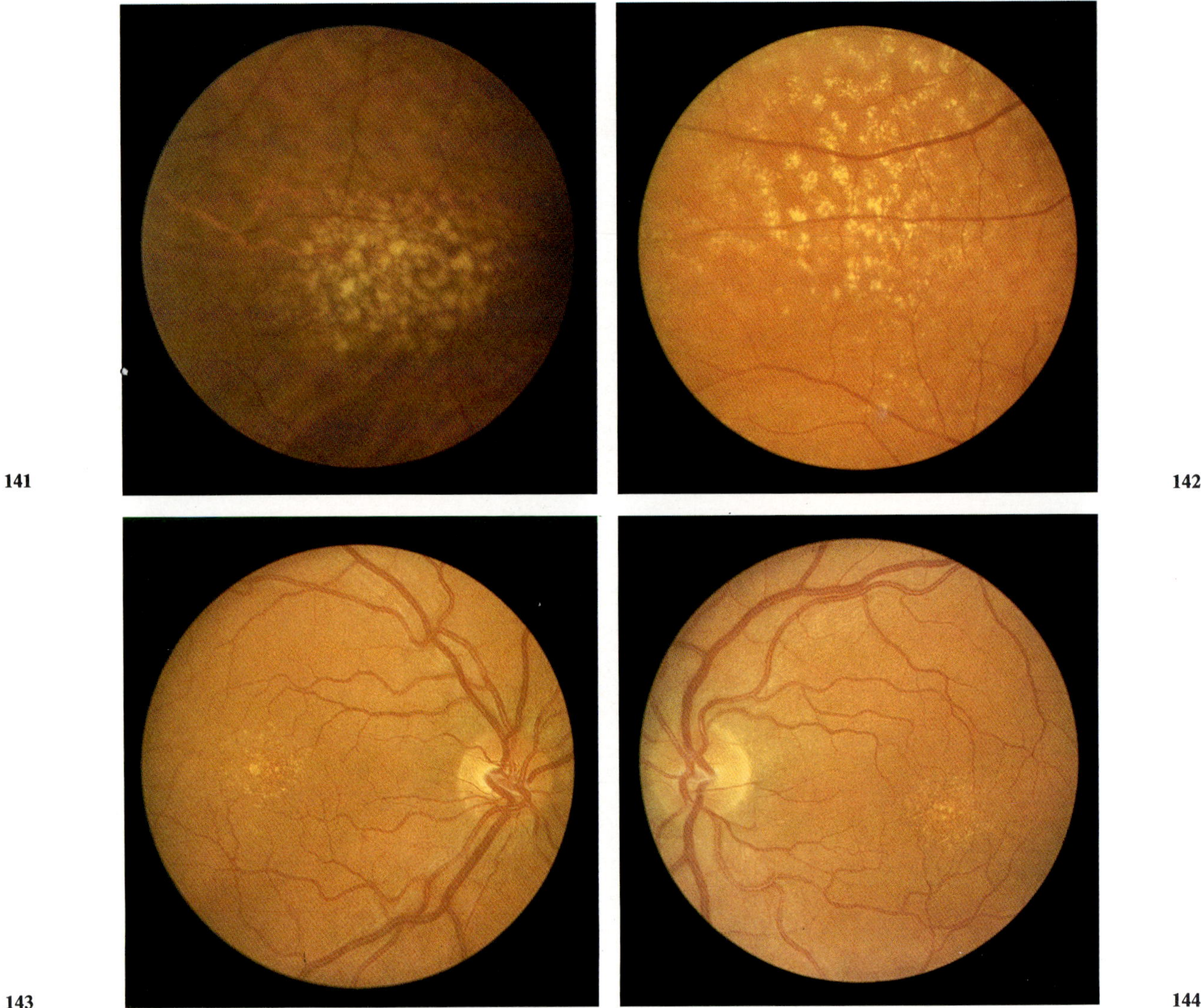

Figure 141. Right eye of a 53-year-old male patient with drusen of Bruch's membrane.

Clinical Findings

The refraction in the right eye was −1.0 cylinder, axis 5°, and in the left eye +0.25 sphere, −1.0 cylinder, axis 175°. Visual acuity in both eyes was 20/25, and the refractive media were clear. Visual fields and mesopic vision were normal.

Figure 142. Right eye of a 48-year-old male patient with bilaterial drusen of Bruch's membrane.

Clinical Findings

The eyes were emmetropic. Visual acuity was 20/20 and the refractive media were normal. Visual fields, color vision, and dark adaptation were normal.

Figures 143 and 144. Right and left eyes of a 38-year-old male patient with drusen of Bruch's membrane.

Clinical Findings

Refraction in the right was +0.25 sphere and in the left eye +0.75 sphere. Visual acuity in the right eye was 20/20 and in the left eye 20/25. Refractive media were clear. Visual fields and color vision were normal. Amsler's test revealed a central metamorphopsia. Mesopic vision was normal and dark adaptation was not affected. The family history could not be explored due to reduced patient compliance. Neither an EOG nor an ERG could be performed. Differential diagnoses include fundus albipunctatus and retinitis punctata albescens (progressive albipunctate dystrophy).

Clinical Course

The macular lesions did not show any progression over a period of 10 years.

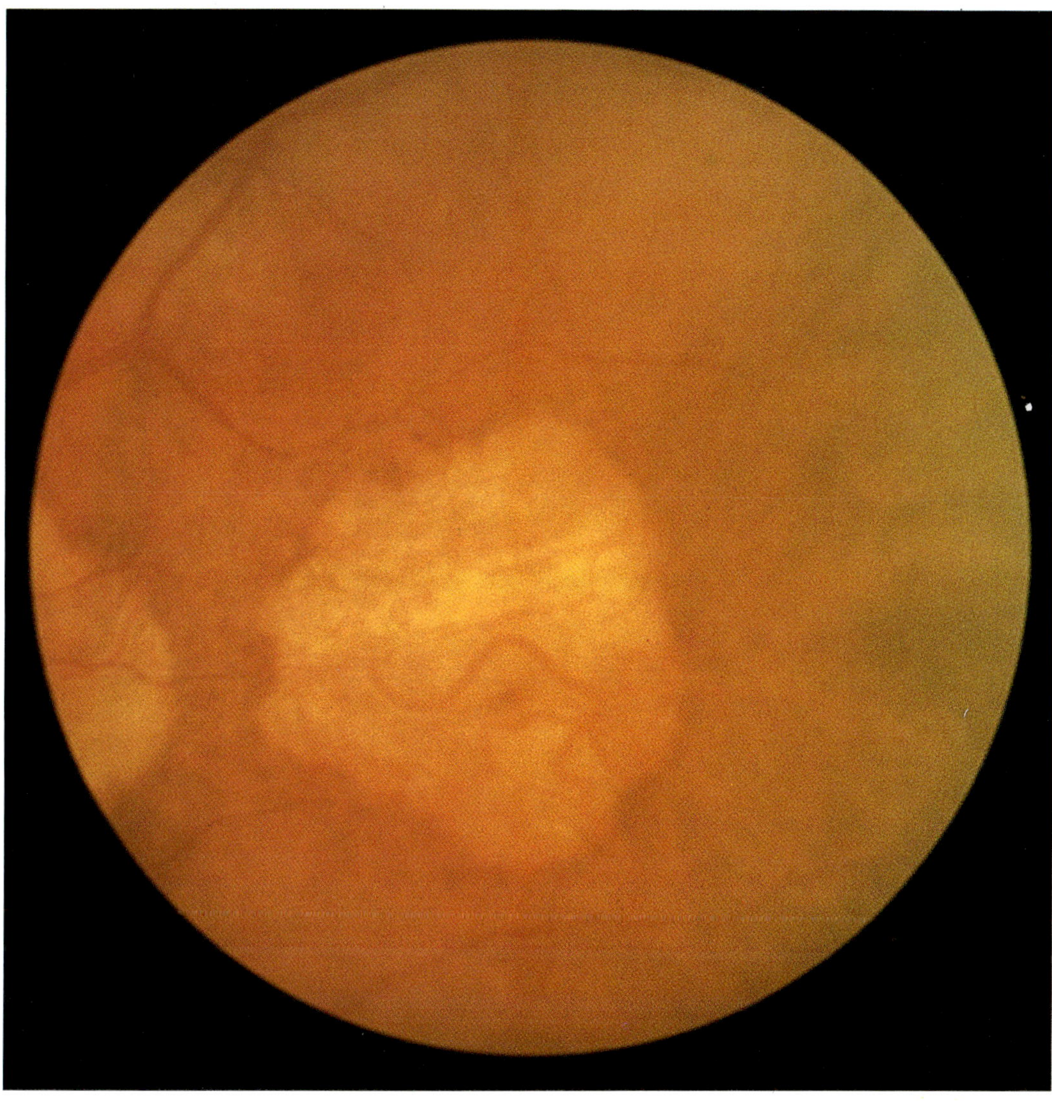

145

Figure 145. Left eye of a 70 year old male patient with bilaterial central choroidal atrophy.

Clinical Findings

The refraction in both eyes was −3.25 sphere. Visual acuity was 20/700. The patient had a subcapsular posterior cortical cataract. Intraocular pressure in both eyes was 16 mm Hg. Visual field testing showed a central scotoma in both eyes with normal outer margins. Mesopic vision was affected. Color vision could not be evaluated.

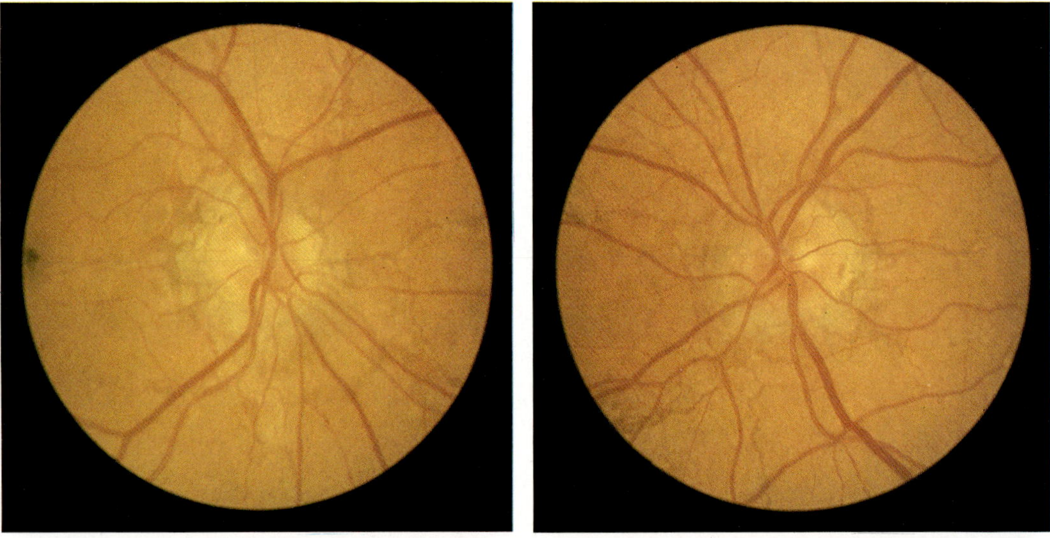

146

147

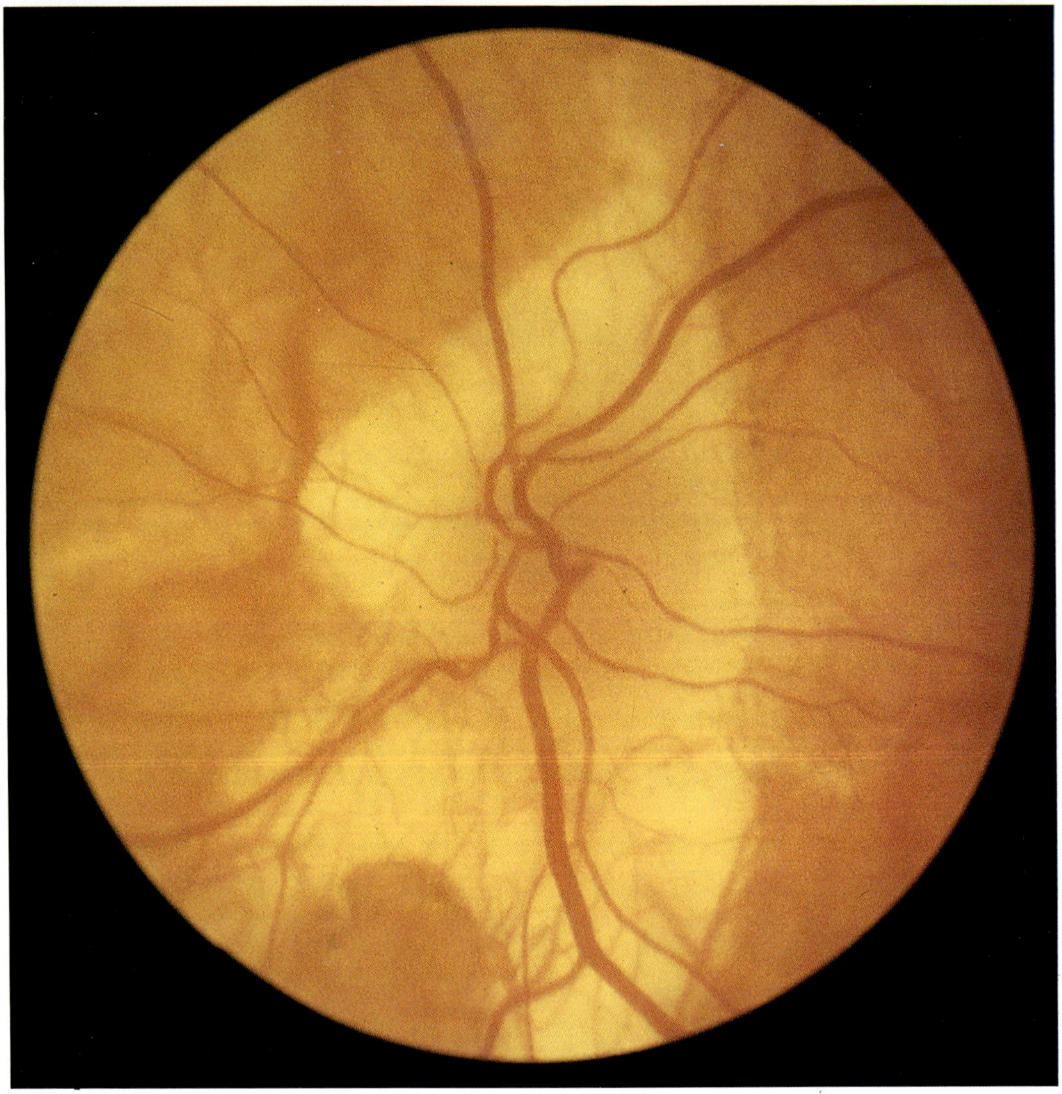

148

149 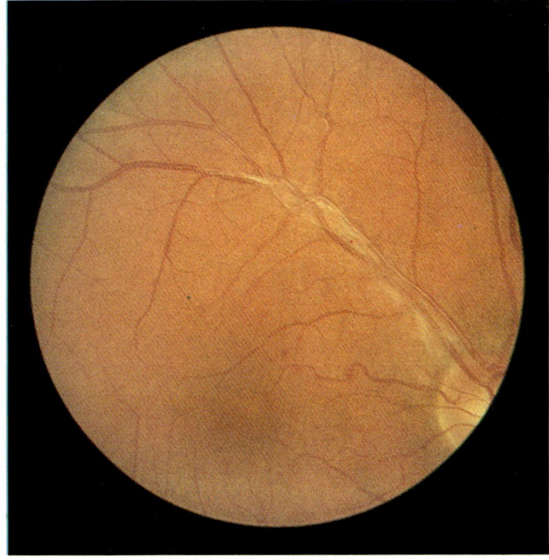

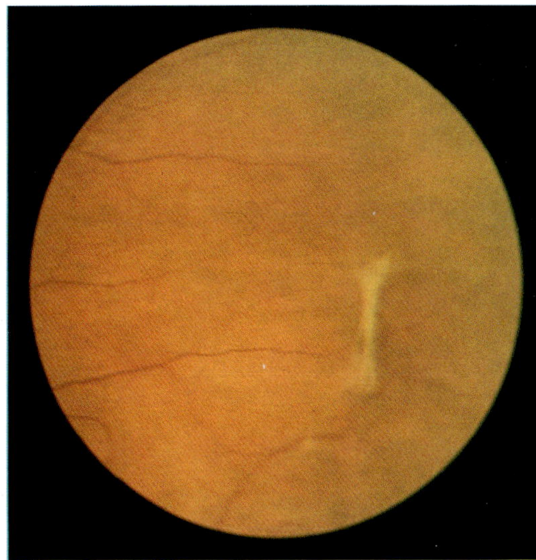 150

Figures 146 and 147. Right and left eyes of a 50-year-old male patient with angioid streaks and age-related macular degeneration in the right eye.

Clinical Findings

Both eyes were hyperopic with a refraction of +2.50 sphere. Visual acuity in the right eye was 20/25, and 20/100 in the left eye. Intraocular pressure in both eyes was 14 mm Hg, and visual fields were normal. Slitlamp examination did not reveal any abnormal findings. A yellow to red-brown peripapillary ring-shaped structure can be seen in the left fundus that mimics retinal vessels. Radial red-brown structures originating from this ring and extending toward the periphery are also visible. These structures do not follow the normal course of retinal vessels, and even cross such vessels at some sites. The right eye (Fig. 146) shows angioid streaks that are most prominent temporally, close to the papillary margin. The macular region shows pigment irregularities.

Figure 148. Right eye of a 72-year-old female patient with serpiginous chorioretinitis.

Clinical Findings

The refractive error in the right eye was +2.5 sphere, −0.5 cylinder, axis 90°, and in the left eye, +2.0 sphere. Visual acuity acuity in both eyes was 20/30. Refractive media were clear with normal visual fields. Mesopic vision was distorted, but color vision was normal. Fundus examination revealed a vital optic disc with blurred margins. There are peripapillary wing-shaped areas of chorioretinal atrophy that extend from the disc peripherally. These white areas do not follow the normal retinal vascular branching pattern. The left eye showed less characteristic findings and could have easily been mistaken for an atypical peripapillary atrophic crescent.

Figure 149. Right eye of a 39-year-old female patient with the proliferative form of Eales' disease.

Clinical Findings

With a correction of −0.75 sphere, −0.5 cylinder, axis 0°, visual acuity of 20/20 could be obtained. Refractive media were clear. Intraocular pressure was 14 mm Hg, and no visual field defects were present. The fundus shows white-gray veil-like ensheathing of the superotemporal vein and its side branches. These abnormalities were first seen during a routine examination. Note the presence of a small punctate hemorrhage superonasal to the macular region.

Serological Findings

Toxoplasmosis, complement fixation titer 1:5, indirect fluorescent antibody (IFA test) titer 1:128. Syphylis, *Treponema pallidum* hemagluttination test negative, cardiolipin flocculation test negative. Listeriosis, complement fixation test H titer 1:400, Gruber-Widal reaction titer 1:400. Rheumatoid factor negative. A neurologic consultation ruled out any indication for multiple sclerosis. ENT and internal examinations were unremarkable.

Clinical Course

The fundus changes in this patient remained stationary for 1 year with a regimen of sulfamethoxazole and pyrimethamine.

Figure 150. Right eye of a 41-year-old male patient with the proliferative form of Eales' disease.

Clinical Findings

Visual acuity was 20/20 and refractive media were clear. Intraocular pressure was 16 mm Hg, and there were no visual changes.

Clinical Course

The patient remained without any complications for 2 years following light coagulation of the proliferative lesion.

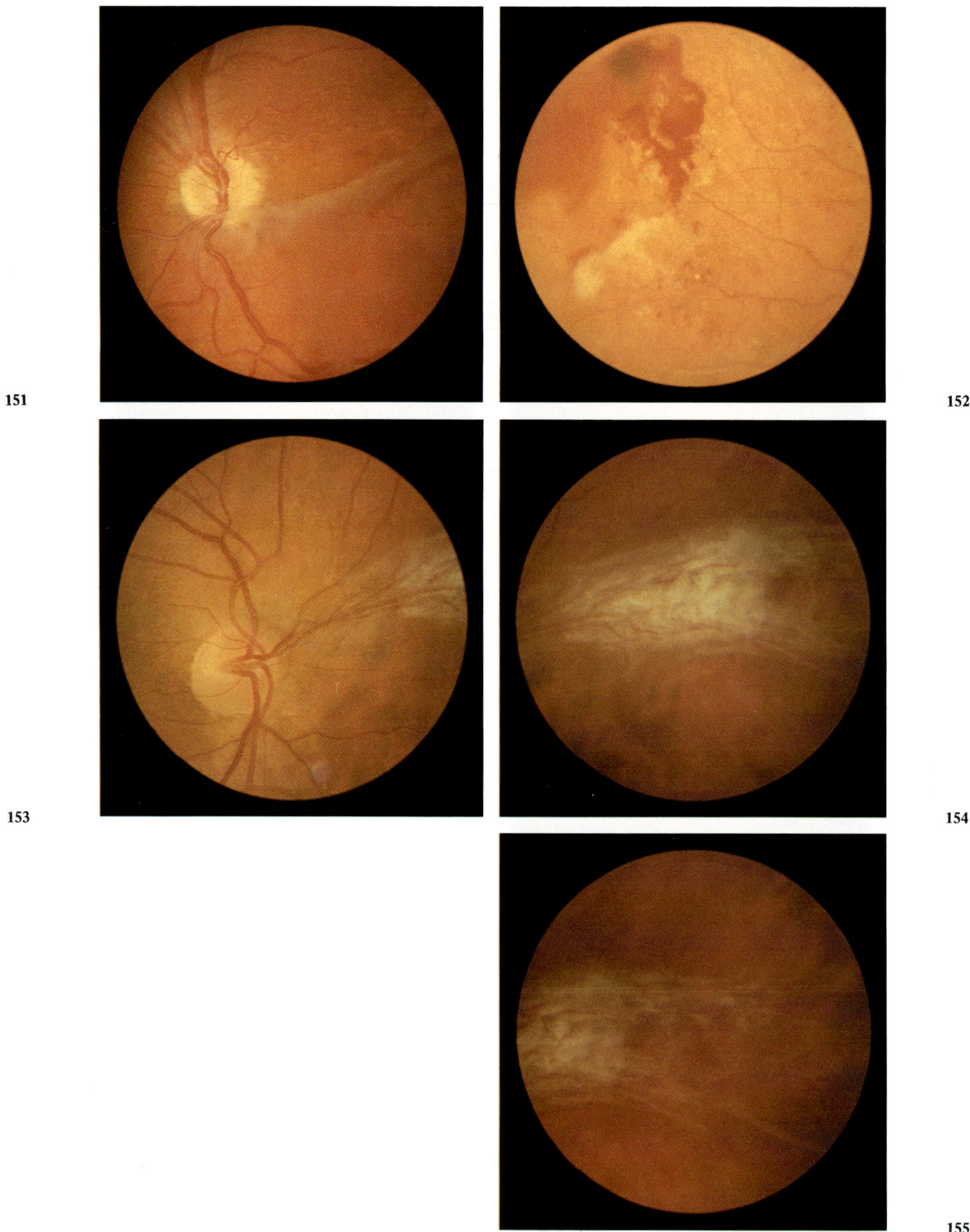

151

152

153

154

155

156 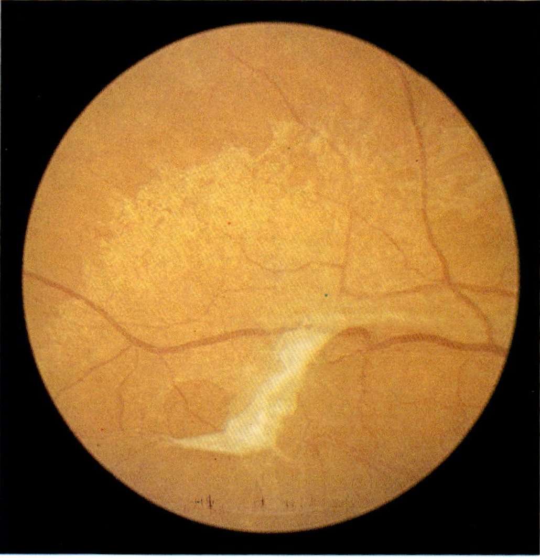

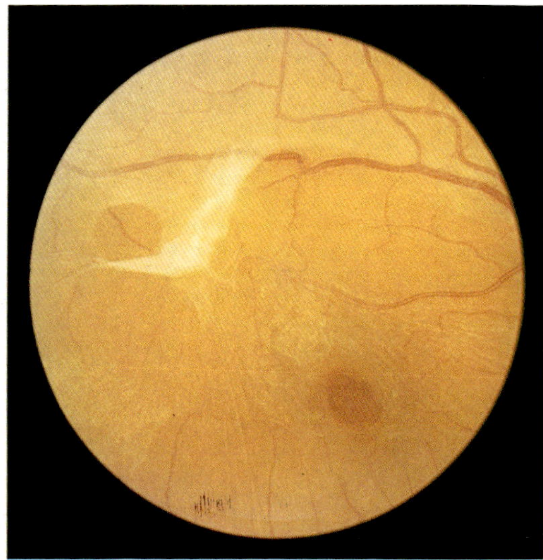 157

Figure 151. Left eye of a 7-year-old male patient with the proliferative form of Eales' disease. Recurrent vitreous hemorrhages are present.

Clinical Findings

The eye was hyperopic (+3.5 sphere) and visual acuity was 20/400. Refractive media were clear, intraocular pressure was 14 mm Hg. There was a central scotoma. A fundus examination showed a proliferative membrane extending from the inferior vascular trunk and optic disc margin toward the macular region, covering large areas of the posterior pole. Extensive medical screening and laboratory testing revealed only normal findings.

Figure 152. Right eye of a 45-year-old female patient with the hemorrhagic form of Eales' disease.

Clinical Findings

The eye was emmetropic. Visual acuity in the phases between hemorrhages and prior to light coagulation was 20/25. Blood pressure was 140/85 mm Hg; blood sedimentation rate, 16/28 mm. Doppler sonography was unremarkable. An extensive medical workup, including a glucose tolerance test, blood cell count and blood coagulation parameters, and liver enzymes, cholesterol, and triglycerides were all normal.

Clinical Course

Following light coagulation, no more hemorrhages occurred during an observation period of 4 years.

Figure 153–155. Right eye of a 45-year-old female patient with proliferative retinopathy.

Clinical Findings

Visual acuity in the emmetropic eye was 20/25, and refractive media were clear. Intraocular pressure was 16 mm Hg, and the visual fields were normal. Blood pressure was 140/80 mm Hg, and sedimentation rate was 12/20 mm. There is an extensive proliferative membrane extending from an area centrally (at a distance of two disc diameters from the optic disc) along the superonasal vessels toward the midperiphery of the fundus (Figs. 154 and 155). There was no history of trauma or other ocular diseases. General screening and laboratory diagnostic tests were unremarkable.

Clinical Course

The patient refused to undergo any treatment.

Figures 156 and 157. Right eye of a 42-year-old female patient with proliferative retinopathy associated with Eales' disease. Supratemporal traction has caused a partial macular hole.

Clinical Findings

Visual acuity in the emmetropic eye was still 20/40, and refractive media were clear. Intraocular pressure was 14 mm Hg. There was a central scotoma. A proliferative sheath extending from the supratemporal vein caused tractional folds that extend into the macula leading to the secondary hole formation.

Clinical Course

Therapy initially consisted of regular checkups.

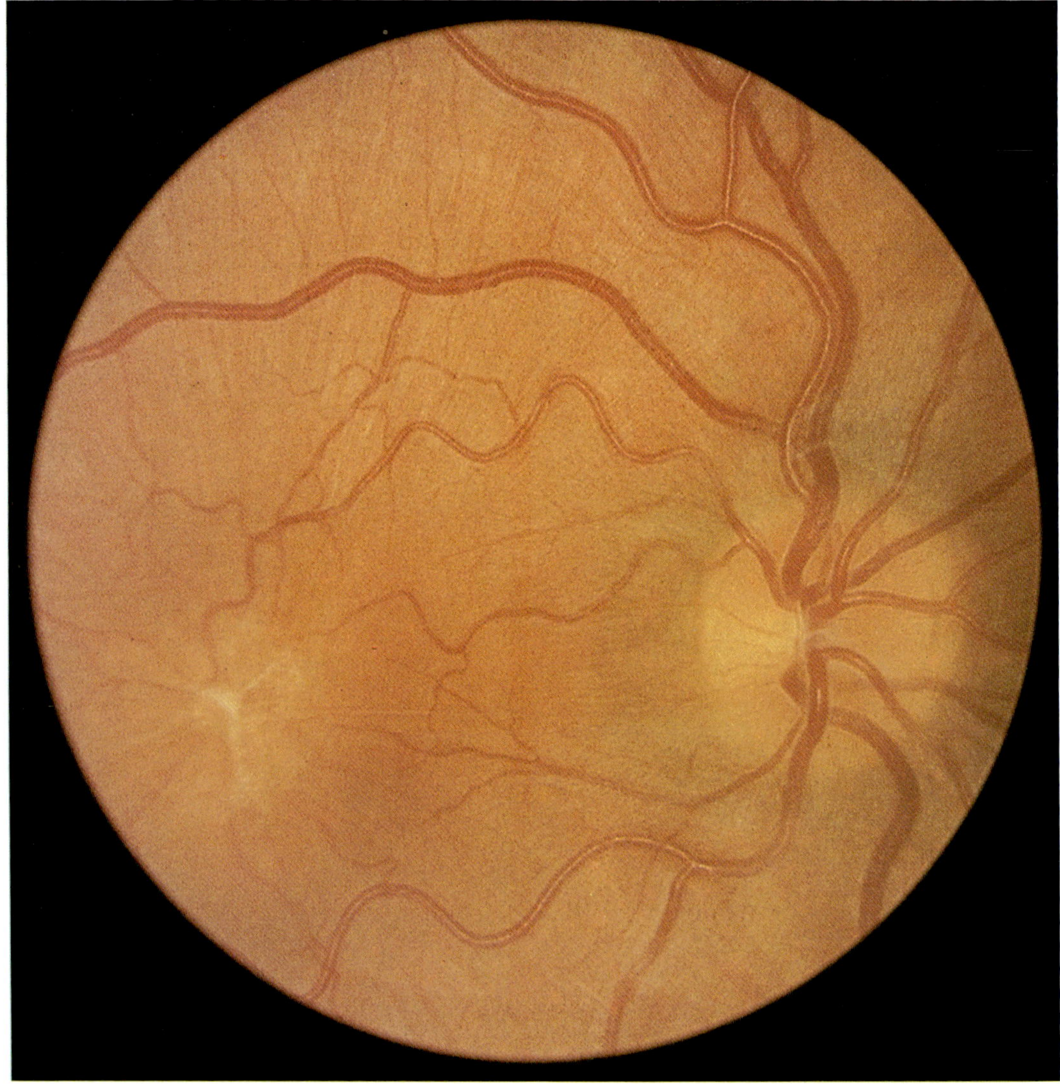

158

Figure 158. Right eye of a 5-year-old female patient with epiretinal membrane of the macular region. Rudimentary retrolental fibroplasia was ruled out because birth was normal in the 10th gestational month with a birth weight of 2920 gm and with no complications. No oxygen therapy was necessary.

Clinical Findings

Both eyes were hyperopic with +3.0 sphere as measured by objective refraction. Visual acuity in the right eye was 20/60, and 20/20 in the left eye. The optic disc is normal. The vessels show increased tortuosity in areas adjacent to the optic disc. There are vascular caliber irregularities. The veins are engorged and there are isolated microaneurysms. The epiretinal membrane has caused the macula to be ectopic with deviations of the vessels in the direction of the traction. Radial folds within the macular region are easily visible.

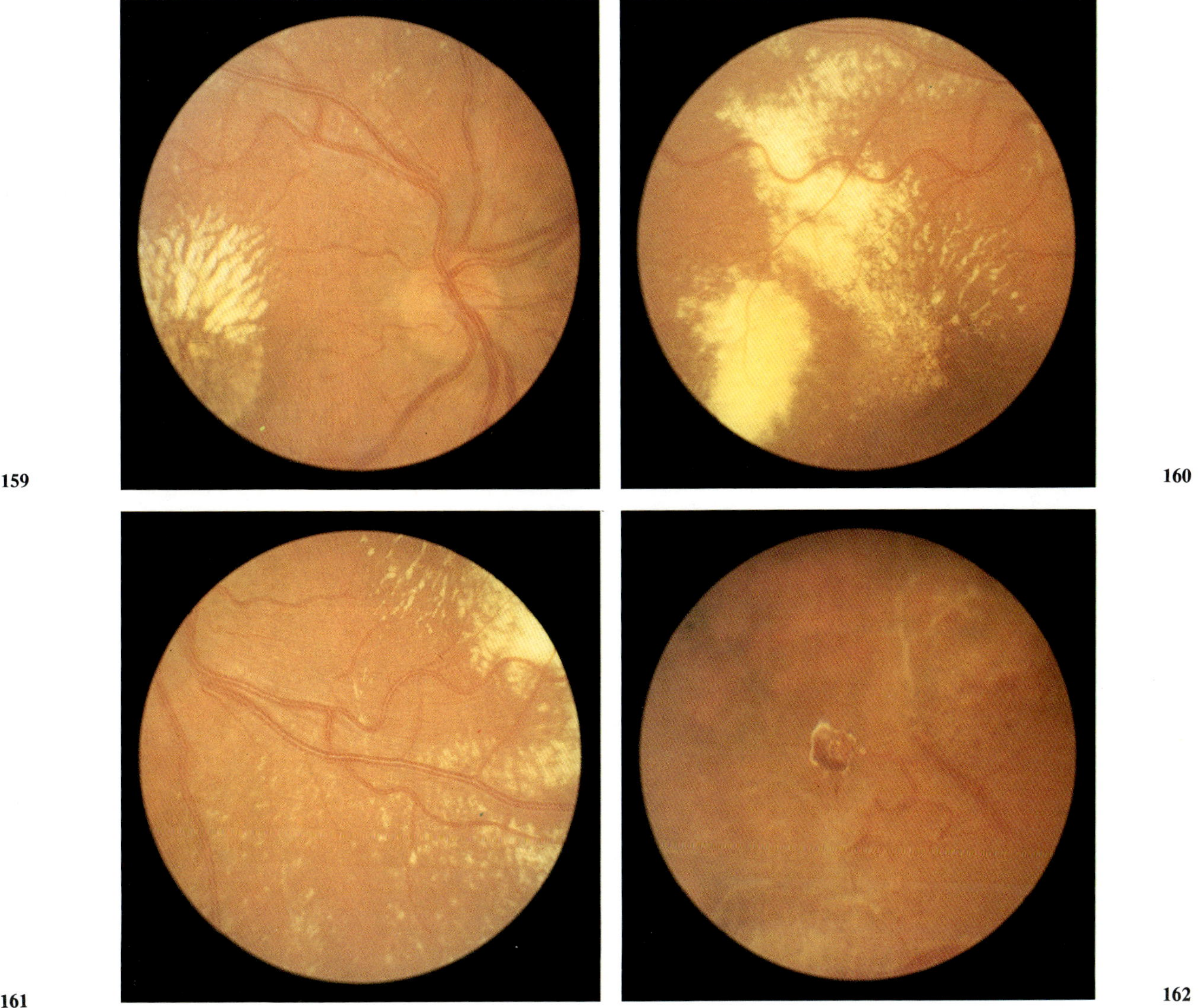

159 160

161 162

Figures 159-162. Right eye of a 6-year-old male patient with Coats' disease.

Clinical Findings

With a correction of +4.25 sphere, −2.0 cylinder, axis 0°, visual acuity in the right eye was 20/1000. With a correction of −0.5 cylinder, axis 0°, visual acuity in the left eye was 20/20. Refractive media were clear.

Laboratory Findings

Erythrocytes 4.9 million, leukocytes 6000, platelets 220,000, blood sedimentation rate 3/10 mm, eosinophils 4, basophils 8, monocytes 2. Electrolytes and a serum electrophoresis were normal. Alkaline phosphatase 304 units/liter, triglycerides 44 mg/100 ml, total cholesterol 142 mm/100 ml, 17-hydroxycorticosteroids 1/39 mg/24 hours excretion in the urine.

Serologic Findings

Toxoplasmosis dye test (Sabin-Feldman dye test) titer 1:64; complement fixation titer 1:5 (when repeated later, there was no titer elevation); rheumatoid factor test negative; anti-streptolysin titer 320 E/ml. Mononucleosis and Epstein-Barr virus tests were IgM negative; an immune fluorescence test for IgF titers was 1:16.

Therapy

The underlying symptoms were treated with supplements.

Clinical Course

The macular star figure (Figs. 159-161) improved, and lipid exudations resolved over a period of 6 weeks. Visual acuity improved to 20/700. The patient refused to undergo light coagulation therapy. (Figure 161 is inverted.)

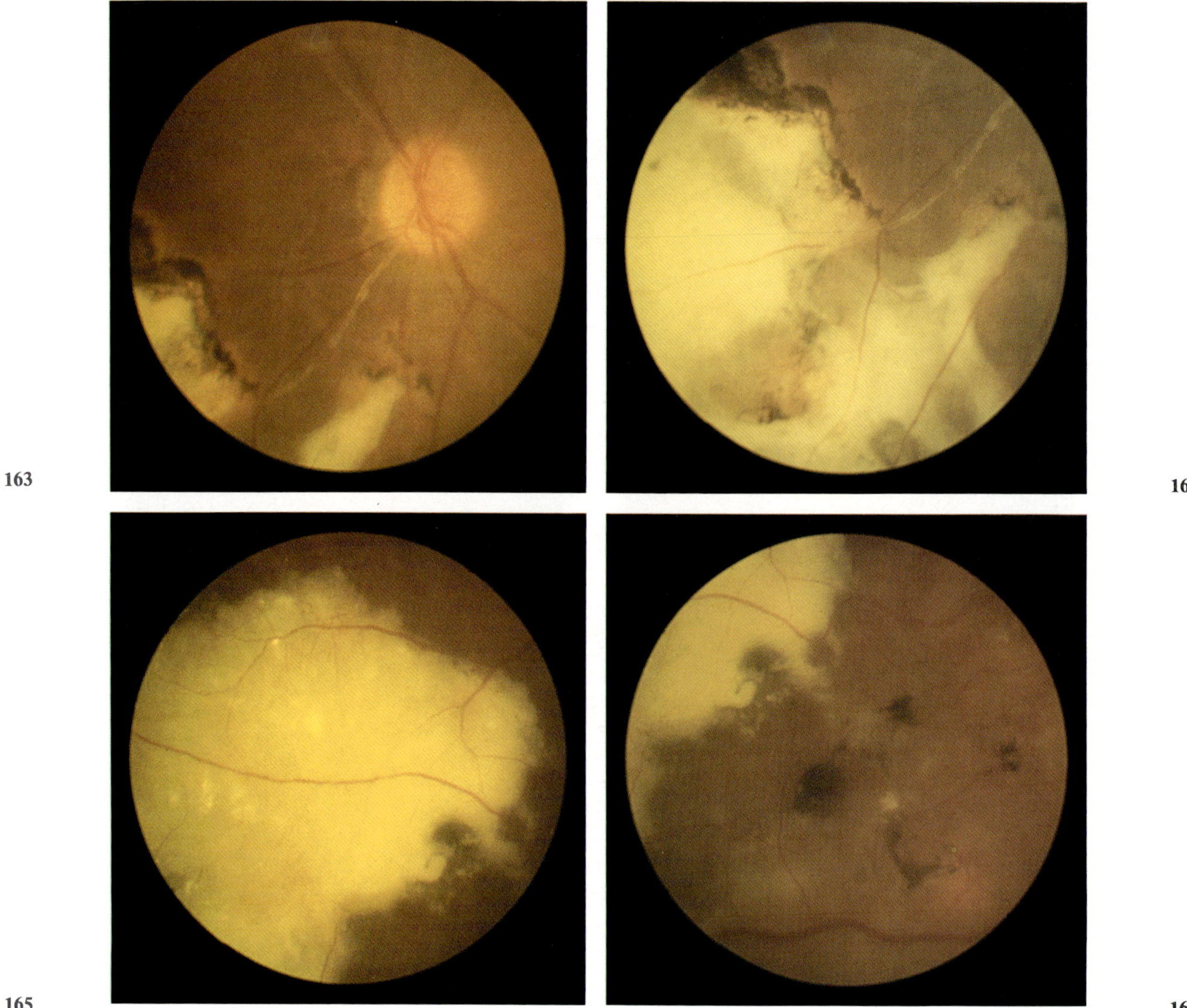

Figures 163–166. Left eye of a 49-year-old female patient with Coats' disease.

Clinical Findings

Both eyes were hyperopic with a refractive error of +2.75 sphere. Visual acuity in the right eye was 20/20, and 20/400 in the left eye. Refractive media were clear, and intraocular pressure was 14 mm Hg. Visual field testings showed a central scotoma and concentric constrictions of the outer margins, leaving a residual temporal visual field remnant. Blood pressure was 165/80 mm Hg, and sedimentation rate was 28/43 mm.

Laboratory Findings

Erythrocytes 4.27 million, leukocytes 6800, differential blood cells counts were normal, serum cholesterol was 543 mg/100 ml, triglycerides were 150 mg/100 ml. Note the extensive areas of white retinal exudation in the fundus that mask large portions of the retina.

Figures 167 and 168. Right eye of a 30-year-old female patient with hypopyon neuritis (Fig. 167).

Clinical Findings

The cardinal ocular finding of hypopyon neuritis confirmed a diagnosis of Behçet's disease in association with other ocular and skin symptoms. The patient suffered from recurrent iritis, and at a later stage, recurrent retinal periphlebitis. Figure 168 shows the fundus of the amaurotic right eye with complete optic atrophy, which was the final outcome of the disease in this patient.

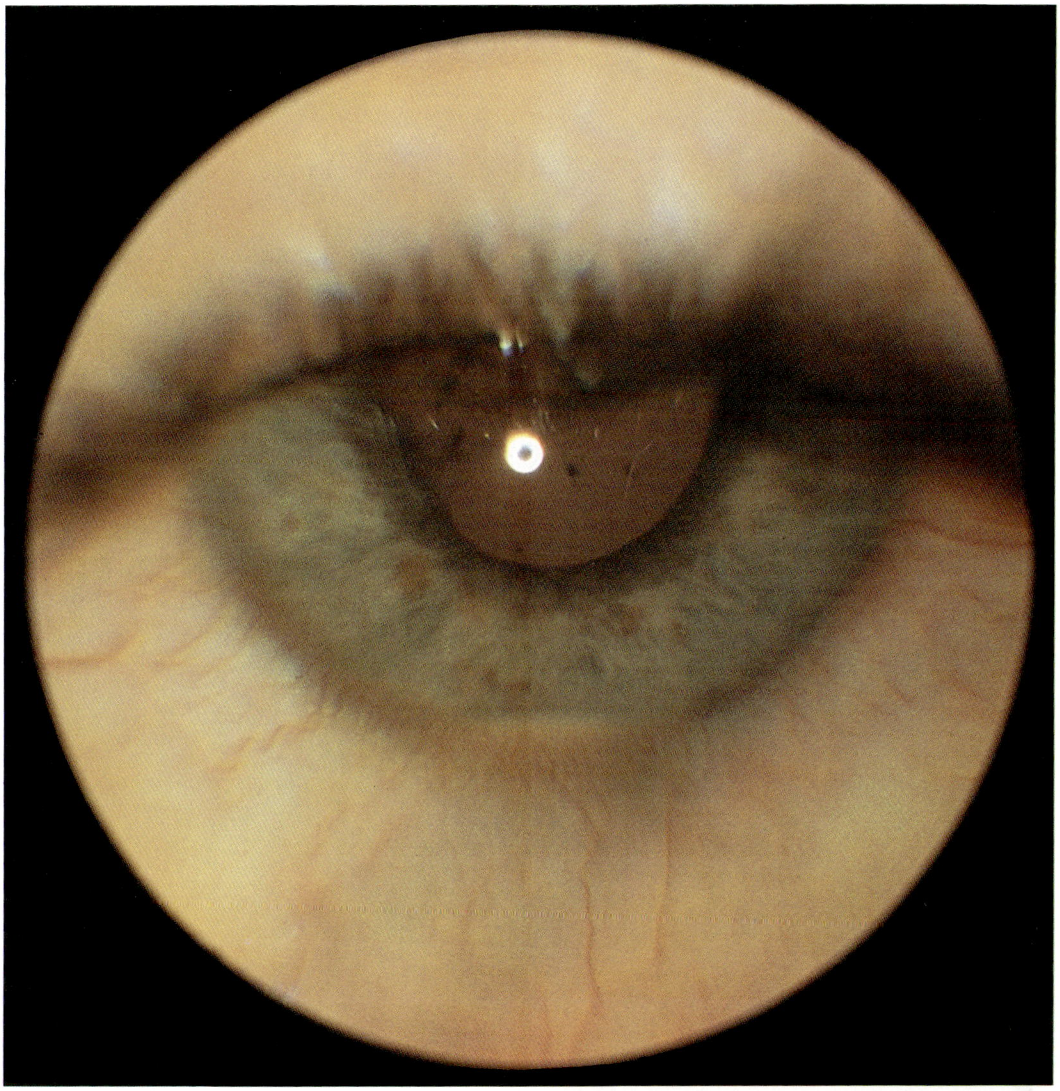

167

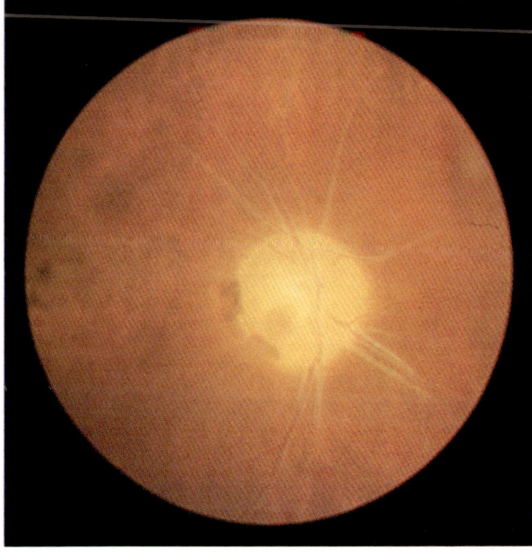

168

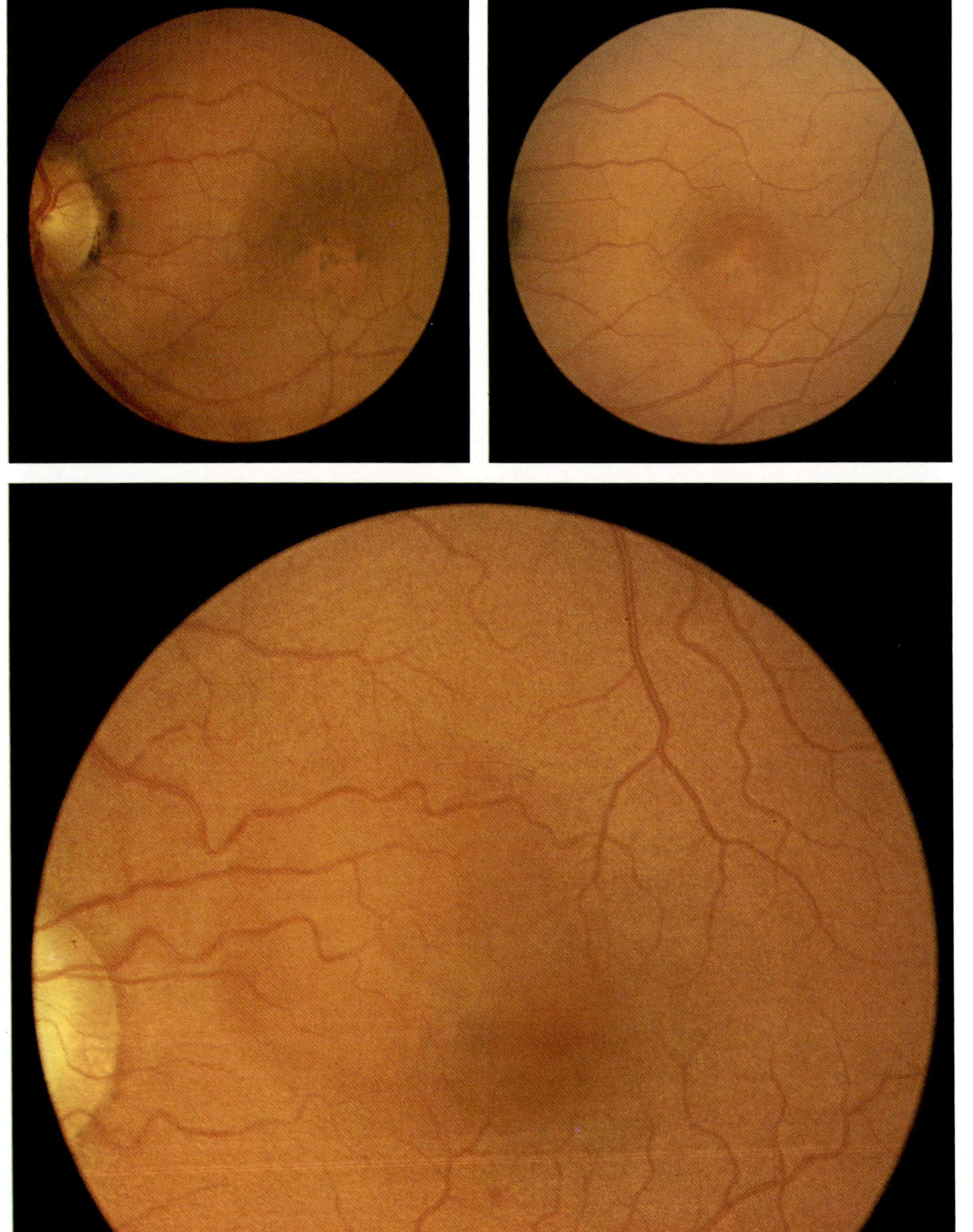

169

170

171

172

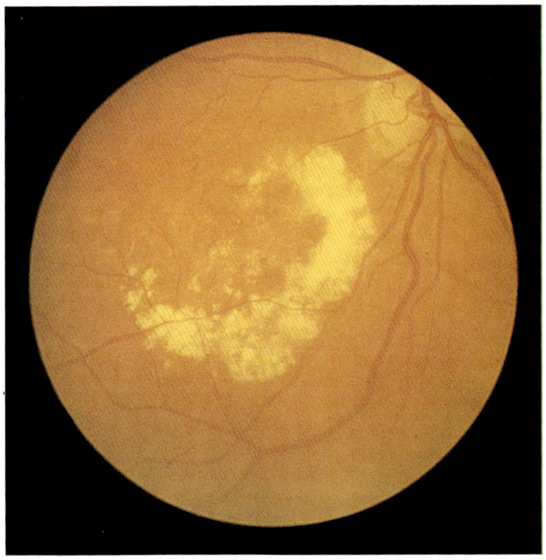

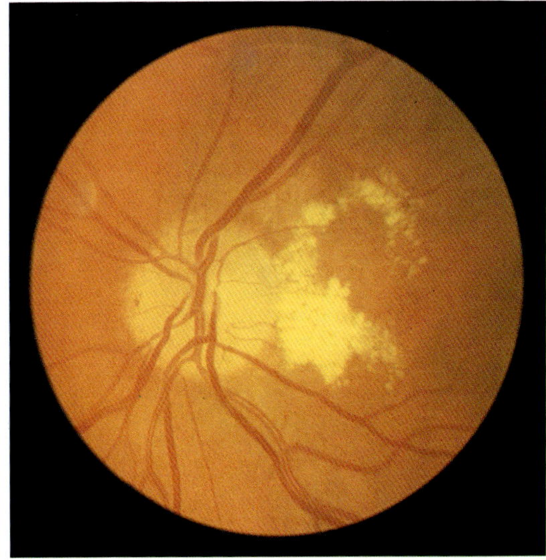

173

Figures 169 and 170. Left eye of a 35-year-old male patient with central serous chorioretinopathy.

Clinical Findings

Visual acuity in the right eye was 20/20, and 20/200 in the left eye. Refractive media were clear, and intraocular pressure in both eyes was 16 mm Hg. The central visual field, as evaluated by the Amsler chart, showed a central scotoma. The peripheral visual field was normal. Figure 170 shows the eye 6 weeks after the onset of central serous chorioretinopathy. Slitlamp examination revealed normal anterior segment with no cell or flare. There is macular edema in the fundus (Fig. 169) with irregularly shaped pigment deposits, especially underlying the serous exudation. The remaining fundus is unremarkable.

Therapy

The patient was treated with localized radiation therapy.

Clinical Course

The central serous chorioretinopathy disappeared 12 weeks after the onset of the first symptoms. Visual acuity recovered to 20/20.

Figure 171. Left eye of a 32-year-old male patient with central serous chorioretinopathy.

Clinical Findings

Visual acuity in the right eye was 20/20. Visual acuity in the left eye with a correction of −0.75 cylinder, axis 145°, was 20/50. By adding +1.0 sphere to this correction, visual acuity could be improved to 20/25. Visual field testing showed a relative central scotoma and normal outer margins. The central scotoma was confirmed using an Amsler chart. Intraocular pressure in the right eye was 14 mm Hg, and in the left eye was 16 mm Hg. Metamorphopsia was present. Slitlamp examination was unremarkable. Fundus examination shows elevated macular edema that measured 2 optic disc diameters and extended between the optic disc and macular region. A small punctate hemorrhage is present inferiorly.

Therapy

The patient was treated with localized radiation therapy.

Clinical Course

The lesion resolved within 6 weeks.

Figure 172. Right eye of a 60-year-old female patient with circinate retinopathy.

Clinical Findings

Visual acuity in this eye was 20/200. Visual field testing revealed the presence of a central scotoma with an incomplete paracentral ring scotoma. Ophthalmoscopically, the fundus showed the typical circinate pattern of lipid deposition in the retina. Note the garland-shaped, irregular lesion that partially encircles the macular area inferiorly. The macula shows signs of cystic degeneration.

Figure 173. Left eye of a 58-year-old female patient with circinate retinopathy.

Clinical Findings

Visual acuity was 20/30, and visual field testing showed an incomplete paracentral ring scotoma. Ophthalmoscopically, the circinate lipid deposition extends from an area immediately adjacent to the optic disc in a horseshoe-shaped pattern toward the macular area.

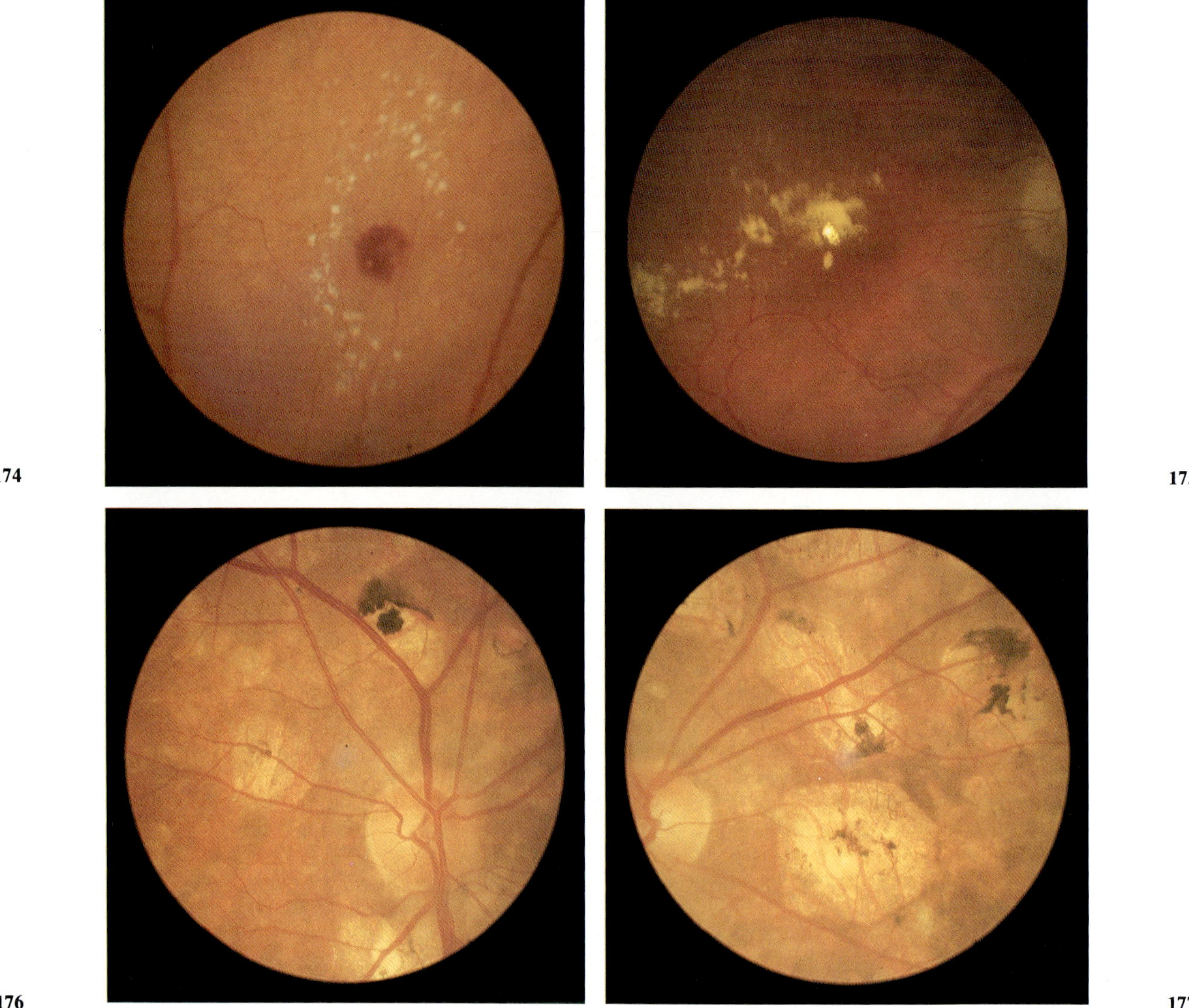

Figure 174. Right eye of a 75-year-old female patient with circinate retinopathy.

Clinical Findings

The patient had a history of diabetes and arterial hypertension. Visual acuity in this aphakic eye with correction was 20/25. Note the atypical location of the lipid deposits in a peripheral part of the retina surrounding a dot-shaped hemorrhage.

Figure 175. Right eye of a 65-year-old female patient with circinate retinopathy.

Clinical Findings

The patient had a history of arterial hypertension and hypercholesterolemia. Visual acuity in this eye was 20/25. Fundus examination revealed a circinate lipid deposit located inferior to the fovea. There are cholesterol crystals within the exudative material.

Figures 176 and 177. Right and left eyes of a 50-year-old female patient with retinal choroidal atrophy following disseminated choroiditis.

Clinical Findings

This patient had a history of tuberculosis of the bone, involving the right knee. With a refraction of 1.5 sphere, −0.5 cylinder, axis 90°, visual acuity in both eyes could be corrected to 20/30. Refractive media were clear in both eyes. No anterior or posterior synechiae were present. Gonioscopic findings were normal. Fundus examination revealed chorioretinal scars that exceed 1 optic disc diameter and differ slightly in size. The scarred areas partially accrue and show irregular, clumped pigmentations. The retinal vessels, which are not affected, cross the chorioretinal lesions.

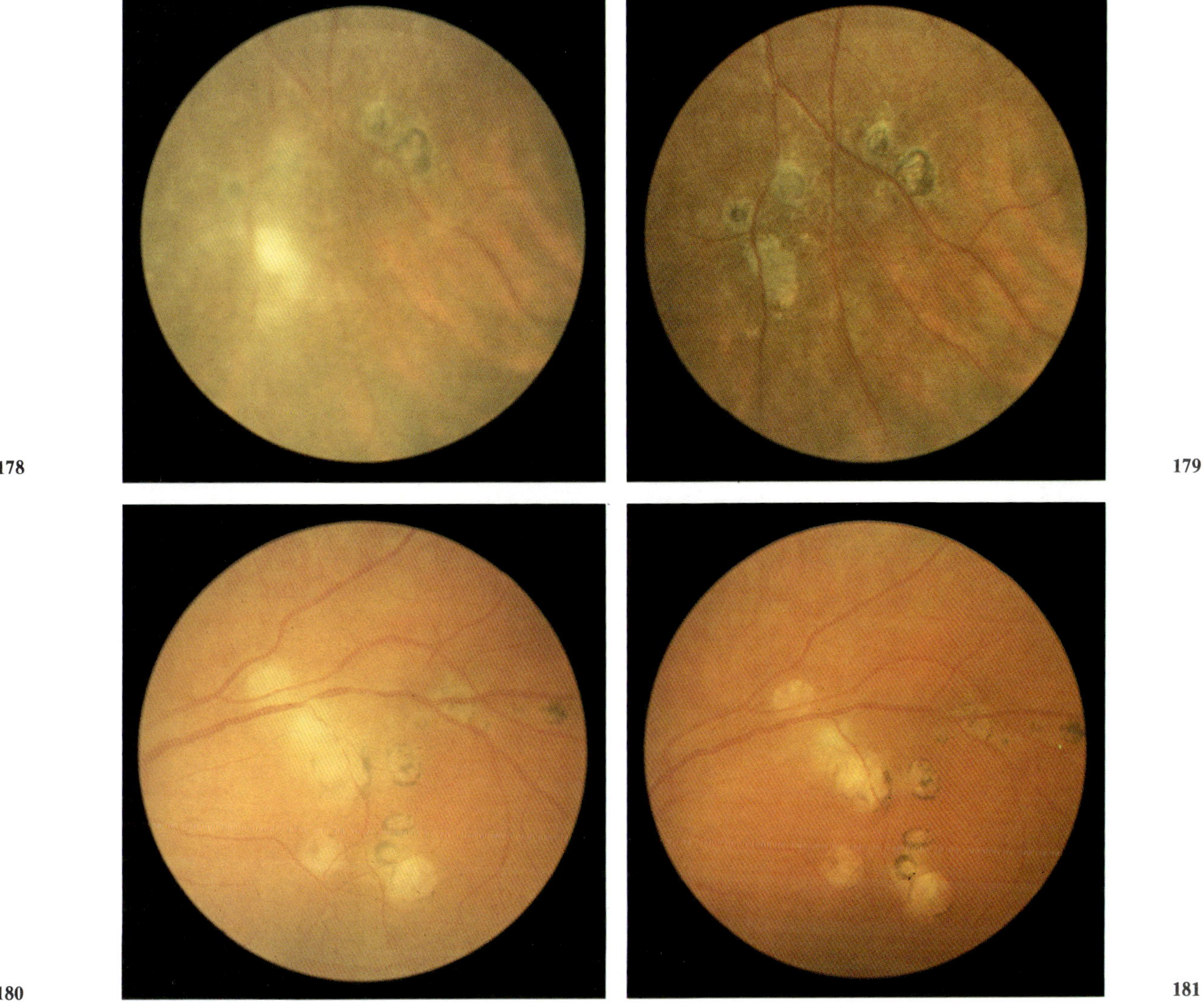

Figures 178 and 179. Left eye of a 21-year-old female patient with subacute chorioretinitis.

Clinical Findings

With a correction of −2.75 sphere, visual acuity was corrected to 20/50. There was 1 to 2+ cell and flare present. There were also cells in the vitreous humor. Groups of partially pigmented, not clearly demarcated chorioretinal lesions of varied size and age were present along the vessels.

Laboratory Findings

Blood sedimentation rate was 38/63 mm. Toxoplasmosis dye titer was 1:1000, and complement fixation titer, 1:5, which did not show any increase in subsequent examinations at 4 and 8 weeks. Tests for leptospirosis, tuberculosis, and syphilis were negative. A general medical examination was unremarkable.

Therapy

The patient was treated with pyrimethamine and doxycycline in combination with systemic prednisolone.

Clinical Course

The acute inflammation subsided and periretinal scars remained. Visual acuity in both eyes recovered to 20/20.

Figures 180 and 181. Left eye of a 13-year-old female patient with subacute chorioretinitis.

Clinical Findings

The eye was emmetropic, and visual acuity was 20/40. There was 1 to 2+ cell and flare present. There were also cells in the vitreous humor.

Laboratory Findings

Blood sedimentation rate was 32/56 mm. Toxoplasmosis dye titer 1:256, complement fixation titer 1:5, which increased in a subsequent examination at 4 weeks to toxoplasmosis titer 1:1000, complement fixation titer 1:10. Tests for leptospirosis, tuberculosis, and syphilis were negative. A general medical examination was unremarkable.

Therapy

The patient was treated with pyrimethamine and doxycycline in combination with systemic prednisolone.

Clinical Course

The acute inflammation subsided and peraretinal scars remained. Visual acuity in both eyes recovered to 20/20.

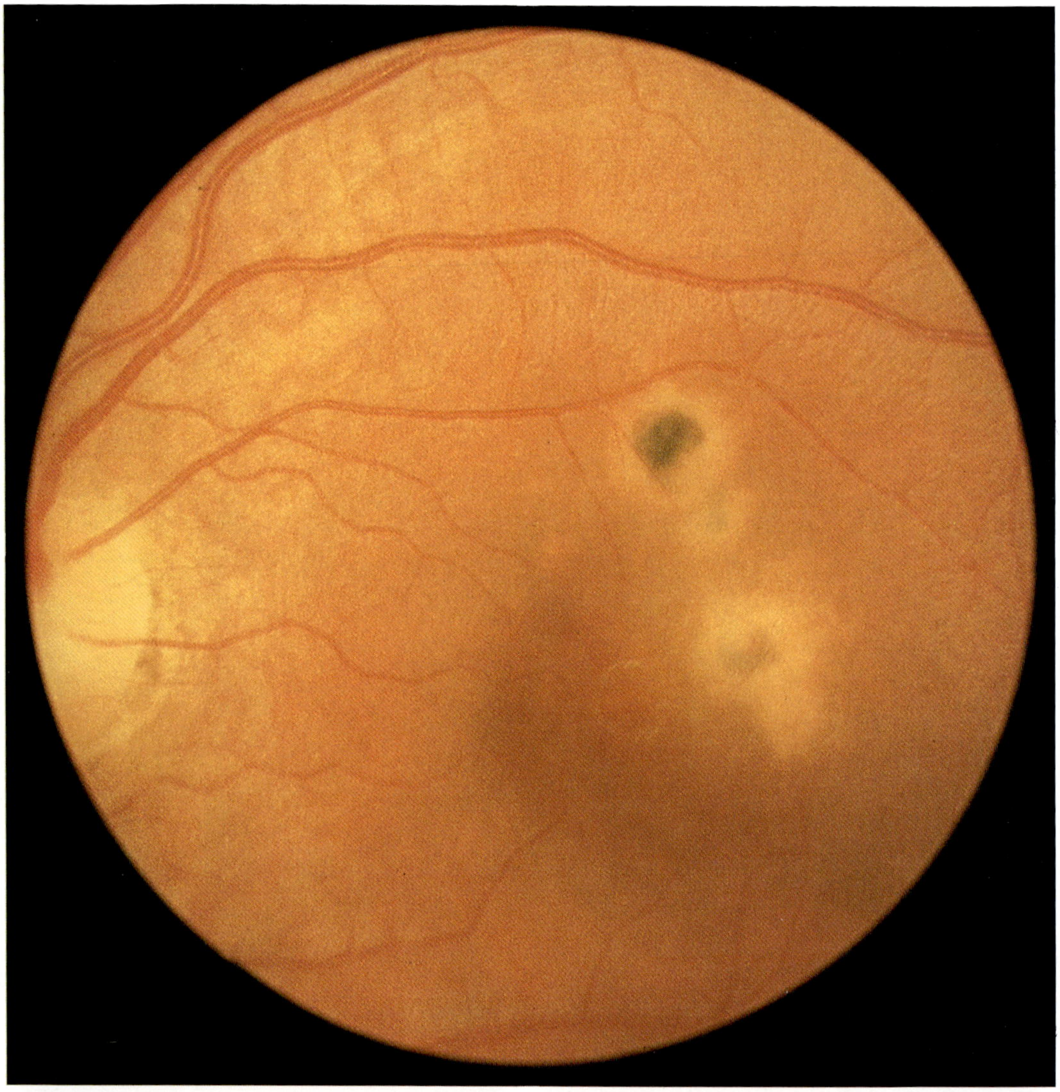

182

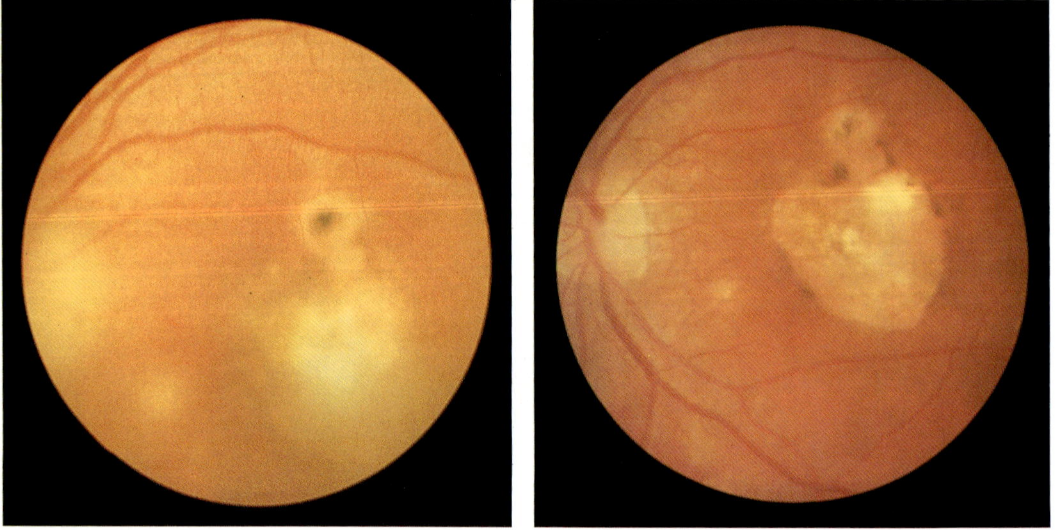

183

184

185 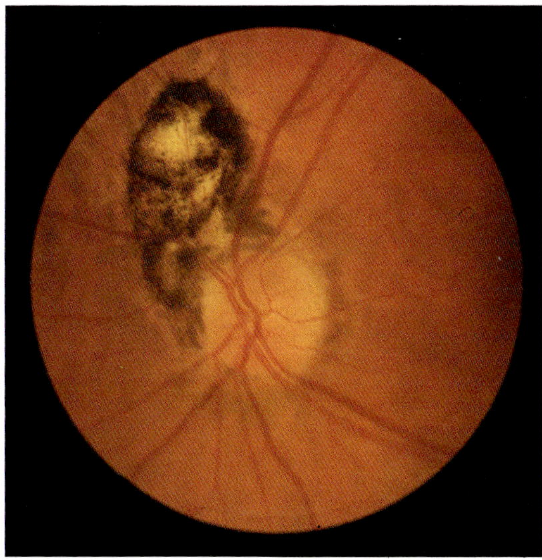

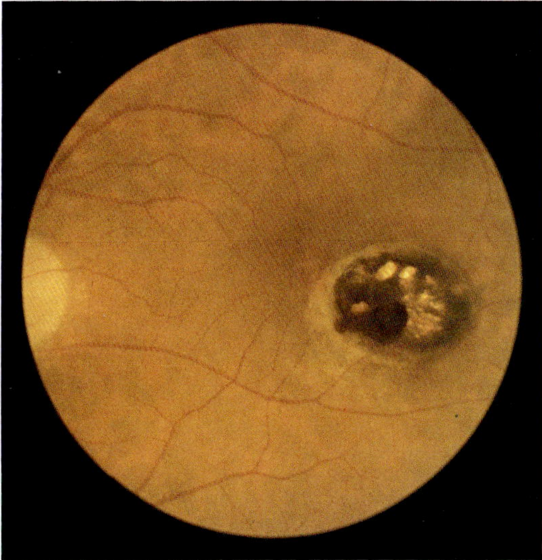 186

Figures 182–184. Left eye of a 12-year-old male patient with recurring paracentral chorioretinitis.

Clinical Findings

Figure 182 shows the posterior pole at this patient's first examination at the age of 7. The objective refraction in both eyes at that time was +1.75 sphere, with visual acuity of 20/20. The lesion was found during a routine ocular examination following a corneal injury to the right eye. After 5 years, visual acuity in the left eye rapidly decreased to 20/200. Blood sedimentation rate was 12/28 mm. An ophthalmoscopical examination showed an optic disc with blurred margins and an acute inflammation involving the posterior pole that also caused the macular edema seen in Figure 183. An ENT and internal examination did not reveal any additional pathology.

Serologic Findings

Toxoplasmosis dye test titer 1:256, complement fixation test was negative. Indirect fluorescent antibody test titer 1:1000 (no titer elevation after 4 weeks). Tests for tuberculosis, *Mycoplasma pneumoniae* disease, and listeriosis were negative.

Therapy

The patient was treated with a regimen of pyrimethamine and doxycycline in combination with systemic prednisolone.

Clinical Course

The inflammation subsided, leaving a chorioretinal scar (Fig. 184). Final visual acuity was 20/100.

Figure 185. Left eye of a 56-year-old male patient with Jensen's juxtapapillary retinochoroiditis.

Clinical Findings

The eye was emmetropic with visual acuity of 20/25. Visual field testing revealed a comet-shaped defect originating from the blind spot. Fundus examination revealed a chorioretinal scar with dark irregular pigmentations. Note the localization of this lesion immediately adjacent to the optic disc.

Serologic Findings

Toxoplasmosis dye test titer 1:256, complement fixation test titer 1:10.

Figure 186. Left eye of a 51-year-old male patient evaluated following central chorioretinitis.

Clinical Findings

Best visual acuity with a correction of +1.75 sphere was 20/200. Visual field testing showed a central scotoma. Note the central chorioretinal scar with dark hyperpigmentations.

Serologic Findings

Toxoplasmosis dye test titer 1:256, complement fixation test titer 1:5.

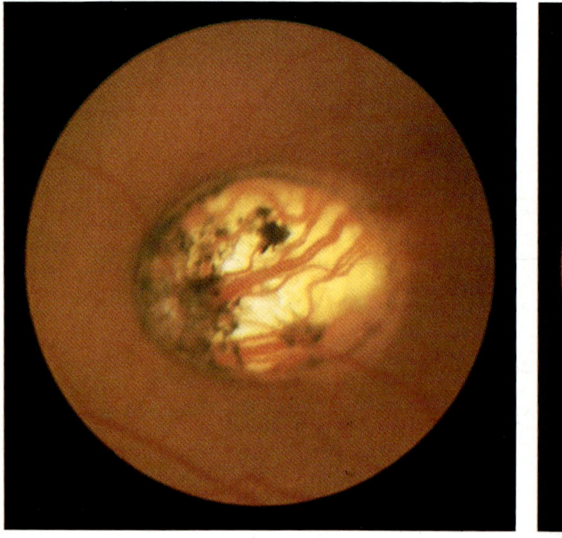
187

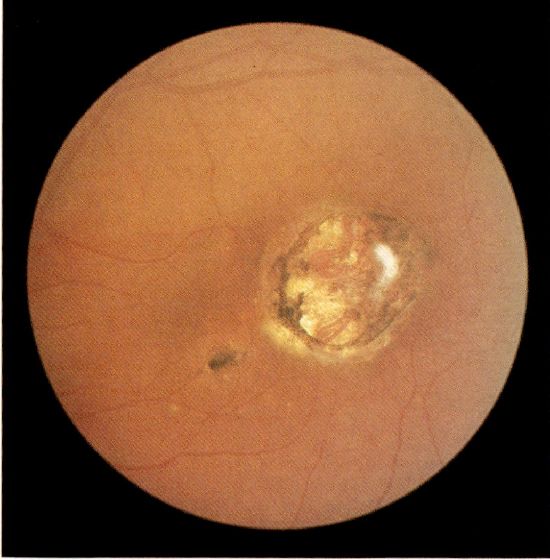
188

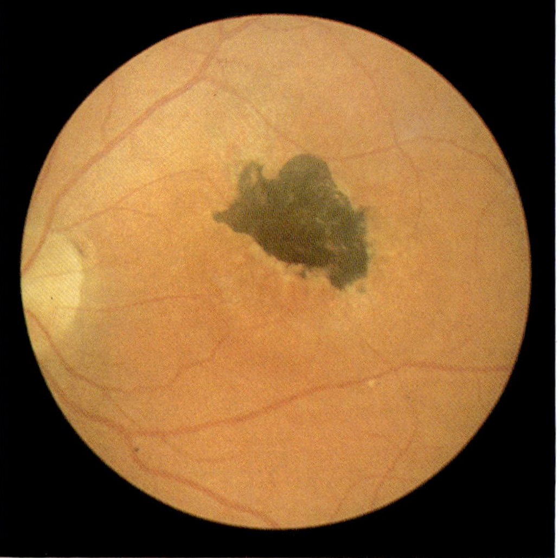
189

Figure 187. Left eye of a 22-year-old male patient with a central chorioretinal scar following central chorioretinitis.

Clinical Findings

A congenital toxoplasmosis infection was presumed. Visual acuity of 20/50 could be achieved with a correction of +6.75 sphere, −2.75 cylinder, axis 10°. Refractive media were clear. A central scotoma was present. A pseudocoloboma of the macula is present in the fundus.

Serologic Findings

Toxoplasmosis dye test titer 1:256, complement fixation test titer 1:5.

Figure 188. Left eye of a 45-year-old male patient with a central chorioretinal scar following central chorioretinitis.

Clinical Findings

The chorioretinitis was presumably caused by a congenital toxoplasmosis infection. With a refraction of +2.25 sphere, best visual acuity was 20/400. Refractive media were clear. A central scotoma was present. The fundus shows a macular pseudocoloboma with a small satellite lesion.

Serologic Findings

Toxoplasmosis dye test titer 1:256, complement fixation test titer 1:5.

Figure 189. Left eye of a 34-year-old female patient with a central chorioretinal scar following central chorioretinitis. A differential diagnosis includes central hemorrhagic choroiditis.

Clinical Findings

The eye was emmetropic and best visual acuity was 20/60. Refractive media were clear. A central scotoma was present. A heavily pigmented scar of the posterior pole is present in the fundus. Note also the gray-white ring-shaped line surrounding the macular area. This line indicates the extension of the previous exudative retinal detachment, which was most likely associated with the acute inflammation.

Serologic Findings

Tests for toxoplasmosis, syphilis, and tuberculosis were negative.

Figures 190–192. Right eye of a 16-year-old patient with a solitary ocular granuloma caused by toxocariasis (*Toxocara canis*).

Clinical Findings

Visual acuity was 20/400 with a central scotoma. Blood sedimentation rate was 3/6 mm.

Laboratory Findings

Erythrocytes 5.1 million, leukocytes 5400, differential blood cell count: eosinophils 8, band neutrophils 6, segmented neutrophils 45, lymphocytes 40, monocytes 1.

Serologic Findings

Microprecipitation tests for living *T. canis* larvae was positive. The infection in the acute phase is shown in Figures 190 and 191. Figure 192 shows the lesion 7 years after the onset of symptoms.

Therapy

The patient was treated with a regimen of tetracycline and sulfamethoxydiazine in combination with prednisolone.

Clinical Course

In the acute phase, there was a cellular reaction within the vitreous. The solitary granuloma then healed, leaving a large chorioretinal atrophic scar.

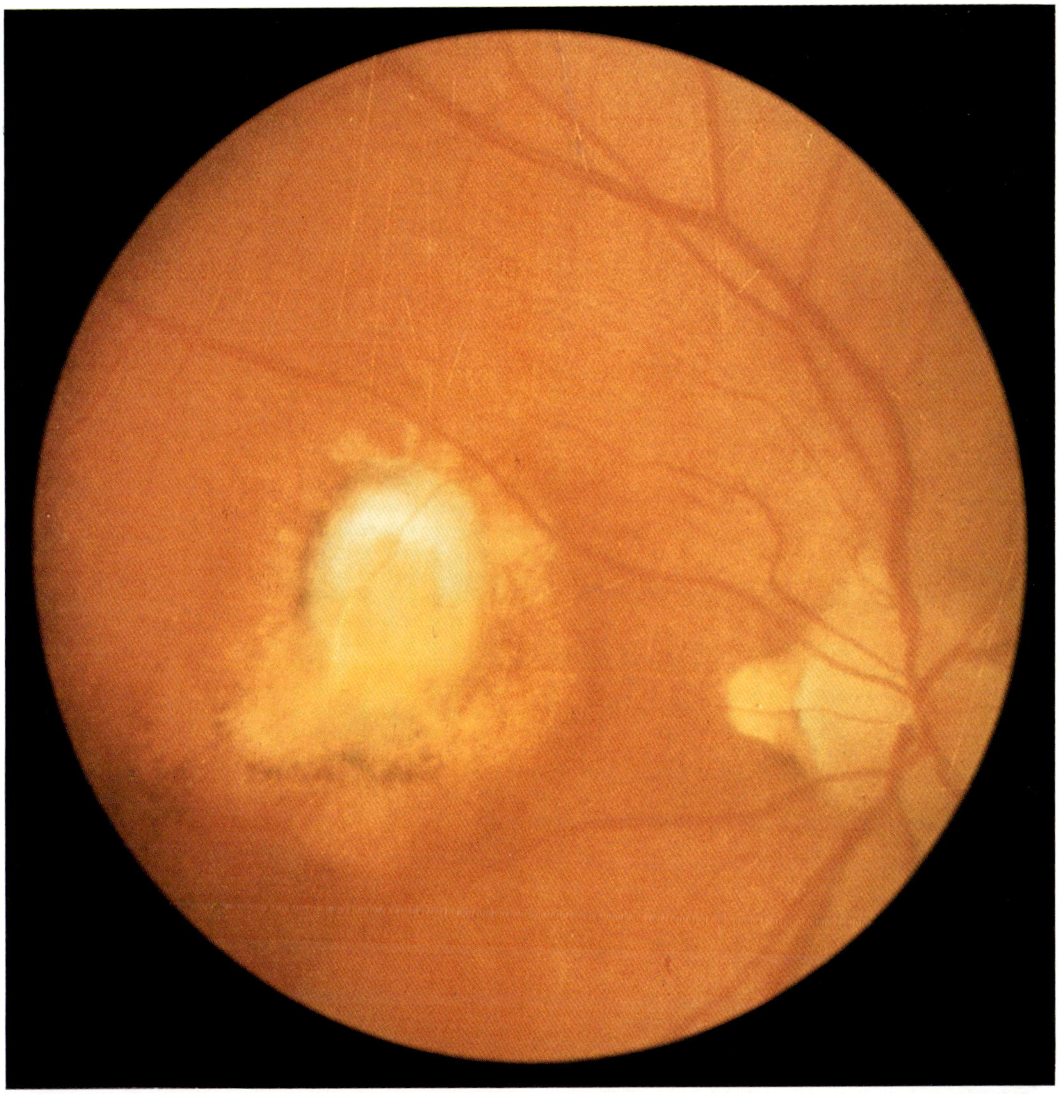

190

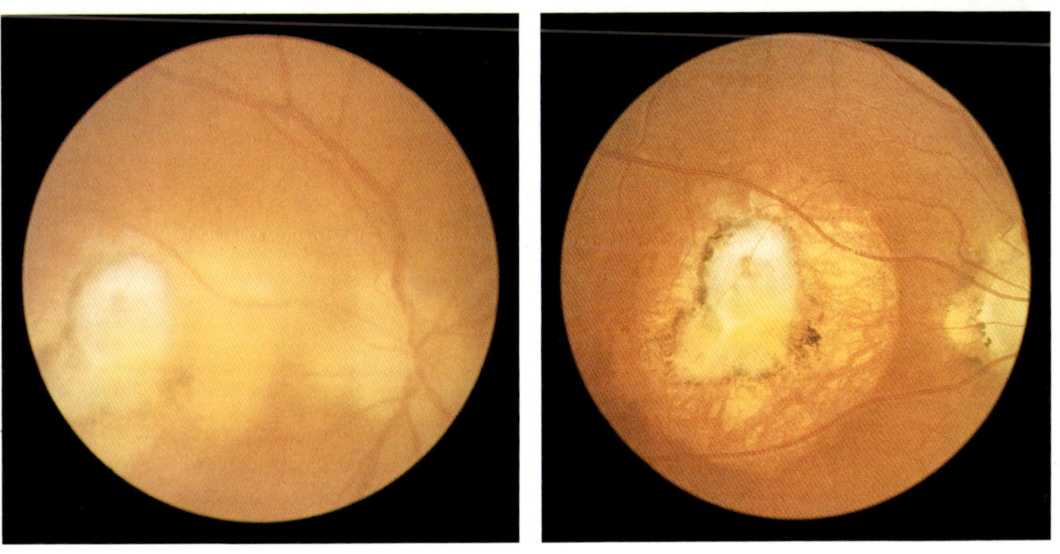

191

192

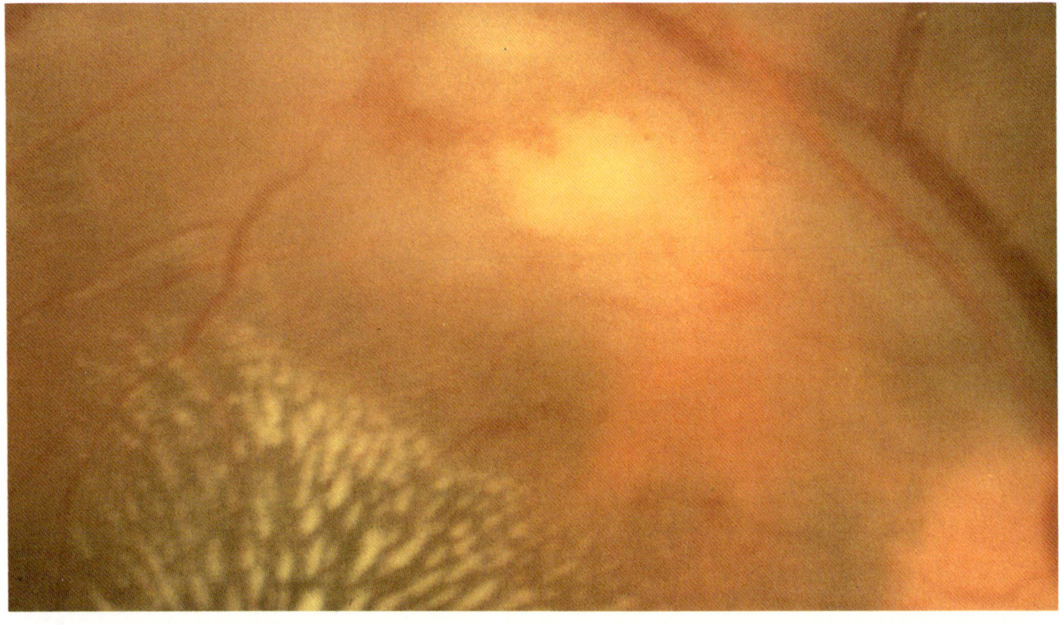

193

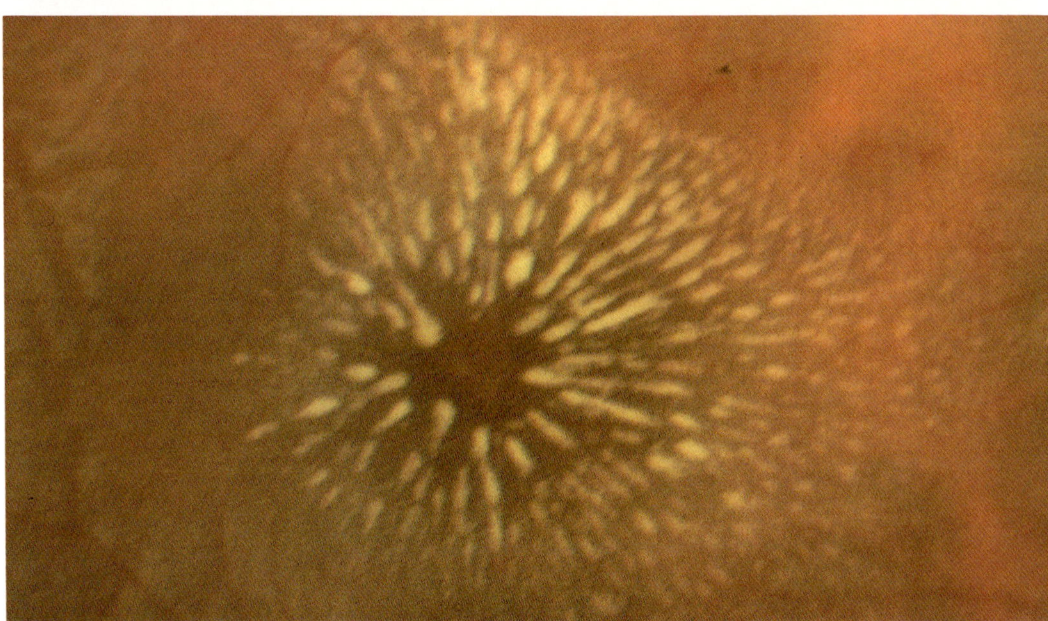

194

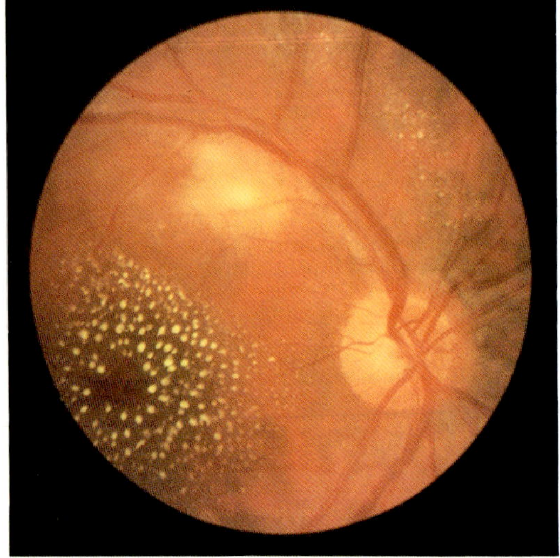

195

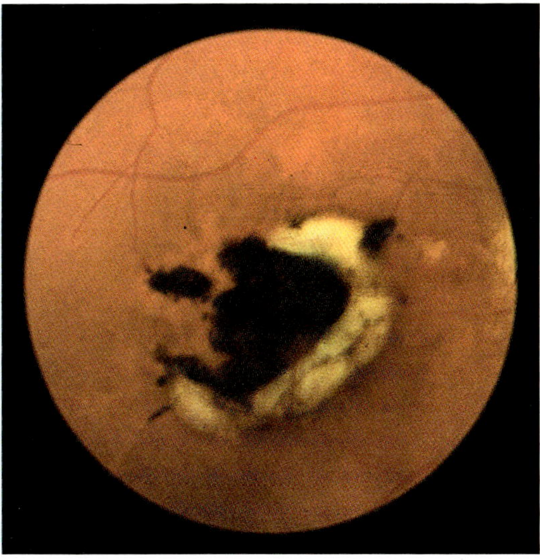
196

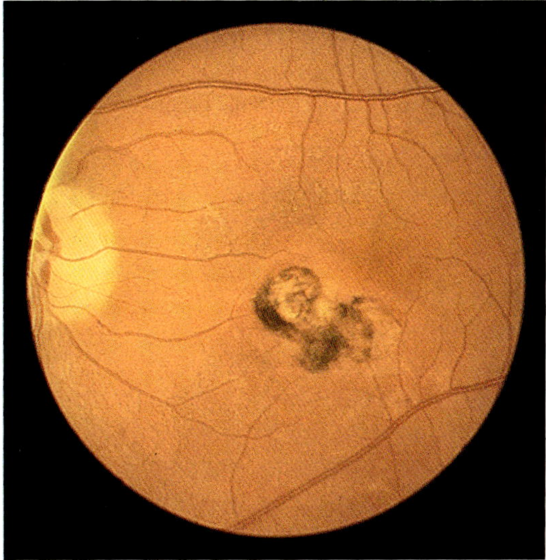
197

Figures 193–195. Right eye of a 16-year-old patient with acute chorioretinitis caused by listeriosis. Four weeks prior to the ocular examination the patient suffered from a influenza-like illness with a severe headache. A decrease in visual acuity occurred in the right eye.

Clinical Findings

Objective refraction in the right eye revealed an error of +0.25 sphere, −0.5 cylinder, axis 115°, for a visual acuity of 20/100. Visual field testing showed an absolute scotoma that originated from the blind spot and extended nasally. The scotoma measured approximately 3 times the size of a normal blind spot. Intraocular pressure was 12 mm Hg. Blood sedimentation rate was 16/35 mm. There were cells in the anterior chamber and vitreous. Acute inflammatory lesions involving both retina and choroid are present in the fundus just inferior to the superotemporal vein at a distance of 2 disc diameters from the optic disc. There is retinal edema and intraretinal hemorrhages around the margin of the lesion. A macular star figure is present.

Laboratory Findings

Hemoglobin 14.5 gm/100 ml, mean corpuscular hemoglobin (MCH) 31.4 pg, hematocrit 45%, erythrocytes 4.61 million, leukocytes 13,000, differential blood cell count: band neutrophils 1, segmented neutrophils 67, lymphocytes 29, eosinophil 1. Stool and urine tests were unremarkable.

Serologic Findings

Toxoplasmosis dye test titer 1:64, complement fixation test titer 1:5 (no titer elevation when controlled 14 days). Leptospirosis antibodies negative, complement fixation test for chlamydial infections negative. See Table 15 for agglutination tests for listeriosis. Figure 193 shows the acute chorioretinal inflammation with the adjacent macular star figure. Figure 194 is a high power photograph of the macular star figure in the acute phase. Figure 195 shows the fundus after antibiotic treatment and after the inflammatory reaction has subsided. The macular star figure appears less prominent and seems to be resolving. Visual acuity was 20/25 to 20/20.

Figure 196. Right eye of a 15-year-old female patient with a solitary ocular granuloma caused by toxocariasis (*Toxocara canis*), and a divergent strabismus.

Clinical Findings

Visual acuity in this eye was 20/200. There was a partial central scotoma.

Serologic Findings

A microprecipitation test for *T. canis* larvae was positive.

Therapy

The patient was treated with thiabendazole.

Clinical Course

The fundus changes remained stationary over a period of 7 years.

Figure 197. Left eye of a 23-year-old male patient with a solitary ocular granuloma caused by toxocariasis (*Toxocara canis*).

Clinical Findings

Visual acuity was 20/30 with a partial central scotoma.

Serologic Findings

A microprecipitation test for *T. canis* was positive.

Therapy

The patient was treated with thiabendazole.

Clinical Course

The fundus changes remained stationary over a period of 6 years.

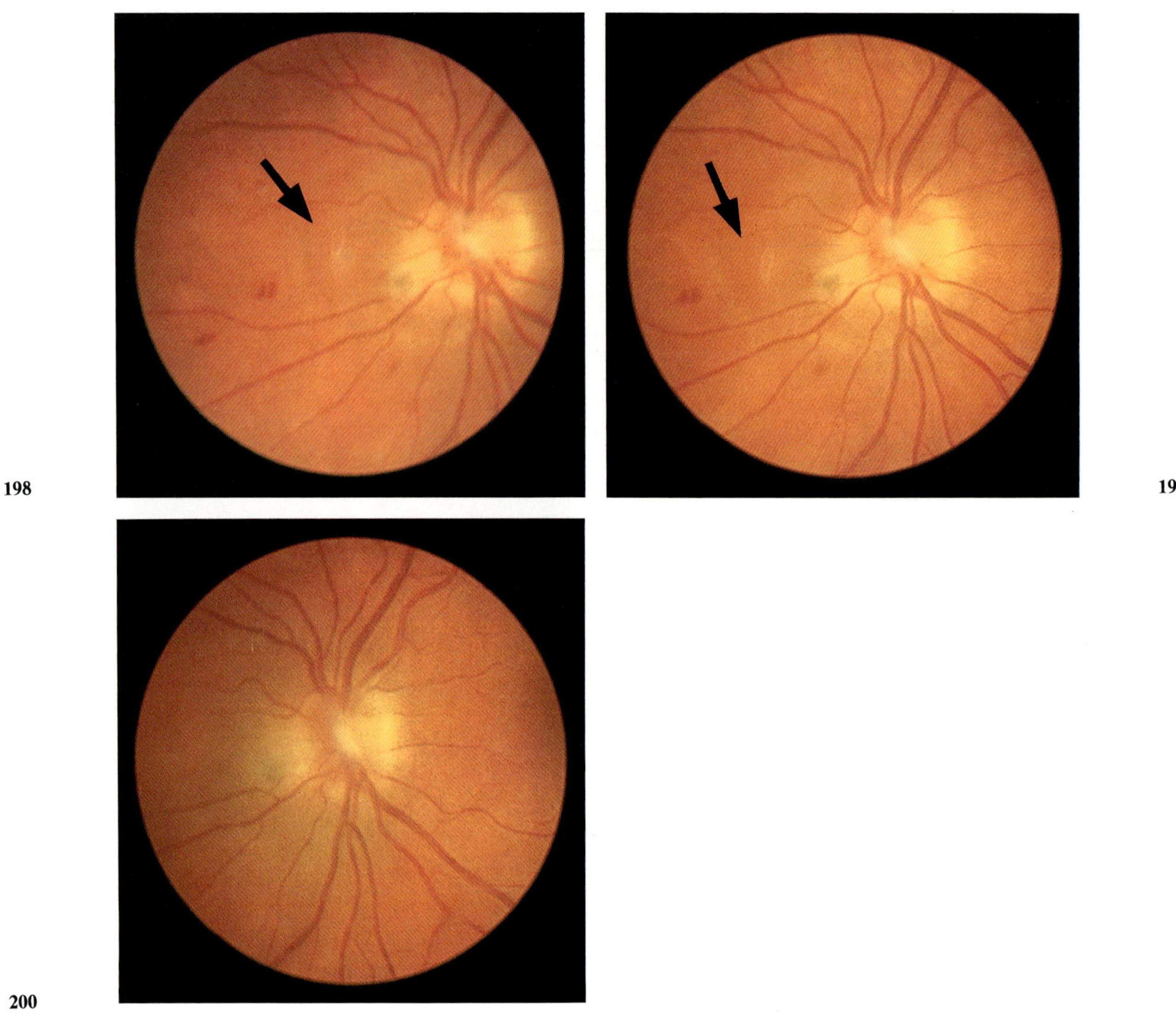

198

199

200

Figures 198–200. Right eye of a 16-year-old male patient with larva migrans visceralis (*Toxocara canis*). The living larva can be seen in the fundus of the right eye (*arrow*). The patient has a history of epilepsy.

Clinical Findings

The patient was examined 6 months after the first cerebral convulsion. Visual acuity at that time was 20/25, and the visual field was normal. There were no cells in the anterior chamber or in the vitreous.

Serologic Findings

A microprecipitation test for *T. canis* was positive, erythrocytes 5.3 million, leukocytes 16,300, differential blood cell count unremarkable (eosinophils 5). Pandy's reaction in the cerebrospinal fluid was positive with a protein concentration of 456 μg and occasional erythrocytes. Computed tomography was unremarkable. An EEG showed rudimentary spikes. Figure 198 illustrates the papilledema and obliteration of the physiologic optic cup. The retinal veins are engorged. There is a juxtapapillary blue-gray pigment spot immediately adjacent to the optic disc at the 7-o'clock position. As mentioned in the text, *T. canis* may mimic a juxtapapillary chorioretinitis. Note the isolated retinal hemorrhages. The *T. canis* larva is visible as a white arcuate foreign body in the retina (*arrow*).

Clinical Course

Figure 199 shows the migrating larvae that changed its position 16 hours after the first photograph was taken (*arrow*). Visual acuity at this time was 20/50.

Therapy

The patient was treated with a regimen of prednisolone, tetracycline, and sulfamethoxydiazine. The previously arcuate appearance of the larva then changed to a more ring-like appearance. Figure 200 shows the optic disc several days later at a time when the inflammation is slowly subsiding. The larva is no longer visible. Three weeks later a complete remission was observed and visual acuity was 20/20. No cerebral convulsions have occurred for several years.

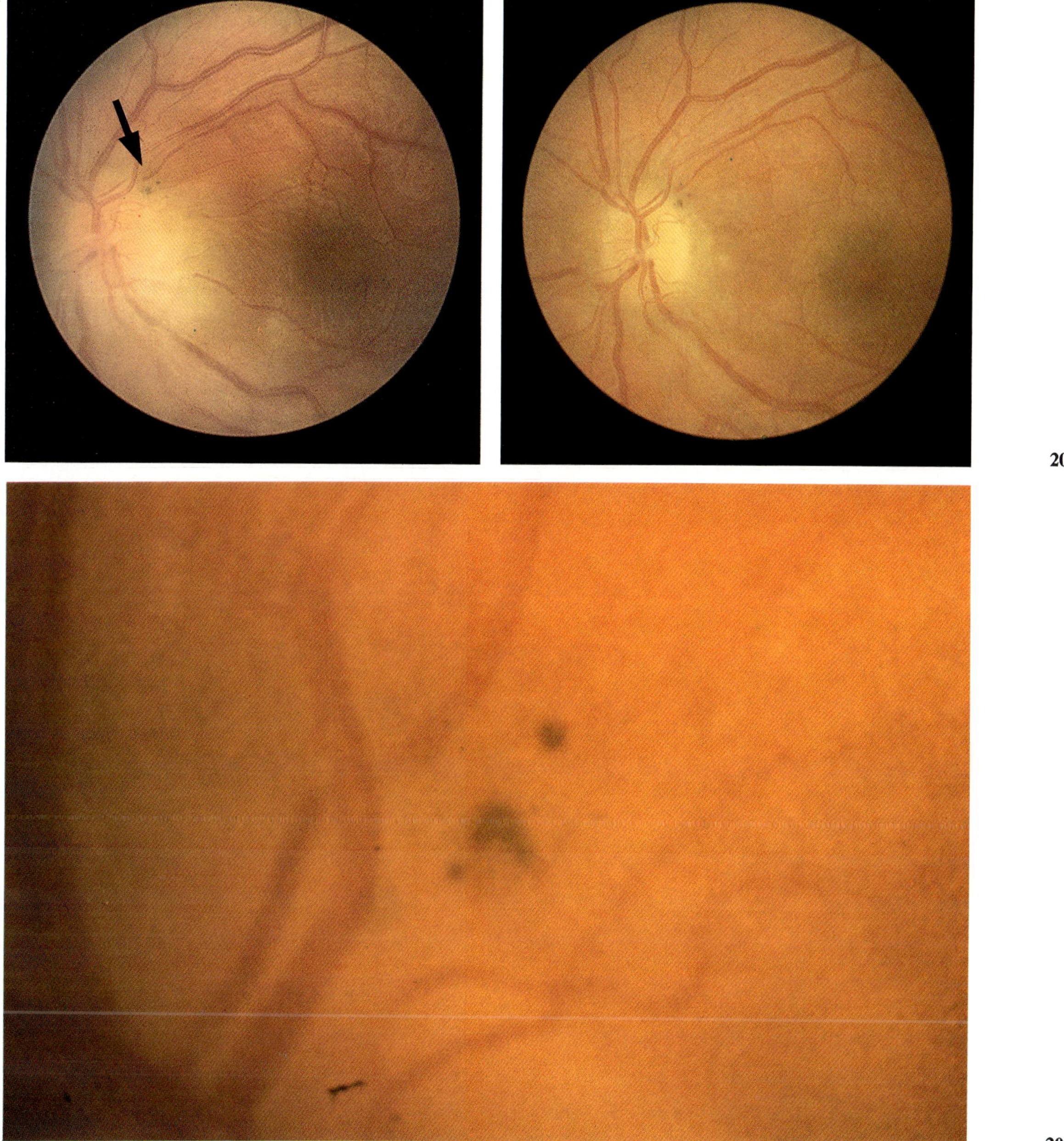

201 202 203

Figures 201–203. Left eye of a 25-year-old female patient with larvae invasion of *Toxocara canis* mimicking Jensen's juxtapapillary chorioretinitis (Fig. 201).

Clinical Findings

Visual acuity was 20/50. There were no cells in the anterior chamber or vitreous. Blood sedimentation rate was 3/12 mm.

Serologic Findings

A microprecipitation test for living *T. canis* larvae was positive, erythrocytes 5 million, leukocytes 7100, differential blood cell count unremarkable (eosinophils 1). Complement fixation test for toxoplasmosis was negative. The Sabin-Feldman test showed a titer of 1:256. Figure 202 illustrates the edematous optic disc with blurred margins (most pronounced in the inferotemporal area). The inferotemporal vessels are partially masked by the overlying edema. Radial folds in the macular edema are also visible. Note the pigmentations adjacent to the optic disc at the 1-o'clock position (Fig. 201, *arrow*). Figure 203 is a high-power fundus photograph of the pigmentations in which two punctate lesions and one arcuate lesion are visible.

Therapy

The patient was treated with a regimen of prednisolone, tetracycline, and sulfamethoxydiazine.

Clinical Course

The inflammation completely subsided and the final visual acuity was 20/20.

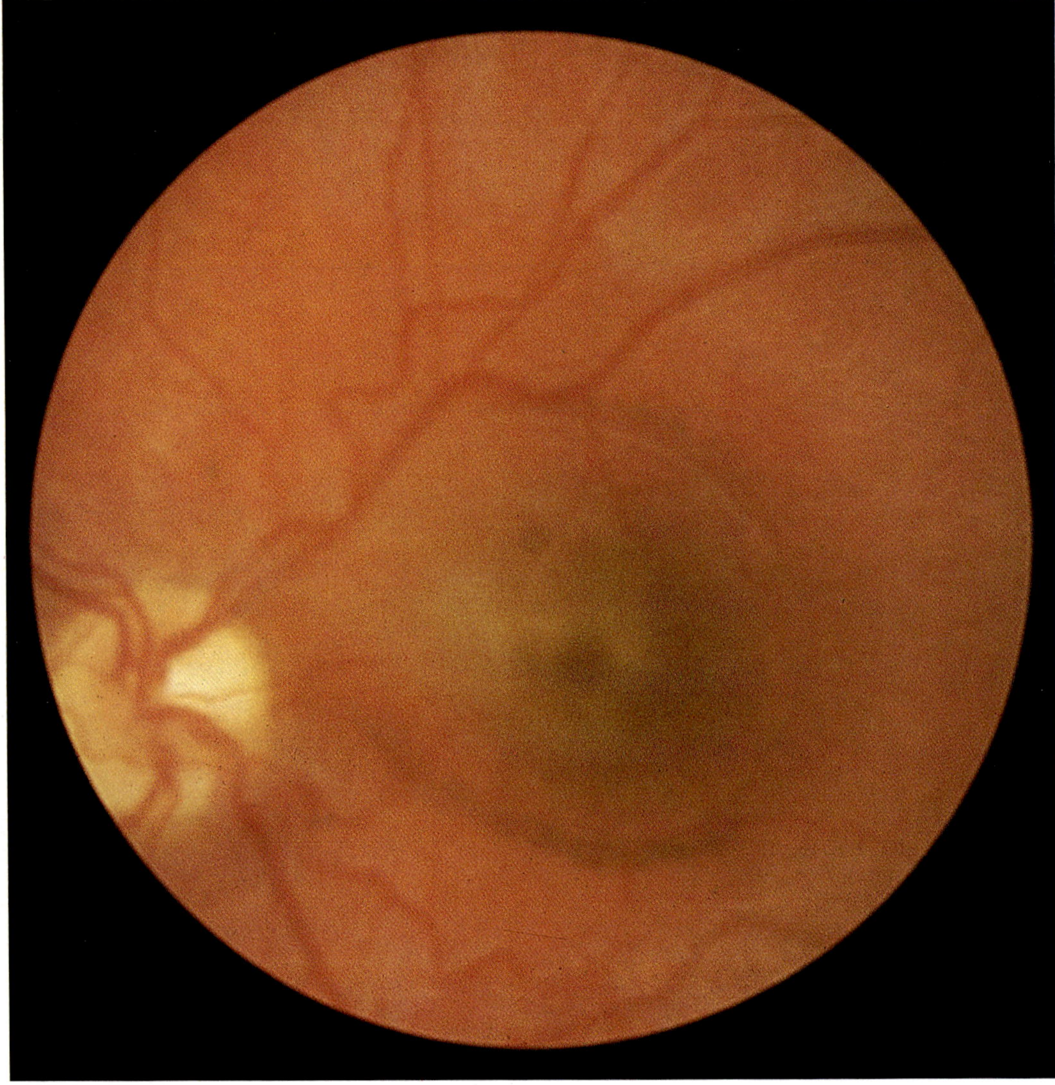

204

Figure 204. Left eye of a 2-year-old child with subretinal hydatid cyst (*Echinococcus granulosus*) and a convergent strabismus.

Clinical Findings

The child did not fixate on any light. The anterior segment was unremarkable and there were no cells in the anterior chamber or vitreous. There was an esotropia of 20°.

Serologic Findings

Tests for cysticercosis and echinococcosis were negative. Erythrocytes 4.8 million, leukocytes 10,200, differential blood cell count unremarkable. Casoni's test was positive.

Clinical Course

The fundus pattern remained stationary over an observation period of 4 years.

Figure 205–207. Left eye of a 50-year-old patient with necrotizing cytomegalic retinitis, diabetes, diabetic retinopathy and Stage 2 of hypertensive retinopathy. The patient's clinical history is the typical example of a consumptive disease with multiple morbidities that created a predisposition for infection by cytomegalovirus. The patient underwent a hysterectomy for uterine carcinoma at the age of 40. Following the surgical intervention, irradiation therapy was performed (pericutaneous cobalt 60 irradiation of the parametria and pelvis for a total dose of 6000 rad). In addition, irradiation with a radium inlay was performed (1400 mg over a period of 20 hours). Six months prior to the onset of the necrotizing retinitis (Fig. 205), the patient was hospitalized. The following internal diagnoses were made: erosive antrum gastritis, anemia, cardiac and renal insufficiency, arterial hypertension, hyperlipidemia, and diabetes mellitus. The neurologic consultant diagnosed an encephalopathy due to hypertension. Cranial computed tomography revealed discreet cortical atropic areas. Immune electrophoresis showed a hypoproteinemia with a reduction of IgG and IgM.

Serologic Findings

Positive antibodies (IgG) were present for cytomegalovirus. The direct identification of the virus in an anterior chamber tap was not possible since the aqueous specimen was not correctly handled. (It was frozen during transport.) Soon a massive vitreous hemorrhage occurred. The differential diagnosis in this case would include such entities as Coats' disease or other forms of exudative retinal involvement.

Therapy

The patient was treated with vidarabin phosphate infusions.

Clinical Course

There was a severe visual loss with visual acuity reduced to hand movements.

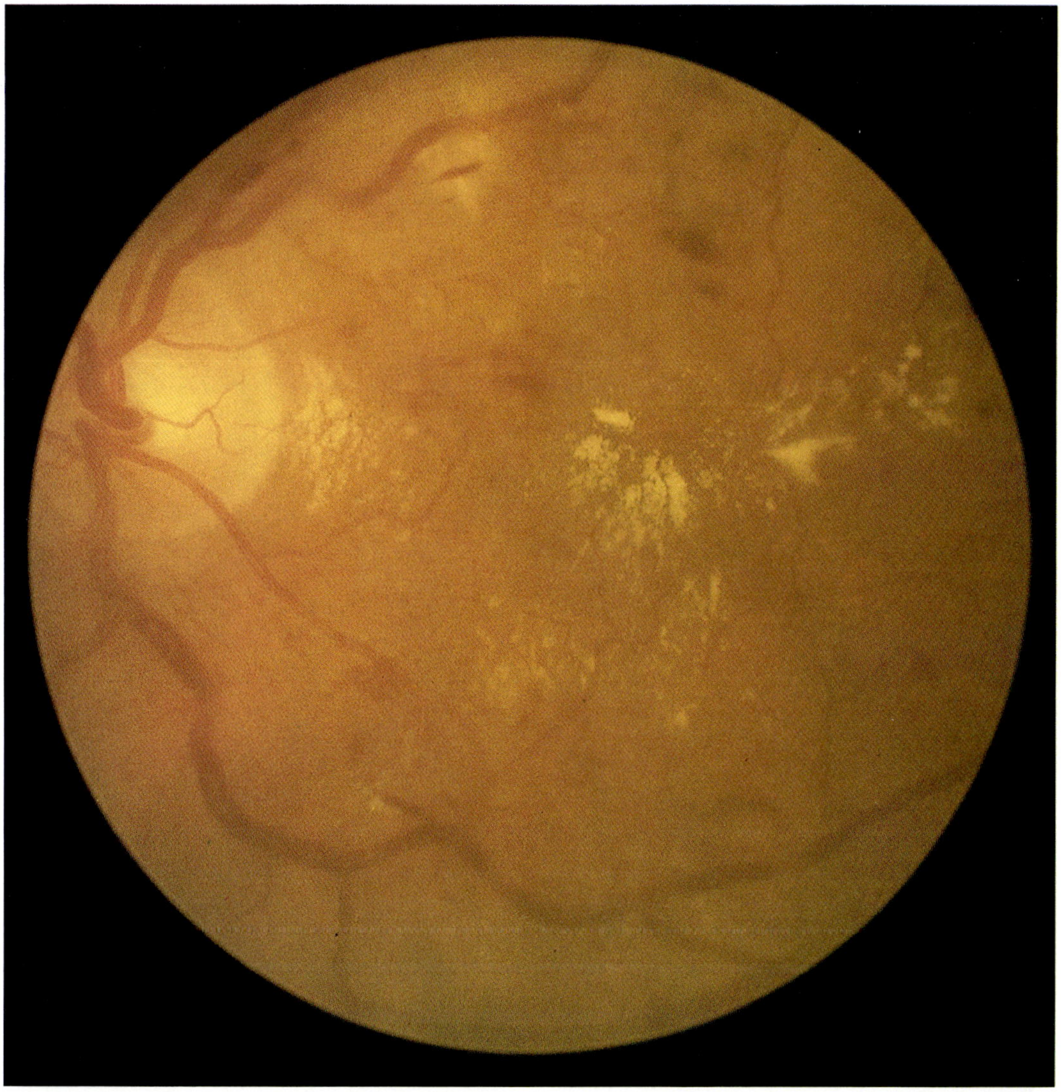

205

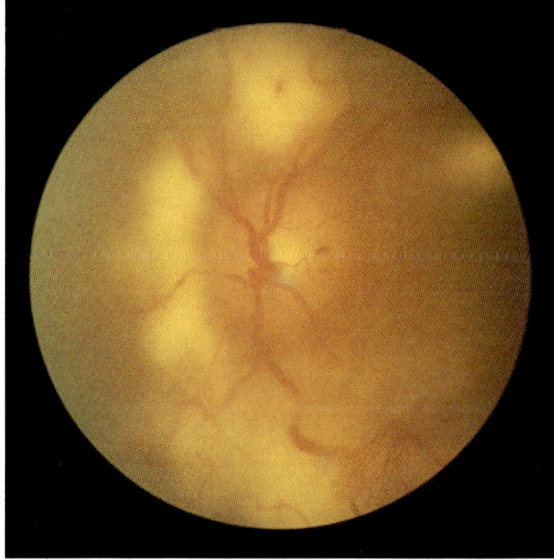

206

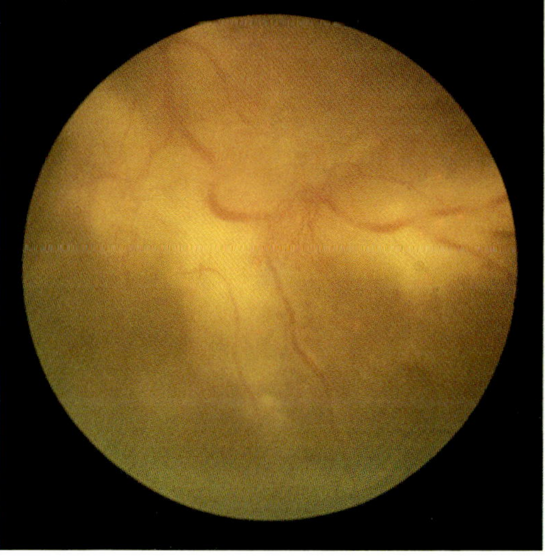

207

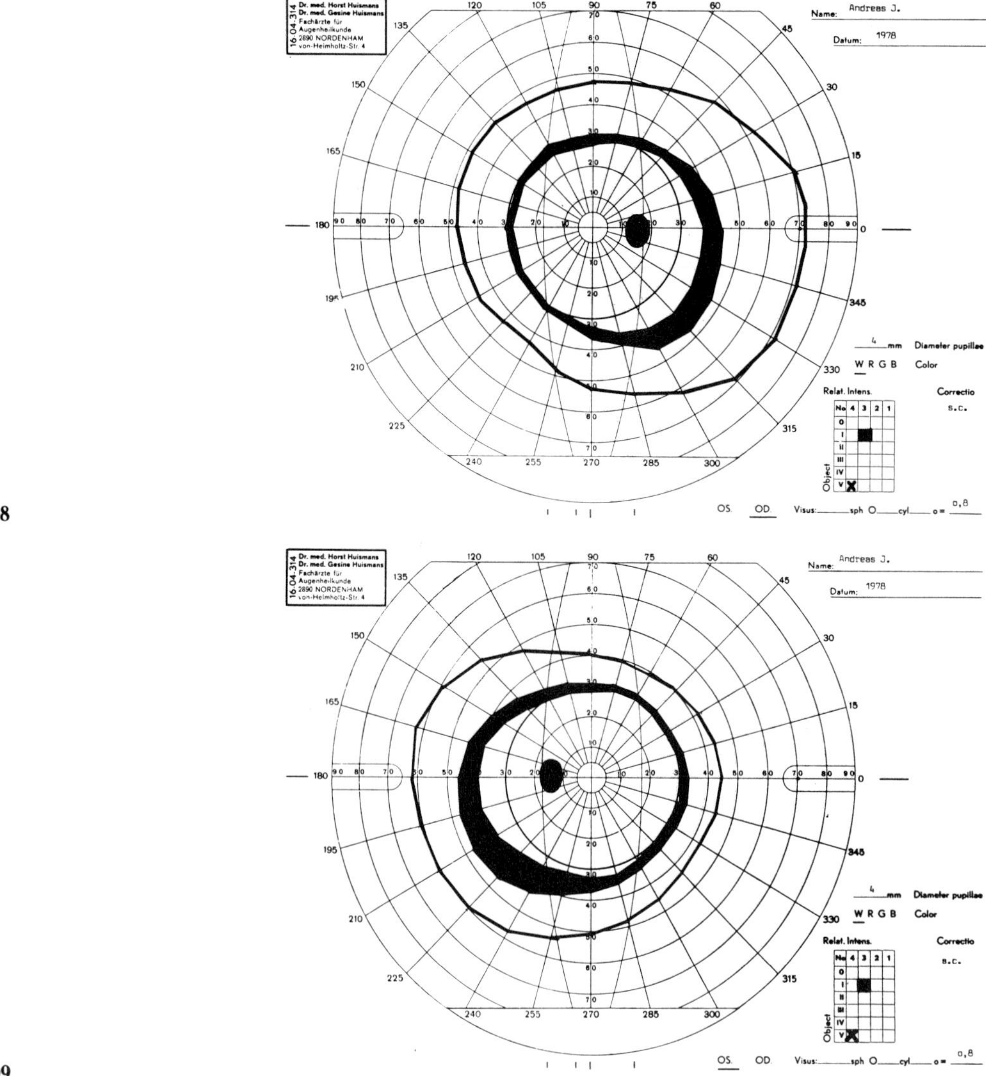

208

209

Figure 208. Goldmann's perimeter chart of the right eye of a 7-year-old male patient with ring scotoma associated with tapetoretinal degeneration. The corresponding fundus lesions are illustrated in Figures 211-215.

Figure 209. Goldmann's perimeter chart of the left eye of the same patient as in Figure 208 with ring scotoma associated with tapetoretinal degeneration. The corresponding retinal lesions are shown in Figures 211-215.

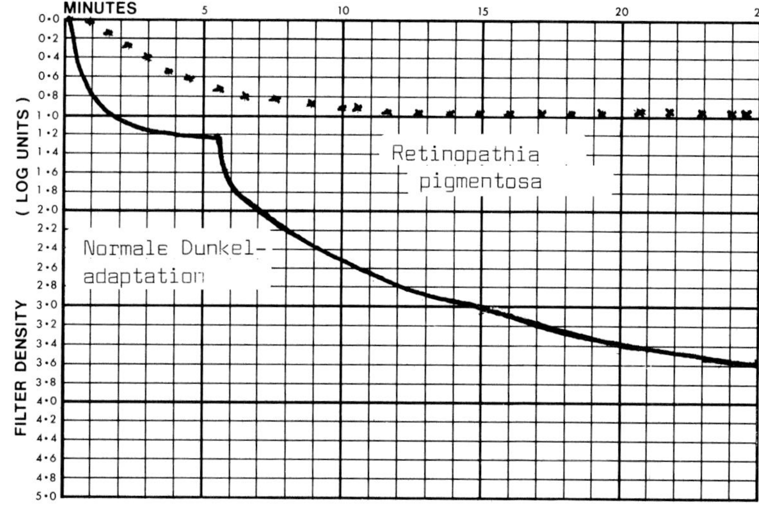

210

Figure 210. Dark adaptation graph prepared with a Friedman central field analyzer of a retinitis pigmentosa patient (*dotted line*) and of a healthy patient (*solid line*). As shown, the normal graph shows a combination of two different cells types resulting in a biphasic graph. The first segment represents the dark adaptation of the retinal cones reaching the adaptation stage after a period of 5–10 minutes. The second segment represents the dark adaptation of the retinal rods. The transition from cone to rod adaptation is clearly shown by a step in the graph. This step is named for Kohlrausch despite the fact that it was first described by Aubert in 1865. The dark adaptation graph in cases of tapetoretinal degenerations is monophasic.

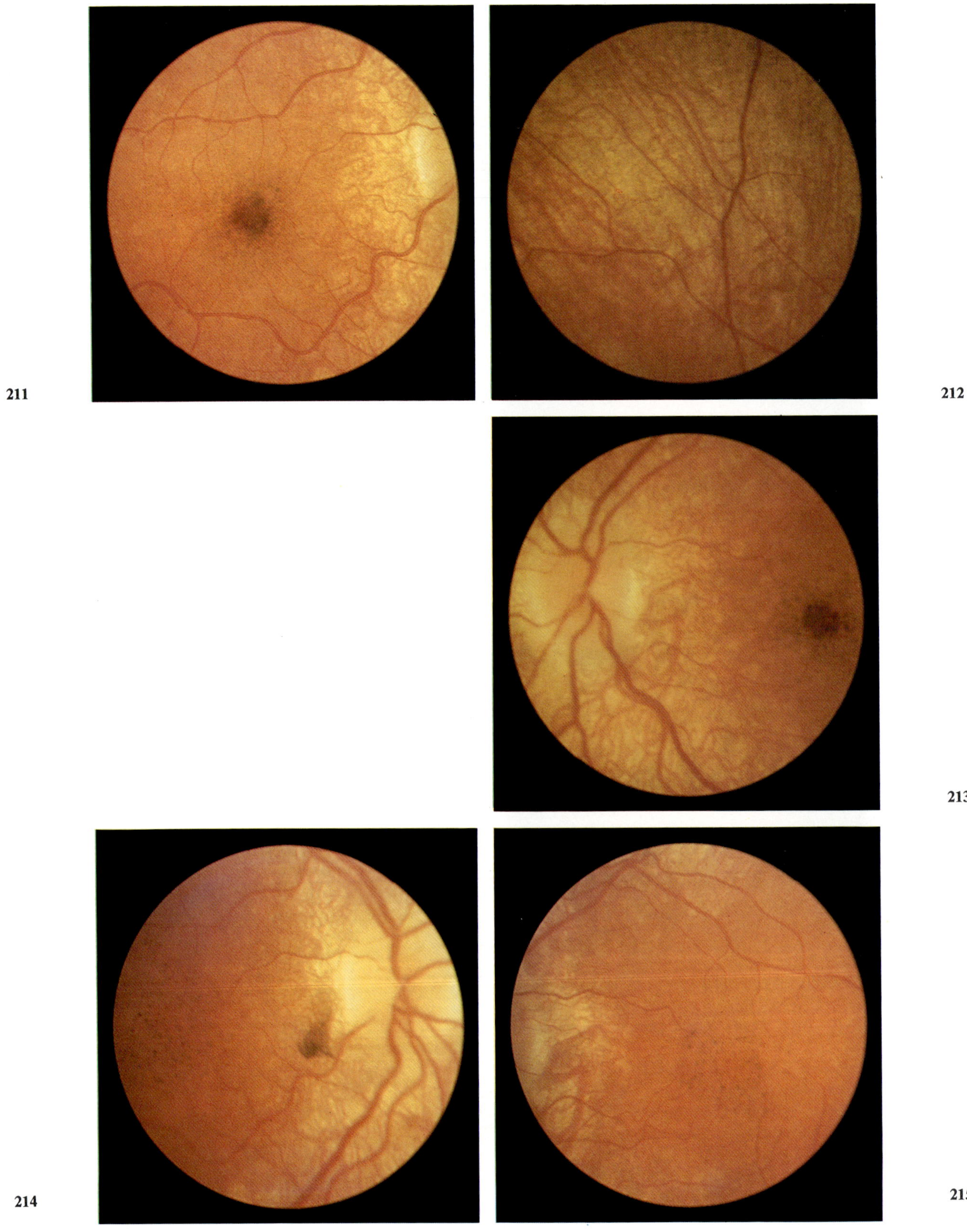

211

212

213

214

215

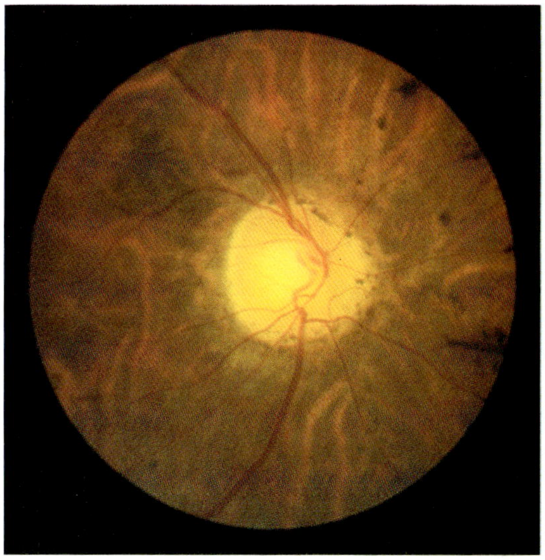

216

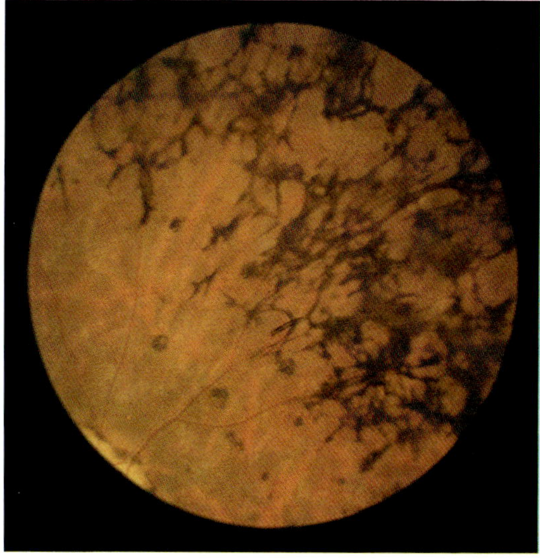

217

Figures 211–215. Right and left eyes of a 7-year-old male patient (same patient as Figs. 208 and 209) with tapetoretinal degeneration (inverse type of retinitis pigmentosa). The right eye had a refractive error of +3.75 sphere, −0.75 cylinder, axis 15°, and the left eye had a refractive error of +3.25 sphere, −0.75 cylinder, axis 155°. Visual acuity in both eyes was 20/25. Visual field testing showed a concentric constriction of the outer margins and the ring scotoma that is illustrated in Figure 209. Mesopic and scotopic vision were affected (hemeralopia). Dark adaptation is illustrated in Figure 210. The anterior segment was unremarkable. The right eye showed a blunt fundus with a yellow-white optic disc. The retinal vessels were unremarkable. The posterior pole showed a pulverulent pigment aggregation. The intermediate retinal area (Fig. 212) has areas of pigment irregularities with hyperpigmentations along the retinal vessels and patchy depigmented areas. The left eye (Fig. 213) shows a similar pigment accumulation at the posterior pole but it appears more clumped. The other findings were identical to the right eye. There was no distortion in color vision and an EEG was normal. An ERG showed only residual A and B waves.

Clinical Course

Figures 214 and 215 show the findings in these eyes 2 years afrer the first photographs (Figs. 211–213) were taken. There is a pigment accumulation immediately adjacent to the optic disc at the 7-o'clock position in the right eye (Fig. 214). Pigmentations of the macular region have largely resolved. The left eye (Fig. 215) shows only discrete pigment irregularities in the macular region that were located in the inner retinal layers as viewed stereoscopically. Visual acuity remained unchanged. However, the ring scotoma in both eyes became enlarged.

Figures 216 and 217. Right eye of a 37-year-old female patient with tapetoretinal degeneration.

Clinical Findings

Refraction in the right eye was −0.25 sphere, −0.5 cylinder, axis 120°, and in the left eye −0.25 sphere, −0.5 cylinder, axis 60°. Visual acuity in both eyes was 20/50. Visual field testing showed a central visual field remnant extending to a point 10° off center (Goldmann perimeter test mark III/4). The anterior segment was normal. The optic disc in both eyes appeared waxy and yellow. The arteries are extremely narrow, but the veins are unremarkable. There are pigment irregularities in a bone spicule pattern. The isolated bone spicule like hyperpigmentations accrued and build a net-like pattern. Underlying choroidal vessels are obliterated. The mesopic and scotopic vision was distorted (hemeralopia).

Therapy

No therapy is known to be effective but there have been some drug trials reported.

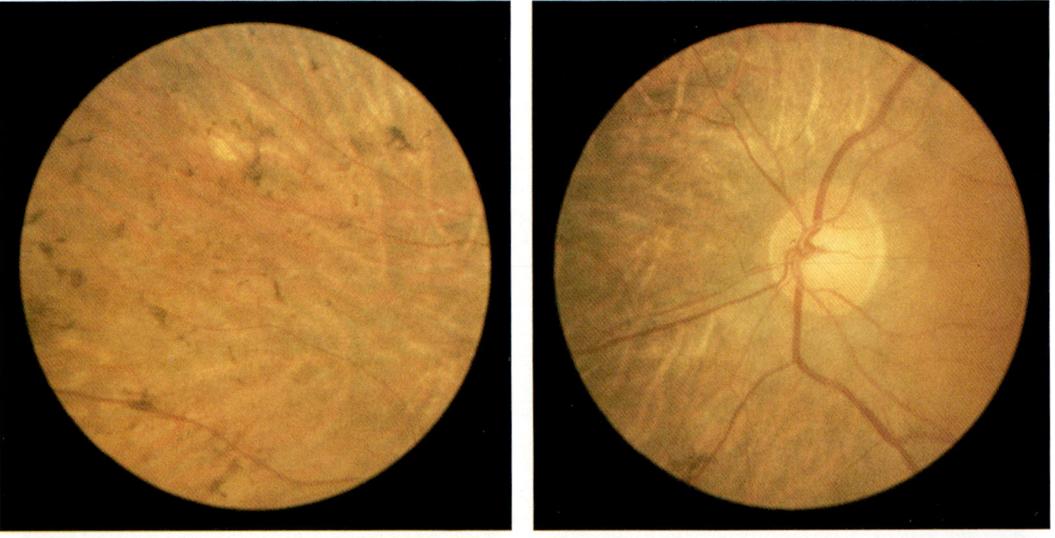

218

219

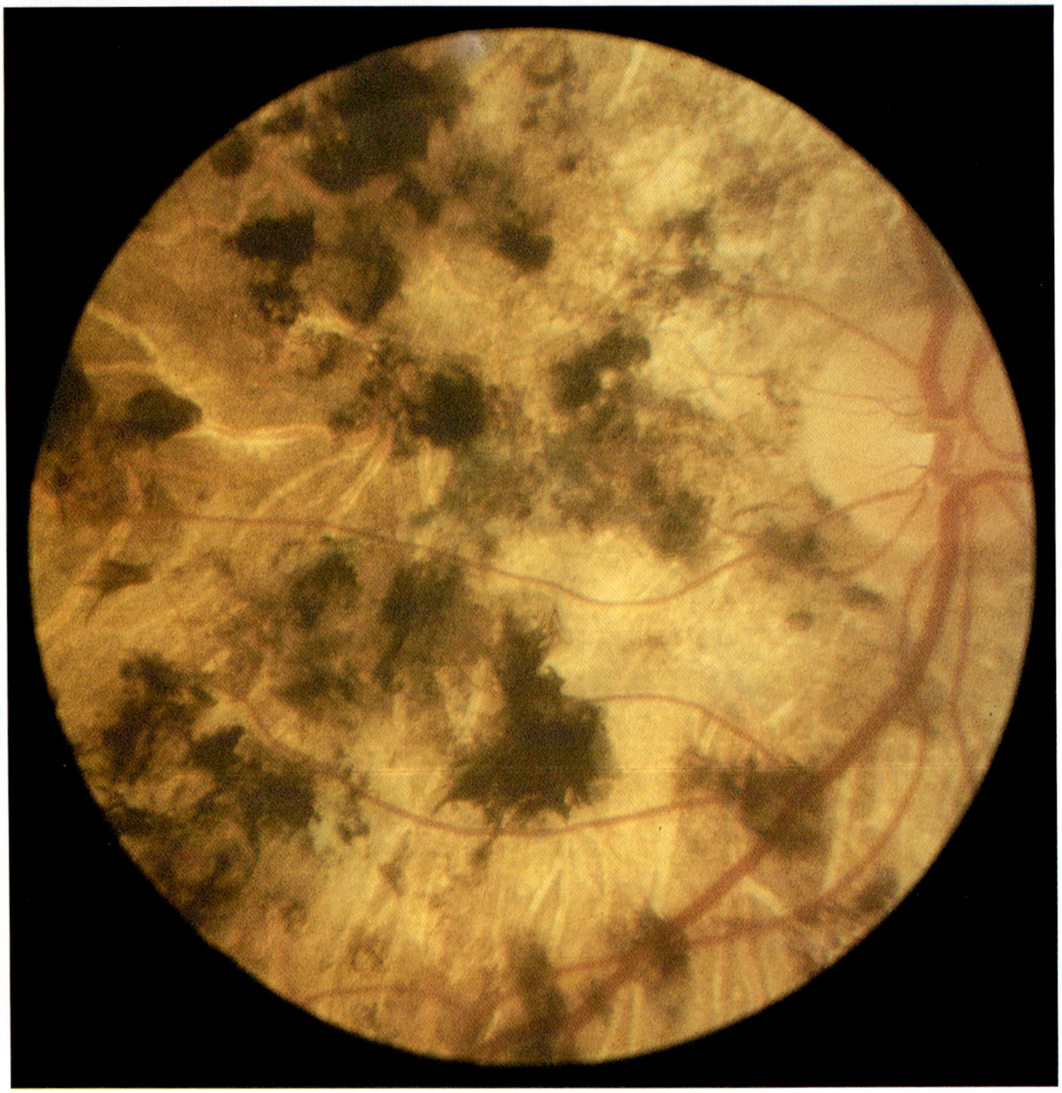

220

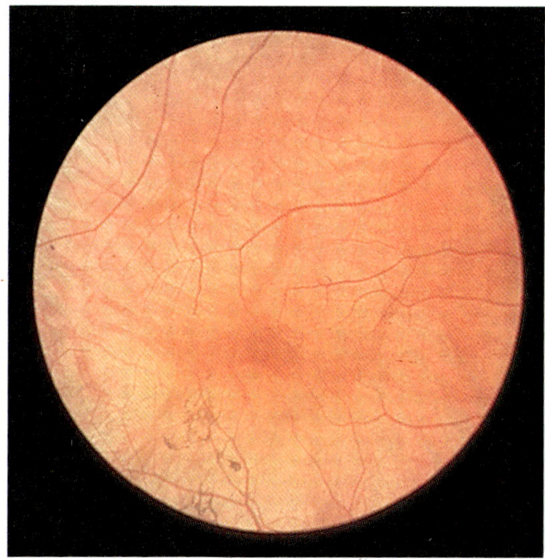
221

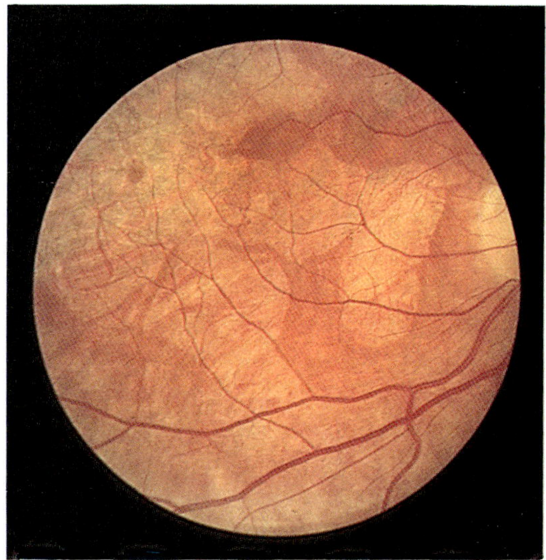
222

Figures 218 and 219. Left eye of a 46-year-old female patient with tapetoretinal degeneration.

Clinical Findings

Refraction in the right eye was −1.25 sphere, −0.75 cylinder, axis 0° for visual acuity of 20/50. In the left eye refraction was −2.0 sphere, −1.25 cylinder, axis 0° with visual acuity of 20/40. Visual field testing showed a central visual field remnant extending up to 5° from the center (Goldmann perimeter test mark III/4). The anterior segment was normal. The optic disc appeared waxy and yellow, indicating the ascending optic atrophy. The arteries are extremely narrow and straight. The temporal branches of the central retinal vein are normal; all other branches appear narrow. There are multiple obstructions of the choroidal vessels. Note the bone spicule-like pattern of hyperpigmented areas in the midperiphery of the retina (Fig. 218). The scotopic and mesopic vision was distorted.

Laboratory Findings

Cholesterol 267 mg/100 ml, triglycerides 115 mg/100 ml, very low density lipoprotein (VLDL) cholesterol 30 mg/100 ml, low density lipoprotein (LDL) cholesterol 183 mg/100 ml, high density lipoprotein (HDL) cholesterol 54 mg/100 ml (no abetalipoproteinemia).

Therapy

No therapy is known to be effective but there have been some drug trials reported.

Figure 220. Right eye of a 42-year-old female patient with old diffused chorioretinitis resembling a tapetoretinal degeneration (pseudoretinitis pigmentosa).

Clinical Findings

Refraction in both eyes was −1.0 sphere with visual acuity of light projection. Refractive media were clear. The optic disc was symmetrically waxy. The retinal veins are normal, but the retinal arteries are markedly narrowed. Note the diffuse partially accruing pigment irregularities that vary markedly in size and shape. There are round pigment clumps at the posterior pole, whereas the equatorial region has a more bone spicule-like pattern. The choroidal vessels are partially obliterated. The intervascular pigment has mostly disappeared.

Figures 221 and 222. Right and left eyes, respectively, of a 45-year-old female patient with gyrate atrophy.

Clinical Findings

The right eye had a refractive error of +1.0 sphere, −0.5 cylinder, axis 0° that corrected to 20/25. The refractive error in the left eye was +0.5 sphere, −1.0 cylinder, axis 0° for visual acuity of 20/100. Refractive media were clear and intraocular pressure in both eyes was 14 mm Hg. Both visual fields were concentrically constricted (35°). There was a hemeralopia and a distortion in color vision (tritanomaly (Panel D-15 test)). Fundus examination in the right eye shows isolated chorioatrophic lesions in the midperiphery and pericentral areas. These areas partially accrue, thus creating garland-shaped formations. The rarification of the retinal pigment epithelium and choroidal intervascular pigment allows a view of the choroidal vessels. Note the presence of partially obliterated choroidal vessels. The retinal arterioles are narrowed. The left eye (Fig. 222) shows similar findings. Note also the yellow, waxy appearance of the optic disc.

Laboratory Findings

Total cholesterol 181 mg/100 ml, HDL cholesterol 56 mg/100 ml, LDL cholesterol 115 mg/100 ml, triglycerides 49 mg/100 ml. The latter value was reconfirmed and was definitely too low, with the normal range between 74 and 172 mg/100 ml. The ornithine level was 2.2 mg/100 ml (normal value < 1.8 mg/100 ml).

Diseases of the Optic Nerve

Optic Neuritis

The term "neuritis" does not necessarily imply an inflammation. Through common usage the term has come to include a diverse group of entities caused by inflammation, vascular disease, or degeneration. The focus in this section is on inflammations affecting the optic nerve. All age groups can be affected. If the inflammation takes place anterior to the lamina cribrosa (in the immediate surroundings of the optic nerve head), the neuritis is defined as a prelaminar or intrabulbar neuritis. If located posterior to the lamina cribrosa, the inflammation is defined as a retrolaminar or retrobulbar neuritis (Figs. 223–226).

The etiology for optic disc involvement remains unknown in a high percentage of cases. Some of the possible causative factors are listed in Table 17. A careful review of the literature revealed the remarkable fact that most of the knowledge about optic neuritis is based on case reports.

Table 17. Factors That May Cause Inflammation of the Optic Nerve

Diseases of the central nervous system
Acute disseminated encephalomyelitis, neuromyelitis optica, polyradiculitis, syphilis of the central nervous system, arachnoiditis affecting the optic nerve and chiasmata

Infectious disease
Diptheria, spotted fever, influenza, congenital syphilis, malaria, mumps, typhus, paratyphus, rickettsial infections, scarlet fever, toxoplasmosis, tuberculosis, cytomegalic inclusion disease
(Occurrence in childhood is not necessarily associated with encephalitis. Occurrence is most often bilateral with a good prognosis when associated with measles, rubella, or chickenpox.)

Diseases extending onto the optic nerve
Orbit: orbital phlegmon, orbital cellulitis, subperiostal abscess
Paranasal sinuses: sinusitis, in particular, orbital infections that are derived from the posterior ethmoidal sinus
Central nervous system: meningitis (arachnoiditis, encephalitis, brain abscess)
Eye: neuroretinitis with accompanying inflammation of the optic nerve, e.g., associated with iritis, or choroiditis

Focal infections
Pyogenic infections involving tonsils, teeth, adnexa, uteri, gall bladder, urogenital tract

Prelaminar Optic Neuritis

Synonym: Papillitis.

Clinical Appearance. Clinically, this entity becomes manifest with a sudden acute or subacute visual loss, or at times complete amaurosis. Macroscopically, the eye appears quiet. Slitlamp examination, however, reveals mild to moderate vitreous infiltrates, depending on the intensity of the inflammatory process.

Ophthalmoscopical Appearance. Initially, the optic nerve head is hyperemic and therefore appears gray-red. The optic disc margins are blurred and indistinct, and the edema extends into the peripapillary areas. The central excavation may contain a grayish white exudate. The lamina cribrosa is not visible, and the optic disc may be elevated (up to 2 diopters). The retinal veins show increased tortuosity, and wide white ensheathing may be present. The arteries remain unchanged. Small, radial flame-shaped venous hemorrhages, overlying the optic disc and extending into surrounding area, may be seen.

In the late stage of postneuritic optic nerve atrophy, the optic disc is gray-white and the lamina cribrosa is masked by an avascular glial proliferation. The optic disc margin is indistinct, especially in the nasal half. Venules surrounding the optic disc remain ensheathed, but normal caliber is restored in the perimeter. In contrast to the veins, the arteries show a decreased diameter.

Differential diagnosis includes papilledemas of different etiologies, pseudopapillitis, optic nerve drusen (Table 18), and syphilitic neuroretinitis. Eye motions that cause pain may indicate myositis or a supraclinoidal aneurysm.

Retrolaminar Optic Neuritis

Synonym: Retrobulbar neuritis.

The term retrobulbar neuritis implies that the pathologic process has attacked a portion of the optic nerve behind the globe, sparing the intraocular segment. This condition is characterized by an acute onset and unilateral involvement. If the central axial part of the optic nerve (maculopapillary bundle) is affected, the condition is termed axial retrobulbar neuritis. If a complete cross section of the optic nerve shows inflammation, it is referred to as transverse retrobulbar neuritis.

Clinical Appearance. There are no external ocular changes. The disease is characterized by a temporary visual loss (sometimes amaurosis). The majority of affected patients complain of spontaneous retrobulbar pain that may be increased during eye movements or by light pressure on the globe through the closed lid. Evoking the Marcus-Gunn pupillary sign is a simple diagnostic test that indicates a retrobulbar distortion in the normal transmission of impulses between the optic disc and the optic chiasmata. This test should be used only if the refractive media are clear and other retinal diseases have been ruled out. If the patient's face is evenly illuminated—this may be determined by using a Goldmann perimeter—both pupils are equally dilated. If the healthy eye is then covered, the pupil of the affected eye dilates; when the affected eye is covered, the pupil of the normal eye does not dilate.

Ophthalmoscopical Appearance. Initially, the fundus appears normal. At times a mild hyperemia of the optic disc may be seen. In late stages, a partial temporal (in cases of axial neuritis) or complete (in cases of transverse optic neuritis) optic nerve atrophy with sharply demarcated margins can be found. In some cases, a temporal pallor of the optic disc may be observed as early as 3 weeks after the onset of symptoms (descending optic nerve degeneration). In addition to the degeneration of the optic nerve fibers, the pale discoloration of the optic nerve head is also caused by the loss of capillaries and by formation of avascular glial scar tissue.

Differential Diagnosis. The differential diagnosis of this disease includes congenital and hereditary optic atrophies (Leber's optic atrophy), as well as tumors within the medial cranial excavation (Figs. 227 and 228).

Multiple Sclerosis

Synonyms: Disseminated encephalomyelitis, polysclerosis.

Multiple sclerosis is the classic example for a disease associated with optic neuritis. Since the axons of the optic nerve posterior to the lamina cribrosa acquire a myelin sheath, the retrobulbar portion of the nerve, like white matter elsewhere throughout the central nervous system, is vulnerable to the demyelinating process that characterizes multiple sclerosis. In about 50% of cases of multiple sclerosis, retrobulbar optic neuritis is the isolated initial symptom.

Approximately twice as many women as men are affected by this quite common neurologic disease. Sixty-five percent of first manifestations are diagnosed between the 2nd and 4th decade of life, but only rarely before 20 years of age or in patients older than 50 years (Mumenthaler, 1976).

The etiology of this disease is unknown. However, several possible mechanisms, including virus infection and autoimmune disease, have been suggested as being causative. Multiple sclerosis represents an inflammatory disease of the central nervous system. Macroscopically, several irregularly disseminated demyelinated foci can be found in the brain and spinal cord. These demyelinated plaques or, in late stages, glial scars may be found within both the cortex and the white substance of the brain. They are regularly found within the ependyma surrounding the brain ventricles (especially around the bottom of the fourth ventricle and surrounding the aqueduct of the cerebrum).

New lesions show inflammatory perivascular infiltrates consisting of lymphocytes and plasma cells. The oligodendrocytes and myelin sheaths surrounding these lesions are swollen. While the axons slowly recuperate, degeneration of the myelin sheaths progresses. The ganglion cells are often undamaged. The firm consistency and gray discolorations of the well-demarcated focal lesions are caused by glial proliferation and increase of reticular fibers. The typical glial scars prompted the name "multiple sclerosis."

Involvement of the Optic Nerve. In approximately one-third of patients suffering from multiple sclerosis, the systemic clinical symptoms develop several years (sometimes up to 20 years) after optic neuritis. In other cases, optic neuritis is a secondary symptom, but in some instances the optic nerve may never be involved. Optic neuritis is primarily a retrobulbar manifestation and, rarely, takes the form of a papillitis. The inflammation is characterized by spontaneous remissions and exacerbations that are usually monocular and may vary in intensity. Paresis of the III, IV, and VI cranial nerves, most often the abducent nerve (nervus abducens), are often characteristic findings. A posterior internuclear ophthalmoplegia and a dissociated nystagmus are other ocular findings that may help in the differential diagnosis when paralysis of the eye muscles is present.

Diagnosis. In cases with optic neuritis, the etiology can not be determined solely by the presence of inflammation. An extensive exploration of the patient's medical, social, and family history is important. An occupational history should be evaluated to discover any possible environmental intoxications, and the family history should be examined for hereditary optic neuritis.

In special cases, e.g., if the patient's symptoms indicate an inflammation of the perinasal sinuses, an otolaryngologist should be consulted. Consultation with an internist may also be useful. Consultation with a neurologist is always indicated. If multiple sclerosis is suspected, magnetic resonance imaging (MRI) can now almost always provide a definite diagnosis (Rosner and Ross, 1987). In areas where an MRI is not available, some special ophthalmic methods may also be helpful in reaching a final diagnosis:

Visually evoked potentials
This test may show the impaired conductivity of the affected axons. A delay in the transmission of stimuli may also be found in patients with multiple sclerosis without a preceding optic neuritis.
Ultrasound
This test may reveal thickening of the dura mater.
Computed tomography (CT)
This test may show thickening of the optic nerve.
Fluorescein angiography
Pathologic changes may be present, especially in cases with intrabulbar optic neuritis or papillitis (Table 18).

Toxic Optic Neuritis

Synonyms: Chronic bilateral retrobulbar neuritis, intoxication amblyopia, toxic neuropathy of the optic nerve.

The term "toxic optic neuritis" includes several toxic or nutritional diseases of the optic nerve. Both eyes are usually affected, most commonly in the form of a retrobulbar neuritis. Typical examples of toxic agents that affect the optic nerve are intoxication with methyl alcohol, tobacco, and some drugs, e.g., quinine-intoxication (Figs. 227 and 228). Other pharmacologic agents that may have deleterious effects on the optic nerve are chloramphenicol, ethambutol, isoniazid, salicylic acids, some ergot-alkaloids, streptomycin, and sulfonamides.

Autointoxications may be caused by diabetes mellitus or extensive skin burns, or during menstruation, pregnancy, or lactation. The products released during severe tumor cachexia may also cause intoxication of the optic nerve.

Hereditary Optic Neuropathy

Synonym: Hereditary optic nerve atrophy.

Hereditary diseases of the optic nerve, similar to toxic optic neuritis, are not true inflammations. They actually represent primary degenerations of the retina and optic nerve. Typical examples of hereditary retinal and optic nerve atrophy are Leber's optic atrophy and Behr's optic atrophy.

Papilledema

The term "papilledema" was coined by von Graefe in 1866. Clinically, this entity most commonly indicates a rise in intracranial pressure that may be caused by a cerebral neoplasm or intracranial space-demanding abnormalities such as a brain abscess, an epidural or subdural hematoma, or syphilitic or tuberculosis granulomatosis. Primary inflammatory processes are usually absent. Functional abnormalities are also not present in the early stages, but may develop later. The German definition of the papilledema ("Stauungspapille") is limited only to diseases caused by increased intracranial pressure. In English-speaking countries, papilledema simply refers to the edematous swelling of the optic disc, and therefore also includes primary inflammatory affections of the optic nerve. In the German literature, the term "Papillenschwellung" was suggested to include a description of the edematous swelling of the optic nerve rather than increased intracranial pressure (Huber, 1956).

Papilledema represents a late symptom in cases of intracranial neoplasm (Figs. 236 and 237). This symptom may be observed in 70% of cases with tumors located inferior to the tentorium cerebelli, and in 60% of cases with tumors located superior to the tentorium cerebelli. Absence of a papilledema does not rule out brain tumors, e.g., it is absent with hypophysial tumors. The symptom of papilledema also does not allow identification of the location of the tumor (left or right brain hemisphere), and no conclusions regarding the type of tumor are possible with this finding. A papilledema is usually bilateral, but rare cases of unilateral involvement have been reported.

Fanta (1973) described an incidence of papilledema in 40.3% of 1704 cases of brain tumor. Huber (1956) reported an incidence of 59% in evaluating a series of 1166 cases. Stärk (1968) evaluated 61 cases of brain tumor in children, and found a 84% incidence of papilledema in patients with cerebral neoplasms.

In contrast to optic neuritis, papilledema does not usually cause severely impaired visual acuity. However, premonitory, transient attacks of blurred vision or amblyopic attacks may occur. These transient attacks may occur spontaneously or during body movements, e.g., while bending over. They usually last between 1 and 3 seconds and seldom exceed 30 seconds. If this time is exceeded, it is likely that a migraine headache will result. The patient may see fogged images with blurred contours, and for short periods a transient amaurosis may occur. Colorful objects are perceived differently because the color intensity and quality may be distorted, and colors are often seen as lighter and more washed out. Severe headache and optic hallucinations (perception of lightning-like flashes, sparkling stars, bright circles or rings) are sometimes seen before or after an attack.

Mild Beginning Papilledema

Signs of early papilledema or a papilledema that only partially develops include an increased hyperemia of the optic disc that causes a darker red color on the nasal side. This is basically a capillary hyperemia caused by the venous stasis. The papillary margins are slightly blurred, beginning superiorly and inferiorly and later involving the nasal and temporal areas. A translucent nasal papillary and peripapillary edema without severe elevation develops. A central excavation is still present and does not show any exudation. At this early stage, the retinal veins may show congestion and tortuosity, indicating the decreased venous outflow. The arteries usually are not changed at this early stage. Later, small linear radial hemorrhages may appear adjacent to the optic disc. A small reflex may be seen in close proximity to the papillary margin. A change in the distance of this reflex from the papillary margin may indicate a worsening of the papilledema (Vodovozov, 1981) (Figs. 229–235).

Fully Developed Papilledema

The increased capillary stasis leads to a reddish discoloration of the entire disc. Some capillaries become easily visible. Huber (1956) called this stage the papillary "plethora" (hypervolemia). The edema causes the disc margins to become increasingly indistinct and blurred. The optic disc diameter is increased, and the gray-white nerve fiber layer is accentuated. The edema overlying the nasal half of the optic disc develops faster than on the temporal side, causing a characteristic kidney-shaped appearance. During a later stage, the entire disc is more or less elevated, and it sometimes mushrooms out into the vitreous. The elevation may measure up to 9 diopters (average 2–5 diopters; 3 diopters correlate to approximately 1 mm). A periodical rhythm (within 24 hours) may develop (Fanta, 1973).

The optic cup appears narrow or may be level with the other disc tissue. The central vessels may show gray ensheathing caused by the dilatation of the perivascular lymph spaces. The papillary margin and peripapillary area may show radial dot and blot, linear, or fan-shaped hemorrhages. Less frequently, flame-shaped hemorrhages can be seen. The retinal veins are engorged and show increased tortuosity, while the arteries usually maintain their normal caliber. Therefore, the ratio in caliber of arteries and veins decreases and may become 2:5. The arteries are deflected over the disc margin and partially disappear within the edema. The presence of a positive venous pulsation does not rule out papilledema. In addition, whitish degenerative areas on the disc and surrounding tissues may be present, which can be histologically identified as cytoid bodies. According to Huber (1956), such cytoid bodies, combined with the hemorrhages, occur frequently in patients with cerebellar tumors or tumors located in the occipital part of the brain. The retina adjacent to the optic disc can have a radial fold formation that may extend into the macular region.

If the intracranial pressure is extremely elevated, a full-blown papilledema may develop within a few hours. In a patient with a medulloblastoma, a bilateral papilledema developed within 3 hours, extending to an elevation of 3 diopters (Fanta, 1973). Similarly, the development within 2 hours of a papilledema of 1 diopter elevation was observed by Zehetbauer (1977). In his case the underlying cause was an extensive intracranial hemorrhage. On the other hand, Fanta (1973) described a case in which a papilledema of 5 diopters elevation fully resolved within 10 hours. Often a papilledema caused by a cerebral tumor may develop at a very late stage, and it may take months to years before the optic nerve becomes affected.

Chronic Atrophic Stage of Papilledema

If the elevated intracranial pressure persists and no operative reduction of the pressure is achieved, the disc eventually shows a gray-white discoloration caused by a reactive glial proliferation. The disc elevation slowly decreases and the optic cup disappears. The venous stasis resolves, arteries and veins show white ensheathing, and the arteries may become narrow. The ophthalmoscopical picture is that of an optic nerve atrophy. Fanta (1973) observed that this final stage may develop within 6–8 weeks. Formation of a vascular network or growth of optociliary shunts can occur within the optic disc (Fig. 231). If the elevated intracranial pressure is released in time, the papilledema may fully resolve without causing any significant permanent damage.

As mentioned, visual acuity usually remains intact over a long period. The most important neurophthalmologic examination is visual field testing. There is a gradual, concentric enlargement of the blind spot because of an increase in the size of the edematous nerve head. Initially, the optic disc becomes enlarged horizontally rather than vertically. A vertical enlargement may be caused by angioscotomas. If macular edema is present, a relative central scotoma and sometimes a centrocecal scotoma may develop. If the papilledema progresses to the chronic, atrophic stage, the visual field becomes concentrically constricted, starting nasally (binasal hemianopsia). Later sector-shaped defects ensue. Dubois-Poulsen (1952) described as another characterisic finding an alteration in the addition of isopters surrounding the blind spot.

Measurement of the elevation of the optic disc may be performed ophthalmoscopically or retinoscopically (Heinz, 1956). Ophthalmoscopially, one has to focus on the most elevated area of the optic disc and note the diopter reading. Then a nonelevated area adjacent to the optic disc has to be measured in the same way. The difference in diopters correlates with the optic disc elevation. Retinoscopically and by using a Maddox rod, various retinal areas are measured, starting temporally, crossing the disc toward the nasal area. A diagram of the optic disc elevation is the result.

Fluorescein angiography reveals vascular abnormalities and alterations in vascular permeability. However, this method does not allow for an exact etiological differentiation of the papillitis.

Alterations in Vascular Permeability and Vascular Leakage. These abnormalities represent the cardinal symptom and are found usually in an early stage of the disease.

Vascular Changes. Dilatation of the optic disc capillaries and the area immediately surrounding the disc is found. The capillaries are markedly tortuous, and variciform dilatations and microaneurysms are often present. The arterial phase and the venous phase of the angiography are more prolonged than normal. Because of the vascular leakage, there is a homogeneous fluorescence of the optic disc that persists for several hours.

Neurological and neurosurgical consultations are always necessary. The neurologic examination should include such tests as an EEG, echoencephalography, electronystagmography, specific neurologic roentgenograms of the cranium and the vertebral column, examinations using radiopaque material (i.e, pneumoencephalography, ventriculography, cerebral angiography, pneumomyelography, angiography of the vertebral column and spinal cord), computed tomography, magnetic resonance imaging (MRI), radioactive tests, and special laboratory diagnostic tests.

Other nonocular symptoms that frequently occur as the disease progresses are beyond the scope of this atlas textbook.

Differential Diagnosis. The differential diagnosis includes a variety of diseases such as prelaminar optic neuritis (papillitis), central retinal vein occlusion, pseudoneuritis or pseudopapilledema, optic disc drusen, hypertensive retinopathy, eclamptic retinopathy, pseudotumor cerebri, vascular pseudopapillitis, and papilledema associated with blood disorders (anemia, leukemia, polycythemia). Other causes include pulmonary disorders (emphysema associated with chronic bronchitis, cardiac insufficiency, bronchiectasia associated with cardiac insufficiency), stenosis of the pulmonary artery, diseases of the heart (severe congenital or acquired heart malformations), tumors of the optic disc (glioma, melanoma, melanocytoma, meningioma, neurinoma, neurofibroma), asssociated with anomalies of the retinal vessels (Wyburn-Mason syndrome), and retinitis and choroiditis of different etiologies.

Therapy. Once identified, the underlying disease should be treated first. In patients with chronic papilledema, i.e., with pseudotumor cerebri, the broad excision of the optic nerve sheaths have been reported to be successful (Herzau et al., 1983).

Etiology of bilateral papilledema (the examples are not listed according to their incidence):

Increased volume of the brain substance (the primary lesion is located within the brain, often associated with perifocal edema).

Brain tumor: cerebral neoplasm (primary tumor or metastases).

Brain tumor in its broadest sense: *Abscess:* derived from auricular or nasal infections, either directly spread from neighboring structures, spread via the blood or lymph channels, or traumatically spread. *Aneurysm:* granulomata (tuberculosis, syphilis, reticulohistocytic granulomatous encephalitis, sarcoidosis. *Hematoma:* epidural, subdural, subarachnoidal. *Cysts: Echinococcus alveolaris,* cysticercosis.

Circulatory irregularities of the cerebrospinal fluid and/or changes in fluid resorption. Cervical discus prolapse, tumors of the spinal cord.

Increased volume of the cerebrospinal fluid: hydrocephalus caused by hypersecretions of fluids or reduced resorption, encephalitis, meningitis (infectious, serous, purulent, acute syphilis, tuberculosis, infections caused by trauma).

Reduction of the outflow of cerebrospinal fluid: occlusive hydrocephalus, septic or aseptic thrombosis of the brain veins or the dural sinuses.

Secondary to decreased volume of intracranial space: craniosynostosis (oxycephaly, Crouzon's disease).

Etiology of unilateral papilledema (only rarely associated with intracranial pressure elevation):

Foster-Kennedy syndrome (tumor of the frontal brain), meningiomas of the II cranial nerve and wings of the sphenoidal bone (direct spread into the orbit), brain tumor associated with monocular myopia exceeding 5 diopters, associated with other osseous anomalies of the cranium.

Monocular papilledema may be defined as a process associated with orbital involvement (abscess, aneurysms, edema, phlegm, and tumor), or associated with ocular involvement (papilledema caused by perforating trauma, fistulating operations, or cataract extractions) (see Fig. 316).

Pseudotumor Cerebri

Synonym: Benign (idiopathic) intracranial hypertension.

Although papilledema and increased cerebrospinal fluid pressure usually have an expanding intracranial mass as the common denominator, occasionally there are cases in which no mass or alteration in the composure of the cerebrospinal fluid can be found. Some possible underlying diseases may be sinus thrombosis, multiple sclerosis, eclamptic pseudouremia, blunt head trauma, acute leukemia, pulmonary emphysema, and defects of the parathyroid glands following a thyroid operation (Sachsenweger, 1975). In most cases, however, the underlying etiology remains unclear.

Female patients seem to be most frequently affected. The major clinical symptoms consist of a chronic headache combined with transient attacks of blurred vision occurring at irregular intervals. These attacks may be perceived as blurred or fogged images that last only seconds or for several minutes.

Some cases resolve spontaneously within 1 year, and the intracerebral pressure returns to normal. Other cases have a chronic course that may persist over several years and finally cause irreversible optic nerve damage.

Ophthalmoscopical Appearance. Bilateral papilledema is a major symptom. The transition into the chronic, atrophic stage with associated functional losses affecting visual acuity, visual fields, and dark adaptation is always possible. Characteristic or specific visual field alterations do not exist; however, lesions of the nerve fibers and concentric constriction of the visual field have been most commonly observed.

Therapy. Creating a broad surgical opening of the optic nerve sheaths to release pressure seems to be helpful in cases of pressure-induced optic nerve damage (Herzau et al., 1983). According to the most recent research, a pressure release that involves the entire cerebrospinal fluid system is not necessary.

Optic Disc Drusen

Synonyms: Colloid bodies, hyaline bodies, colloid formations, hyaline excrescences, verrucosités hyalines (French).

The first ophthalmoscopical description of optic disc drusen was by von Liebreich in 1868 (German, "Drusenpapille").

Clinical Appearance. In most cases, no subjective symptoms exist and the drusen are found during a routine ophthalmoscopical examination (Fig. 243). In a few cases, headaches may be an early symptom. Distortions of visual acuity and visual fields are explained by pressure damage of the nerve fibers. A reduced visual acuity is only rarely found in cases of primary idiopathic drusen of the optic disc. Quite often visual field testing reveals an enlargement of the blind spot, sometimes concentric constriction of the visual field, and pericentral scotomas. Sometimes flickering scotomas, transitory blindness, transitory eye muscle paresis, and epileptic seizures may supplement the symptomatology.

Ophthalmoscopical Appearance. Clinical examination frequently reveals an irregular, nodular, mulberry-like appearance of the optic disc surface. The lesions are white or whitish yellow, appear translucent, and may be isolated or in groups. Both monocular and binocular involvement is possible. The drusen material supposedly represents degenerative products of the axoplasm. The drusen may extend onto the retina adjacent to the optic disc and may be associated with retinal hemorrhages (parapapillary, peripapillary, and juxtapapillary). Initially, the blocked lymph flow creates blurred papillary margins, and in later stages may resemble papilledema. The papillary elevation measures between 1 and 3 diopters; in exceptional cases, up to 10 diopters of elevation has been described. It is necessary to differentiate between visible and deeply located ("buried") drusen (Figs. 238–242).

Histopathologically, drusen of the optic disc are composed of concentric laminations with no cellular structure or capsule. These hyaline deposits can be prelaminar or situated within the lamina cribrosa. Frequently the drusen become calcified. Optic disc drusen have an incidence of 3.4% in the general population.

Two types of drusen have been identified by the pathogenesis: (*a*) primary (idiopathic) drusen are stationary lesions and show progression in only 17% of cases; and (*b*) secondary drusen are associated with various ocular disorders, such as juvenile glaucoma, simple glaucoma, absolute glaucoma, buphthalmia, chorioretinitis, optic neuritis, intoxications (ethyl alcohol, lead, tobacco), uveal tumors, circulatory disorders within the optic nerve head, embolic occlusion of the central retinal artery, central vein thrombosis, and trauma. If drusen are associated with tapetoretinal degenerations, a severe visual loss is typical.

To a lesser extent, drusen also can be found in craniopharyngioma, meningioma, and arachnoiditis of the optic nerve and optic chiasma. Occasionally, drusen result from such systemic diseases as bronchial asthma, arterial hypertension, and nephritis. Optic disc drusen

Table 18. Differential Diagnosis Papilledema/Papillitis/Pseudopapillitis

	Papilledema	Papillitis
Etiology	Various causes	Congenital anomaly of optic disc
Location	Most often bilateral (unilateral occurrence may indicate orbital lesions)	Most often unilateral (exceptions: meningitis, infectious diseases of childhood)
Functional disorders (preexisting diseases of the optic disc and retina; opacification of the media and amblyopia are not considered)		
Visual acuity	Initially normal, very slowly progressive loss of visual acuity, often within months. Patient's history: amblyopic episodes	Immediate marked reduction
Visual field	Defects vary according to location and extent of involvement of the visual tract; blind spot enlarged in early phase	Central scotoma
Light perception	Normal	Pathologic
Ophthalmoscopical appearance		
Optic disc		
Margins	Blurred, serous, peripapilledema	Blurred (inflammatory, proteinaceous, peripapillary exudates)
Diameter	Appears enlarged	Appears enlarged
Color	Initially moderate redness (capillary stasis), later gray-red appearance, radial hemorrhages	Dark beefy-red (severe hyperemia), sometimes radial hemorrhages
Elevation	Up to 12 diopters possible Initially edema of the nasal half, translucent, slowly progressive occlusion of optic cup, finally mushroom-shaped elevation into vitreous	Up to 2 diopters Edema appears about 2 weeks after onset without treatment; cloudy, muddy swelling
Optic cup	No exudate; in advanced stages central excavation is leveled	Central excavation leveled early (inflammatory exudates)
Retina		
Vessels	Arteries narrow	Decreased artery diameter indicative for prognosis of final visual acuity
	Veins are dilated; brighter and darker vascular segments can be seen	Venous outflow obstruction; peripapillary vascular ensheathing
Parenchyma	Initially isolated; in later stages multiple radial hemorrhages surrounding optic disc	Hemorrhages, at times adjacent to optic disc
	Exudates (cotton wool spots indicating ischemic areas), degenerative lesions	Exudates, age-related drusen, small punctate exudates
Radial retinal folds	Present	Absent
Fluorescein angiography	Angiogram reveals dilated capillaries overlying the elevated optic disc and its immediate surroundings; capillaries show increased tortuosity and variciform appearance; microaneurysms present, arterial and venous phases are delayed; leading symptom is vascular leakage	Congested capillaries overlying optic disc and immediate surroundings, severe vascular leakage, vessels partially masked by exudates; in late stages details cannot be discriminated
Prognosis	Papilledema may fully resolve if underlying cause is corrected within a few weeks; persistent papilledema will lead to secondary optic atrophy	Often transition into optic atrophy (temporal)

Pseudopapillitis (pseudoneuritis)
Same
Most often bilateral
Not affected; often occurs in hyperopic eyes; pseudoneuritis, hypermetropia also seen
No defects, blind spot rarely enlarged
Normal
Blurred, no edema
Not enlarged
Normal vital disc coloration (tan) depending on number of epipapillary capillaries and blood flow in capillaries
Up to 2 diopters Mild, cone-shaped elevation into vitreous
Central excavation normal
Arteries not affected, sometimes tortuosity of vessels Vascular ensheathing sometimes present
No hemorrhages No exudates
Absent
Well-demarcated papillary margins with no vascular changes or leakage
No transition into optic atrophy

may also be associated with Alport's syndrome, Groenblad-Strandberg syndrome, and Bourneville's disease.

Prognosis. The diagnostic procedure includes a neurophthalmological examination and an extremely thorough ophthalmoscopical examination. Photographic documentation of the lesion, as well as a controlled follow-up, are strongly recommended.

These diagnostic procedures may be supplemented by ophthalmochromoscopy (indirect red light) and fluorescein angiography. These methods may help to detect deeply buried drusen. If indicated, general internal and neurologic examinations, including computed tomography, should be performed. The fellow eye has to be evaluated for anomalies of the optic disc vessels and retinal vessels.

The examination of family members for similar findings may help to confirm the diagnosis.

Differential Diagnosis. The primary differential diagnosis includes such entities as papilledema, papillitis associated with optic disc drusen, and pseudopapillitis (see Table 18, Figs. 244–247).

Therapy. There is no drug treatment that has been shown to have any impact on the formation of drusen. Pharmacologic trials with anabolic hormones and vitamins C and E have been reported in the literature, but long-term results are not available.

Papilledema Associated with Iridocyclitis

Papilledema may be found with several inflammatory disorders such as iridocyclitis (Figs. 248–250), choroiditis, and periphlebitis of the retina.

Ophthalmoscopical Appearance. The optic disc shows a papilledema with elevations between 1 and 3 diopters and, in rare cases, up to 6 diopters. The area involved may measure 2–4 disc diameters. The entire posterior pole may become involved, and an isolated retinal detachment may occur. Once the edema resolves, circular retinal folds, extending between the optic disc and the macular region, and radial folds along the posterior pole may be observed. The optic cup contains exudate, and at times a veil-like white tissue proliferation may be present that resembles an epipapillary membrane. The central retinal vessels may become ensheathed. Papillary and peripapillary capillaries show increased blood filling and microaneurysms. The retinal veins are engorged and show increased tortuosity. Neovascularization and shunts may be observed. Sometimes transient microhemorrhages may be found. A slitlamp examination reveals pigmented, keratic precipitates and, more often, cellular infiltrates within the vitreous. Fluorescein angiography does not permit an accurate differentiation between this entity and a true papilledema. If the papilledema precedes the iridocyclitic inflammation, most cases have a good prognosis. However, the papilledema may persist over years. Visual acuity may be reduced by cystoid macular edema, which sometimes imitates a retinal hole.

Papilledema Caused by Chloroquine Therapy. Side effects of this drug are observed if a yearly dosage of 300 grams is exceeded (Fig. 253, Table 19).

Table 19. Side Effects of Chloroquine and Its Derivatives

Lids
- Ptosis

Ocular muscles
- Strabismus, bilateral paresis of IV cranial nerve

Conjunctiva plica semilunaris, caruncle
- Blue-grayish pigmentation

Cornea
- Gray to gray-brown pigmentations (deposition of chloroquine or its metabolized side products interepithelially, within Bowman's membrane, or in the superficial corneal stroma). These pigmentations are usually located between the palpebral margins or in the lower third of the cornea. Corneal sensitivity is also decreased; corneal nerves are thickened and show small nodules at branchings.

Lens
- Cataract (cupuliform cataract)

Retina, retinal vessels, optic nerve
- Maculopathy ("bull's-eye macula") (Fig. 253), macular edema, peripheral pigment irregularities (differential diagnosis: retinitis pigmentosa), optic nerve atrophy (neurotoxic effect), segmental constriction of the retinal vessels (vasoconstrictive effect)

Visual field
- Pericentral, central, and ring scotomas

Color vision
- Distortion in red-green discrimination

Subjective symptoms
- Perception of glimmer and flicker, perception of colored rings surrounding light sources, photophobia, feeling of pressure within or behind the eye, distortion in visual acuity and accommodation

Acute Ischemic Optic Neuropathy

Synonyms: Apoplexia papillae, arteriosclerotic papillitis, optic nerve infarction, ischemic optic neuritis, ischemic optic neuropathy, vascular pseudopapillitis, anterior ischemic optic neuropathy.

The different etiologies of acute ischemic optic neuropathy are listed in Table 20. In 50% of cases, this condition is unilateral, with bilateral occurrence an exception (Figs. 251 and 252). The interval between involvement of the first and second eye may be 1-7 years.

The patient's history reveals prodromi of short duration including blurred vision or amaurosis fugax that oc-

Table 20. Causes of Vascular Pseudopapillitis (Hayreh, 1975)

Allergic diseases
- Serum sickness (immune complex disease), BCG vaccination, paratyphus A and B, urticaria, Quincke edema

Hematologic diseases
- Several types of anemia including pernicious anemia and sickle cell disease, leukemia, thrombopenia, chlorosis, idiopathic polycythemia

Cardiovascular diseases
- Heart diseases, heart valve malformation, myocardial infarction
- *Vascular diseases:* generalized atherosclerosis, arteriosclerosis, arterial hypertension, arterial hypotension
- *Generalized arteritis (arteriasis):* endangiitis obliterans, Winiwarter-Bürger disease (thromboangiitis obliterans), Takayasu's disease (pulseless disease), Horton's arteritis (temporal or giant cell arteritis).
- *Arteritis associated with connective tissue diseases:* polyarteritis nodosa, lupus erythematosus
- *Vasomotor disorders:* Raynaud's disease, migraine, disorders of the cervical discs (C_4-C_7), stenosis of the internal carotid artery

Metabolic diseases
- Diabetes mellitus

Disorders of the endocrine system
- Graves' disease, and following thyroidectomy and thyrostatic therapy

Infections
- Ocular herpes zoster, syphilis

Posthemorrhagic amaurosis
- Caused by extensive hemorrhage (major sources of extensive blood loss: intestinal tract, uterus, and, less frequently, rhinogenous hemorrhages or hemorrhages from kidneys, lungs, and open wounds)

Ocular diseases
- Glaucoma, including low tension glaucoma, caused by compression of the optic disc blood vessels (peripapillary malignant melanoma, glioma, drusen) or retrobulbar compression of the blood flow (endocrine exophthalmus, retrobulbar tumor, pseudotumor orbita), orbital trauma

cur hours or days before the acute symptoms of the fully developed anterior ischemic optic neuropathy becomes manifest. This enitity is found more often in people of middle age rather than in the elderly. Most cases are seen between 45 and 50 years of age. Predisposing factors are arterial vascular disorders such as arterial hypertension, arteriosclerosis, and diabetes mellitus.

Arteriosclerotic narrowing and/or occlusion is the most common cause of anterior ischemic optic neuropathy, usually affecting the posterior ciliary arteries or the axial vessels of the optic nerve within the segment of the nerve immediately adjacent to the globe.

Ophthalmoscopical Appearance. The acute stage shows a papilledema involving the entire optic disc or a large sector of it. The peripapillary region also becomes edematous, but the optic disc elevation rarely exceeds 2 diopters. The optic disc is initially hyperemic, but often within hours becomes markedly pale ("pale papilledema," François, 1975). This pale stage is followed by a temporary capillary hyperemia that makes the optic nerve pink, but the pale appearance returns. This final stage may also involve only one sector of the disc (sector-shaped papilledema) (Figs. 254–256). The optic cup becomes level with the surrounding disc tissue. Flame-shaped hemorrhages supplement the clinical appearance. Sometimes isolated, soft exudates (cotton wool spots) are seen adjacent to the optic disc. The arteries are narrowed, and the veins are engorged and tortuous. The fellow eye often shows arteriosclerotic or hypertensive vascular changes.

The differential diagnosis may become complicated if the vascular papilledema suddenly affects the otherwise healthy fellow eye. If the patient's history is unknown, the appearance of both eyes may resemble the Foster-Kennedy syndrome. This syndrome, usually associated with tumors of the frontal brain, the II cranial nerve, or the spenoidal bone, is characterized by the simultaneous appearance of papilledema in one eye and optic nerve atrophy in the other eye. If such a combination is observed, caused by a vascular pseudopapillitis, it is more correctly termed pseudo-Foster-Kennedy syndrome.

Diagnostic Procedure and Findings. The sedimentation rate is moderately increased. A temporal artery biopsy should be performed to rule out a hidden temporal arteritis (see "Temporal Arteritis"). While visual acuity remains intact, visual fields may show a variety of defects. Arcuate or sector-shaped defects, mostly in the inferior nasal quadrant, up to a complete hemianopsia caused by a slow extension of the defect, may be found depending on the extent of damage to the nerve fiber layer. The visual field may also show concentric constrictions. A central scotoma may be caused by affection of the macular bundle of nerve fibers or by the associated macular edema. Other cases show a superior hemianopia or superior sector-shaped visual field losses.

According to Reuscher and coauthors (1978), fluorescein angiography is not helpful in locating the vascular occlusive process or rendering a differential diagnosis of optic nerve ischemia versus papilledema caused by different etiologies. As in all papilledema, an increased fluorescence of the optic disc is found. Only rarely, and often only in the initial phase, a sector-shaped, nonprofusive area may be found within the capillary filling of the optic disc. Both ERG and EOG remain unchanged if only the optic nerve is affected, which is most often the case. An ophthalmodynamography reveals reduced pulsation volumes on the affected side. Doppler sonography may be used to rule out a distortion of the blood flow within the carotid artery. Retinal doppler sonography also may be useful.

Therapy. The prognosis regarding final visual acuity is usually poor. One may try a therapeutic regimen of corticosteroids for 2 months. Initially, 18 mg should be given systemically, and the dosage should then be tapered slowly. As previously mentioned, a temporal artery biopsy should be performed. Drugs that increase blood perfusion may be useful (Huismans, 1978a). Acetazolamide (Diamox), administered intravenously or orally, can reduce the intraocular pressure (Hayreh, 1975). The use of anticoagulants also has been proposed (Saraux and Murat, 1967).

Temporal Arteritis

Synonyms: Horton's arteritis, cranial arteritis (superficial, diffuse) generalized granulomatous arteritis, periarteritis segmentalis superficialis, giant cell arteritis, polymyalgia arteritica.

This entity was first described in 1890 by Hutchinson, who correctly termed it "arteritis of the aged." A systematic investigation of this disease, which is a generalized immunologic vasculitis of old age, was performed by Horton and coworkers in 1932. Temporal arteritis usually becomes manifest in the 6th decade of life (Figs. 257–269).

Clinical Appearance. The major clinical symptoms are the triad of headache, prominence and knottiness of the superificial temporal artery, and increased erythrocyte sedimentation rate. The headache is usually severe, and attacks most often occur during the night. The headache is perceived as a diffuse unilateral or bilateral temporal pain with projections into the back of the head, orbit, maxillae, nose, and ears. A typically prominent temporal artery can be found in 40% of cases. The artery appears tortuous, nodular, and thickened and shows no pulsation. It is extremely tender to the touch. The sedimentation rate is markedly increased. A Westergren finding of 90–100 mm within the first hour is not uncommon.

Other clinical findings include a prodromal stage of this disease marked by increased body temperature and general illness (weakness, loss of appetite, weight loss, depression). Soon rheumatoid symptoms such as pain in muscles and joints, especially in the neck, shoulder, and hip, may ensue. Another interesting finding is that the muscles of the jaw and tongue may become tired and painful, causing difficulty with normal articulation and eating. The skin of the head may become tender, and occasionally areas of localized gangrene are seen. Severe complications include myocardial infarction and cerebral apoplexy. In 10% of cases the disease ends in death.

Laboratory tests show an increased α_2-globulin fraction, increased serum copper, and a decreased iron level. These findings indicate an acute inflammation. Furthermore, leukocytosis and sometimes thrombocytosis may be found. The differential white blood cell count shows an eosinophilia. Alkaline phosphatase levels are increased. Other enzyme levels usually are normal. Rheumatoid factor, antinuclear antibodies, and tests for lupus erythematosus are negative. The C-refractive protein is positive.

Mild or occult temporal arteritis is a concealed form of this disease that is often misdiagnosed. In this form, the temporal artery is found to be normal during manual palpation. Other general typical symptoms may be absent or follow the ocular findings at a later stage.

The eyes are involved in 50% of cases. Simultaneous bilateral involvement is only rarely found. The fellow eye usually becomes affected after an interval of 1-3 weeks. Three different ophthalmoscopical appearances may be present: (*a*) the optic disc may appear normal (the vasular occlusion is extrabulbar within the orbital portion of the central retinal artery); (*b*) an ischemic papilledema may be present; and (*c*) there may be a retinal ischemia caused by a branch or central artery occlusion.

The prognosis for retention of good visual acuity is negative in the 25% of cases in which monocular or binocular amaurosis develops. Other ocular findings include eye muscle paresis, mostly affecting the III and VI cranial nerves.

A temporal artery biopsy serves a diagnostic and therapeutic purpose. According to Siegenthaler and Siegenthaler (1961), the vasoconstrictive stimulus that precedes a reduced blood supply within the collateral system is eliminated when the affected portion of the artery is removed. Histopathologically, the biopsy reveals an arterial wall that is thickened by a granulomatous, inflammatory process (eosinophils, lymphocytes, and plasma cells). Characteristic findings are Langhans' giant cells and fibroblasts. The cellular infiltrate extends outwardly, involving the adventitia of the vessel, and inwardly, involving the inner elastic lamina, which becomes thickened and fragmented. The vascular lumen, which is already narrowed by the cellular infiltrates in the vessel wall, often becomes completely occluded by a secondary thrombosis. Ischemic, necrotic areas result.

A false-negative biopsy may be explained by the spotty, segmental occurrence of the infiltrates within the vessel walls. Because of these "skip lesions," it may be necessary to remove several arterial sections to verify the presence of the disease.

Differential Diagnosis. The differential diagnosis includes vascular diseases of different etiologies, malignant tumors, metastases, plasmacytoma, carcinosis of the meninges, chronic meningeal tuberculosis, dermatomyositis, periarteritis humeroscapularis, entrapment neuropathy, polyneuritis, or otitis external maligna.

Therapy. In addition to an arterial biopsy, treatment with prednisolone for 12-18 months is indicated.

Optic Atrophy

The ultimate sequela of progressive optic nerve disorders is optic atrophy. Different diseases may cause this final loss of conductive function of the optic nerve (the III neuron). The type of optic atrophy depends on the pathogenetic factor involved and its location. The two important categories of optic atrophy are an ascending atrophy, in which the primary lesion is situated at the retinal level, and a descending optic atrophy, in which the primary lesion is located intracranially, in the retrobulbar optic nerve, the chiasma, or within the optic tract. Different etiologies for optic atrophy are listed in Table 21.

Ophthalmoscopical Appearance. The physiologic, vital red-yellow color of the optic disc changes to white-gray or yellow-white. This pallor may develop at different times, depending on the underlying cause for the optic disc atrophy. In traumatic cases, for example, it lasts between 3 and 4 weeks until the entire disc or temporal half of the disc undergoes these changes. That this is the most commonly affected site is explained by the anatomical course of the maculopapillary bundle. In extreme cases, the pallescense may cause a stark-white appearance. However, the degree of paleness cannot necessarily be correlated with the extent of functional loss. With visual acuity, in particular, a marked discrepancy is sometimes found. A classic example of this is an optic atrophy caused by multiple sclerosis. With this disease, the degenerative processs primarily affects the myelin sheaths but the axons remain intact for a longer time. Paleness of the optic disc is caused by the degeneration of nerve fibers and subsequent glial proliferation, as well as by the loss of minute capillaries that normally impart a pink color to the nerve head. The glial, fibrous tissue proliferation accentuates the white appearance of the disc because the newly formed tissue lacks vessels and has a very dense scar-like structure. Especially in a patient who has a preexisting large optic cup that shows only a mild glial proliferation, a plate-shaped or cup-shaped atrophic excavation with a visible lamina cribrosa pattern may result. Because it is a part of the brain, the optic nerve has almost no regenerative capacity.

The disc margins may appear well-defined (in cases of a simple optic atrophy) or blurred (in cases of an optic nerve atrophy following papillitis). The latter finding is sometimes seen with retinal optic atrophies. The vasular pattern in optic atrophies of different etiologies is listed in Table 22.

Table 21. Etiologies of Optic Atrophy

Simple, genuine atrophic atrophy (atrophia optici simplex)
Congenital (embryopathy)
Virus infections (infectious hepatitis, mumps, rubella), congenital syphilis, congenital toxoplasmosis. All these conditions represent a postneuritic optic atrophy
Hereditary (hereditary degenerative diseases of the central nervous system
Behr's disease (complicated heredofamilial optic atrophy), Friedreich's ataxia (hereditary spinal ataxia, heredoataxia), Marie's ataxia (hereditary cerebellar ataxia)
Cerebral sclerotic syndromes
Tuberous sclerosis (Bourneville's disease, epiloia), Krabbe's syndrome (diffuse, infantile familial sclerosis representing one form of progressive cerebral leukodystrophies; also called globoid cell leukodystrophy), Merzbacher-Pelizaeus disease (early, infantile form of progressive cerebral leukodystrophy), Schilder's disease (encephalitis periaxialis diffusa), Scholz' disease (subacute, juvenile form of metachromatic leukodystrophy), Unverricht's disease (progressive familial myoclonus epilepsy)
Neural muscular atrophy
Charcot-Marie-Tooth disease (peroneal muscular atrophy), Déjérine-Sottas disease (hereditary hypertrophic neuropathy)
Cranial and skeletal anomalies
Apert's syndrome (acrocephalosyndactyly), Van Buchem's syndrome (familial generalized cortical hyperostosis), Crouzon's syndrome (craniofacial dysostosis), Pyle's syndrome (familial metaphysial dystrophy), Uehlinger's syndrome (generalized hyperostosis, acropachyderma), Albers-Schönberg syndrome (osteopetrosis)
Dermatoses
Bloch-Sulzberger disease (incontinentia pigmenti), Goltz syndrome (focal dermal hypoplasia)
Disorders of the lipid metabolism
Neuroaxonal dystrophy, Tay-Sachs disease (infantile type of cerebral sphingolipidosis)
Leber's disease (heredofamilial optic atrophy)
Acquired optic atrophy
Severe hemorrhage (gastrointestinal tract, pregnancy, abortion)
Pernicious anemia: Biermer's disease
Vascular causes
Arteriosclerosis of the internal carotid artery or ophthalmic artery, central retinal vein occlusions of different etiologies, Takayasu's syndrome, temporal arteritis
Demyelinating diseases
Multiple sclerosis
Infection
Syphilis, tabes dorsalis
Intoxication
Optic nerve neuropathy
Systemic diseases
Paget's disease (osteitis deformans)
Trauma
Fractures of cranial bones, windshield and shotgun wounds
Tumors
Chiasmatic syndrome caused by intra- and extracellular pituitary adenomas, intra- and extracellular cranial pharyngeomas, supracellular meningiomas, supracellular chiasma leiomyoma, supraclinoid aneurysm, arachnoiditis of the optic chiasma, Jacod's syndrome (total ophthalmoplegia, blindness, and trigeminal neuralgia caused by tumors of the epipharynx), foramen lacerum aperture, fasciculitis opticus
Postneuritic optic atrophy
Intrabulbar optic neuritis (papillitis), retrobulbar optic neuritis.
(Note: An identical optic disc appearance also can be found in cases of chronic, atrophic papilledema.)
Retinal optic atrophy
Persistent retinal detachment, severe chorioretinitis, macular diseases, macular degenerations (including Stargardt's disease), excessive myopia, tapetoretinal degenerations
Glaucomatous optic atrophy
Chronic glaucoma, including low tension glaucoma

The abundance of different etiologies and clinical variations preclude a listing of typical subjective symptoms and characteristic findings associated with optic atrophies. Therefore, only a few examples may be mentioned.

Visual Acuity. In cases of ischemic optic neuropathy, the visual acuity is acutely and severely affected. A more slowly progressive visual loss is observed in glaucomatous patients.

Pupillary Reactions. An Argyll Robertson pupil is very suggestive of neurosyphilis associated with tabes dorsalis (70% of cases). An absolutely nonresponsive pupil, which develops immediately, is observed in patients with severe optic nerve trauma.

Visual Fields. Arcuate scotomas are found in glaucomatous eyes, and a "gun barrel" visual field characterizes cases of advanced pigmentary degenerations. A lesion of the optic chiasma is manifest as an almost symmetrical visual field loss that begins superotemporally and advances to a bitemporal hemianopsia. Leber's optic atrophy, however, is typically associated with a bilateral, absolute central scotoma.

Dark Adaptation. Night vision is affected early in retinal pigment degenerations (hemeralopia). The adaptation graph typically lacks the Kohlrausch bend.

Color Vision. In cases of Leber's optic atrophy, deuteranopic changes have been described. In cases of infantile optic atrophy, a pseudotritanopia may be present.

Electroretinogram. In patients with amaurosis caused by total optic atrophy, a normal ERG often can be found. In cases of retinal optic atrophy, the ERG usually shows pathologic changes or it may be extinguished (tapetoretinal degenerations).

Diagnostic Guidelines If Optic Atrophy Is Diagnosed for the First Time

1. Extensive exploration of the patient's own and familial history (may include examination of other family members).
2. Basic ophthalmic examinations: testing of visual acuity, refraction, tests for binocular vision, neurophthalmologic tests (for pupillary

Table 22. Ophthalmoscopic Findings in Optic Nerve Atrophy (Differential Diagnosis)

Different Types of Optic Nerve Atrophy	Ophthalmoscopical Findings: Optic Disc	Ophthalmoscopical Findings: Retinal Vessels (Arteries and Veins)	Ophthalmoscopical Findings: Posterior Pole Retinal Periphery
Simple, complete optic atrophy	Color: all different degrees of pallor, gray-yellow, whitish-gray to bright white Margins: well-demarcated Lamina cribrosa: often visible	Retinal vessels not involved or narrowed and elongated, caliber irregularities of the arteries at times, arteriosclerosis	Vascular optic atrophy, age-related drusen, macular degenerations, macular star figure, O-shaped depigmentations
Partial (temporal or sector-shaped) optic atrophy	Color: temporal or sector-shaped disc paleness		
Postneuritic optic atrophy, papillitis (differential diagnosis), chronic papilledema, or optic atrophy following papilledema	Color: gray-white Margins: blurred or slightly prominent Lamina cribrosa: often not visible Peripapillary area: pigment irregularities at times	Vessels partially constricted, tortuous, vessels may show thickening of walls and white-grayish ensheathings (especially in close proximity to the optic disc)	
Retrobulbar optic neuritis	Findings similar to those described with simple, complete optic atrophy		
Retinal optic atrophy	Color: waxy, yellowish Margins: well-demarcated or slightly blurred Lamina cribrosa: often not visible	All vessels, especially arteries, extremely narrow ("thin as a thread")	Pigmentary degeneration: brown-black bone spicule-like pigmentations
Glaucomatous optic atrophy	Color: gray-white Margins: well-demarcated Lamina cribrosa: visible Peripapillary area: glaucomatous halo Optic cup and vascular trunk: nasal displacement of the central retinal vessels, curving around the margins of the excavated disc		

motility), test for Marcus Gunn pupil, tests for nystagmus, tests of eye motility, exophthalmometer measurements, tests for corneal sensitivity, visual field tests, ophthalmoscopical optic disc evaluation and photographic documentation, slitlamp examination, tomography, tests for dark adaptation, color vision testing, blood pressure measurements on both arms, sedimentation rate, ophthalmodynamography, and doppler sonography (carotid arteries, vertebral arteries), retinal doppler sonography (optional).

3. Examinations by a neurologist and neuroradiologist and by other specialists, if indicated.
4. Clinical ophthalmic examinations: ERG, fluorescein angiography, visually evoked potentials.

Differential Diagnosis of a Pale Optic Disc. The differential diagnosis of a pale optic disc includes optic atrophy, optic disc anomalies (persistent hyaloid artery, disc hypoplasia, atypical microcoloboma, papilledema), physiological paleness of the disc in newborn eyes, paleness associated with senile disc excavation or large physiologic excavation, peripapillary choroidal atrophy in highly myopic eyes, and optic disc drusen.

Therapy. Treatment of the underlying disease, if possible.

Optic Nerve Head Changes Associated with Glaucoma

Glaucomatous Cupping of the Disc

The ophthalmoscopical examination of a glaucomatous eye usually shows a marked difference of the glaucomatous optic cup when compared with the healthy fellow eye. Malformations and high anisometropia must be ruled out. The typical glaucomatous excavation is usually oval with the longest diameter in the vertical direction (96% of glaucomatous eyes). The excavation is also off-center and may show extensions superiorly or inferiorly. The vessels are displaced nasally, a finding that may be normal in highly myopic eyes.

Diagnostic Criteria for Glaucoma

The previously described ophthalmoscopical findings, in combination with the additional increased intraocular pressure, make glaucoma highly suspect. One exception to the rule of elevated intraocular pressure is low tension glaucoma. Radial or flame-shaped retinal hemorrhages surrounding the optic disc, most often in the inferotemporal quadrant (rarely centrally), are indicative of this condition.

Another important criterion for the diagnosis of glaucoma is visual field defects. It has been observed that in most glaucomatous eyes visual field defects develop in a specific sequence. First, the blind spot becomes enlarged, followed by development of Bjerrum's scotoma. Soon a nasal arcuate scotoma develops. The next, more severe, defect is a nasal depression of the visual field connected with an arcuate scotoma (nasal step of Roenne). A ring scotoma that spares the isolated central field follows. In the final stage, even this central field remnant deteriorates.

Ophthalmoscopical Appearance. As the disease progresses, the initial temporal excavation deepens and shows a characteristic cupping. The vessels become displaced nasally and seem to be pressed against the margin of the cup. The affected area of the disc becomes atrophic and pale, and the lamina cribrosa is more exposed (glaucomatous optic atrophy) (Figs. 270–273).

Intraocular Pressure and Risk Factors

Normal Intraocular Pressure Range. An intraocular pressure of 26 mm Hg indicates the upper physiologic limit. If the intraocular pressure is repeatedly measured above this limit, the patient is at high risk for glaucoma. The start of an anti-glaucoma regimen is indicated.

Ocular Hypertension. Leydhecker (1983b) defines intraocular pressures between 21 and 25 mm Hg as ocular hypertension if the following conditions can be shown: risk factors are absent, intraocular pressure is controlled several times during the day, computer perimetry shows a normal visual field, and ophthalmoscopical examination of a dilated pupil reveals normal optic disc findings.

Risk Factors. *Generalized risk factors:* arteriosclerosis, diabetes mellitus, acquired arterial hypotonia, patients older than 60 years, familial history of glaucoma, and glaucoma of the fellow eye. *Morphological ocular changes:* large excavation of the optic disc, peripapillary hemorrhages, and pseudoexfoliation. *Social risk factors (patient compliance):* unreliable patients, patients living far from ophthalmic care (Leydhecker, 1983b).

Upper Limit for Intraocular Pressure in Risk Patients. For patients in the high risk category, intraocular pressure should not exceed 21 mm Hg to be tolerable. Therapy should be started early to lower intraocular pressure by 4–5 mm Hg (Leydhecker, 1983).

Staging of Glaucomatous Excavations

The progression of a glaucomatous cupping can be judged by determining the cup/disc (C/D) ratio. In other words, a comparison must be made of the rim of an excavated cup to the total diameter of the optic disc. According to some studies, an average value of this ratio is 0.2–0.3. Two methods for determining the ratio are: (*a*) stereoscopic fundus photography with evaluation, and (*b*) objective fundus object measurements using the method described by Littmann in 1982. For the latter test, it is necessary to have a telecentric fundus camera and the Littmann ophthalmometer. Another method was described by Kennedy and coauthors (1983) that uses photographic interference lines. This method allows for an absolute measurement of different fundus structures (Tables 23 and 24).

Acute Glaucoma: Hints for the Non-Ophthalmologist

A diagnostic pupil dilation may induce an acute glaucoma (dilatation glaucoma or angle block glaucoma). The glaucoma may develop within several hours or days.

Table 23. Incidence of Glaucomatous Visual Field Losses Compared to the C/D Ratio (Gloster, 1977)

Vertical C/D Ratio	Visual Field Loss, %
0.4	0
0.5	7
0.6	17
0,7	44
0.8	90
0.9	100

Table 24. Extension of Glaucomatous Visual Field Losses (Gloster, 1977)

Average C/D Ratio	Type of Visual Field Defect
0.56 (0.12)[a]	No visual field defect
0.73 (0.10)	Paracentral or arcuate scotoma
0.82 (0.08)	Extension of arcuate scotoma peripherally and loss of nasal quadrant
0.88 (0.07)	Central and temporal visual field remnants

[a] The values in parentheses indicate the standard deviation.

Predisposing Factors. Old age, short globe in hyperopic eyes (narrow anterior chamber angle caused by hypertrophic ciliary body, a relatively large lens that causes narrowing of the anterior chamber, and small corneal diameter), psychic and toxic factors (ethyl alcohol and caffeine, especially if consummed in large amounts), meteorologic-biologic factors (mountain winds). Female patients are most often affected.

Subjectively, patients report fogged vision, perception of rainbow colors surrounding light sources caused by corneal edema, reduced visual acuity (near and distant), epiphora, photophobia, feeling of pressure within the eyes, headache with projection into temporal region, back of the head, and jaws and/or teeth, nausea, abdominal pain, and vomiting.

The most important objective sign is the increased intraocular pressure that can often be appreciated easily by digital palpation on the extremely rigid globe.

Additional objective signs include:
Lids: edema, pseudoptosis
Conjunctiva: hyperemia (congestive hyperemia)
Sclera: ciliary vessels become visible (red lines indicating congestive hyperemia)
Cornea: hazy, epithelial edema, bullous keratopathy
Anterior chamber: narrow
Aqueous humor: cell and flare reaction
Lens: slightly dislocated anteriorly
Pupil: oval and nonreactive to light (Note: iritis is typically characterized by a small pupil. In simple conjunctivitis, the pupil reacts normally. Grayish green pupillary reflex (German, "gruener star").
Iris: muddy, loss of details (hyperemic edema)
Fundus (often the fundus cannot be examined at all): hyperemia and papilledema, sometimes pulsation of the central retinal artery, peripallary hemorrhages. (Note: a glaucomatous excavation may not be present, especially if this is the first glaucomatous attack (Figs. 274 and 275).)

Therapeutic Procedures for Acute Glaucoma. If neccessary, therapy for acute glaucoma should be prescribed by a non-ophthalmologist if the diagnosis is confirmed:

1. Intravenous injection of 500 mg of acetazolamide (Diamox) must be performed carefully, with careful observance of all counterindications.
2. The patient should use pilocarpine eye drops (2–3%) or eye drops containing β-blockers, with careful attention to all possible side effects.
3. Based on the author's experience, application of ocular ointment containing 2% pilocarpine hydrochloride has a positive effect.
4. Corneal edema should be treated with eyedrops containing prednisolone.

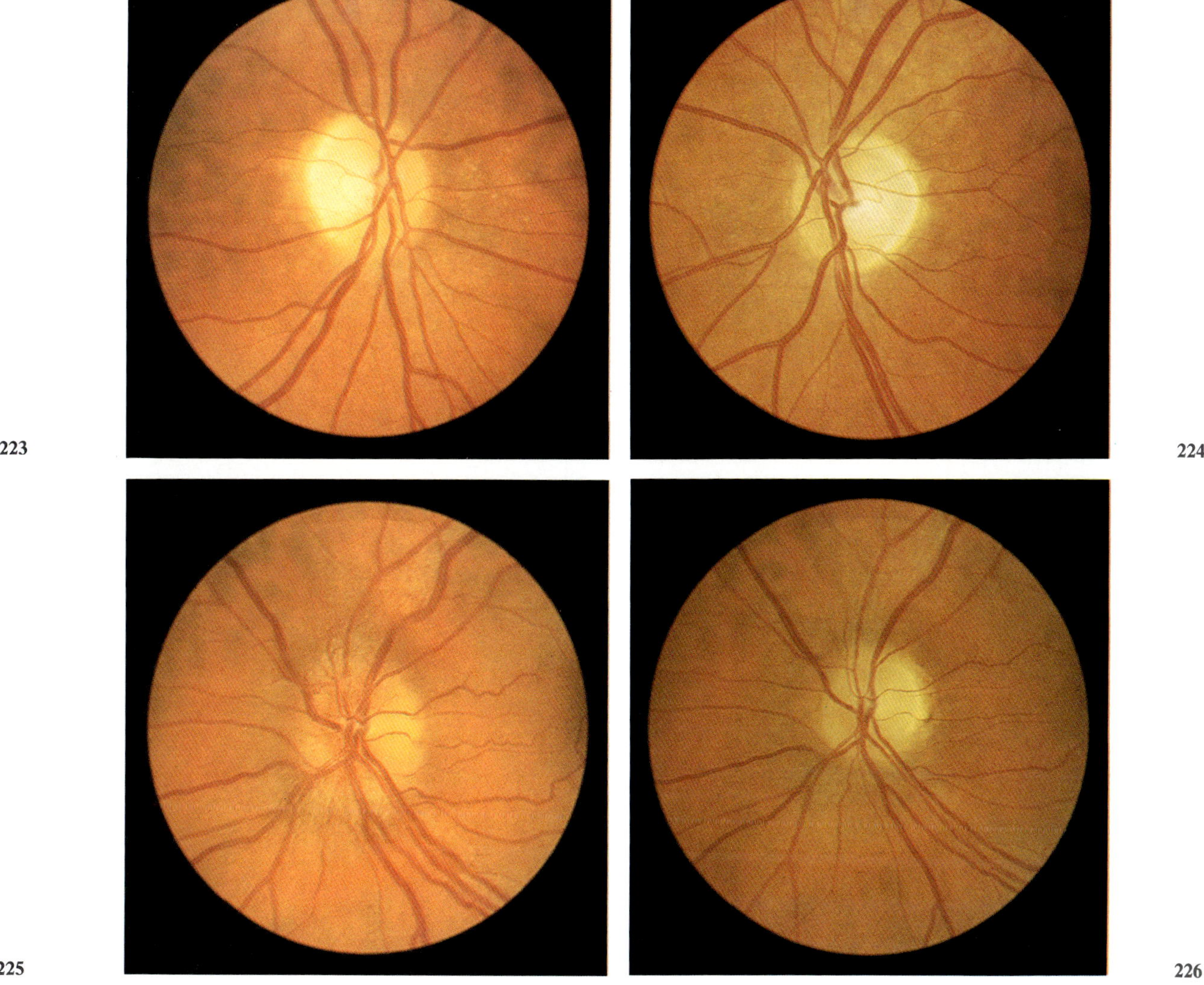

223 224

225 226

Figure 223. Right eye of a 43-year-old male patient with bilateral recurrent retrobulbar optic neuritis, bilateral temporal optic atrophy; possible diagnosis: multiple sclerosis.

Clinical Findings

Objective refraction in the right eye was +0.25 sphere with visual acuity of 20/25. Visual fields were normal. During the acute inflammation, there was a relative central scotoma (Goldmann's perimeter test mark I/4). No other ocular abnormalities were found when the eye was examined after the neuritis subsided. Doppler sonography (Huismans, 1983d) of both supratrochlear arteries was normal. Retinal doppler sonography was also normal. Ophthalmodynamography showed a pulsation volume of 53.9 mm in the right eye and 56.3 mm in the left eye. The pulsation volume ratio was 0.95. An ENT and an internal examination were normal. A neurologic examination was normal except for absent abdominal reflexes. An EEG and cranial x-ray were normal. Computed tomography revealed a mild cortical atrophy of the frontal brain and of the cortex in the region of the sylvian fissure. Total protein in the cerebrospinal fluid was elevated (61 mg/100 ml with IgG of 3.3 mg/100 ml).

Figure 224. Left eye of the same patient as Figure 223 with temporal optic atrophy and all other ophthalmoscopical findings identical to the right eye.

Clinical Findings

Objective refraction was −0.25 sphere with a visual acuity of 20/20.

Figures 225 and 226. Left eye of 44-year-old female patient with recurrent optic neuritis that is a possible side effect of taking a contraceptive drug for over 10 years.

Clinical Findings

Visual acuity was 20/1000 with eccentric fixation. Neurologic, ENT, and internal examinations were normal.

Clinical Course

The first manifestation of this inflammation occurred as a retrobulbar neuritis. After several recurrent inflammatory episodes, it presented as a papillitis leading to a postneuritic optic atrophy.

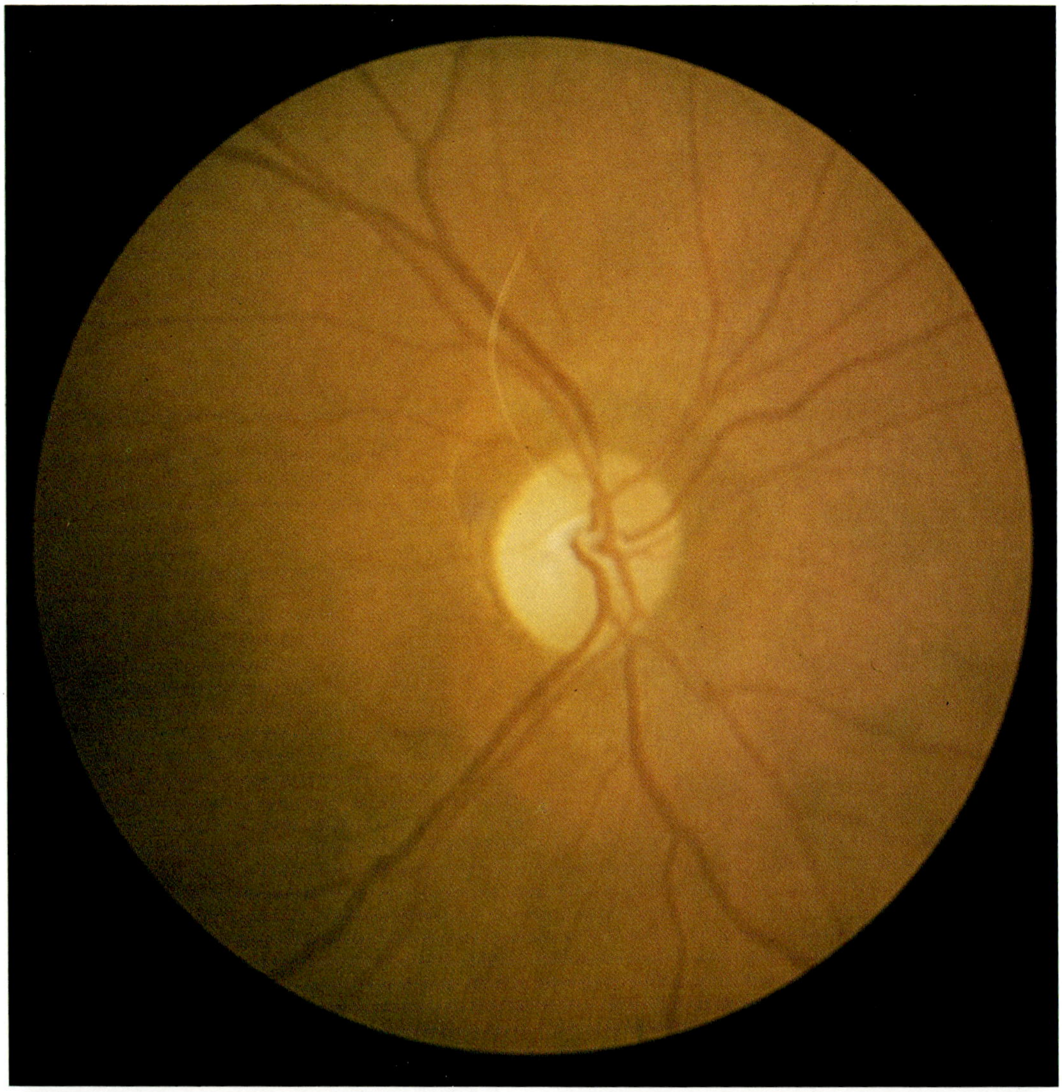

227

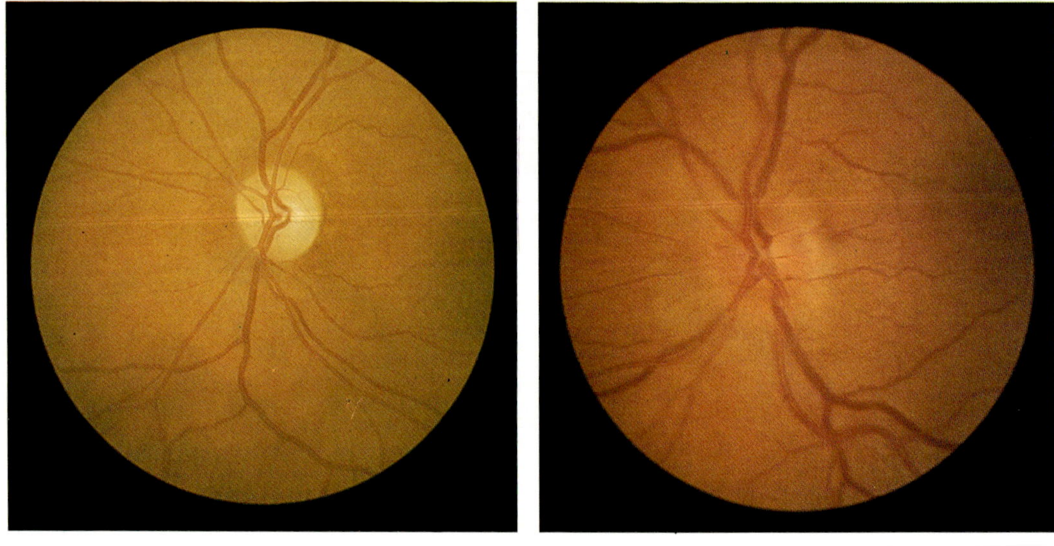

228

229

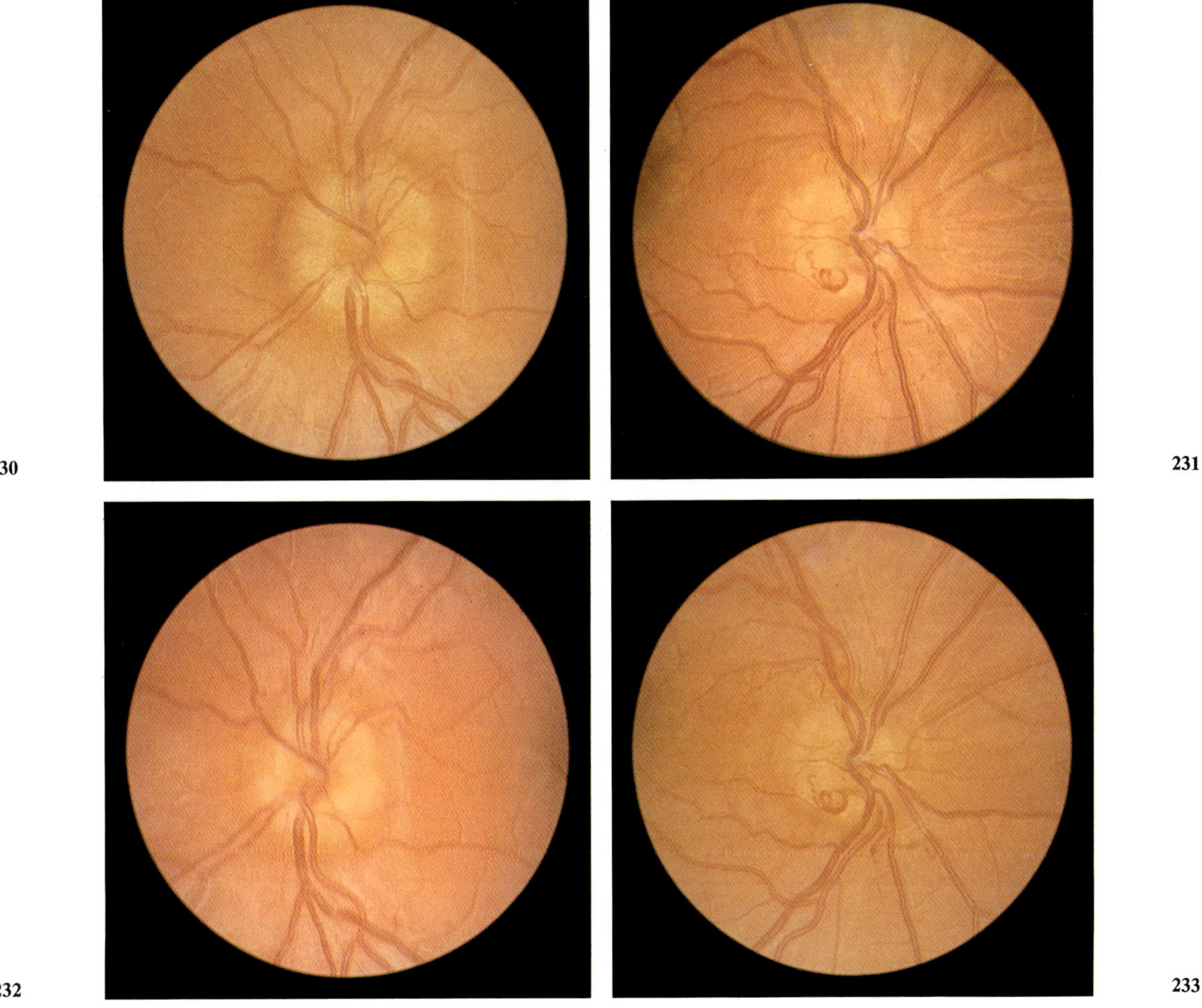

230 231

232 233

Figures 227 and 228. Right and left eyes of a 42-year-old female patient with bilateral optic atrophy.

Clinical Findings

Visual acuity in the right eye was 20/300, and 20/400 in the left eye. Visual field testing revealed a bilateral central scotoma and a concentric constriction of the outer margins. The patient had taken a single dose of 40 quinine tablets in order to induce an abortion during the 2nd or 3rd month of gestation.

Figure 229. Left eye of a 53-year-old female patient with early papilledema.

Clinical Findings

Visual acuity in both emmetropic eyes was 20/20. The refractive media were clear, and intraocular pressure in both eyes was 16 mm Hg. There was no perception of double images and no nystagmus. Pupillary reactions were normal. Visual field testing showed a bilateral enlargement of the blind spot with normal outer borders. An adaptation graph was normal. Neurological symptoms could be explained by the presence of a large brain tumor located in the temporoparietal occipital region of the left hemisphere. The tumor was histologically identified as a glioblastoma.

Clinical Course

The patient died 3 months after an operation for removal of the tumor.

Figures 230–233. Right and left eyes of a 10-year-old female patient with bilateral papilledema.

Clinical Findings

The patient's history showed treatment with hydroxyprogesterone for gigantism for 2 months prior to onset of the papilledema. Such treatment is highly questionable. Growth reduction using medical therapy alone has been achieved in young females with prolonged estrogen therapy, a cyclic estrogen gestagen, or estrogen therapy combined with increased gestagen dose between the 21st and 26th day of the menstrual cycle. At the time of examination at age 10, the patient was 5 feet 7 inches tall. Visual acuity in both emmetropic eyes was 20/20. The refractive media were clear and there was no nystagmus. There was normal motility of the external muscles and of the pupils. There was a bilateral enlargement of the blind spot. An ophthalmoscopical examination revealed bilateral prominent optic discs (Figs. 230 and 231). The elevation of the right disc was 1.5 and the left disc 0.5 diopters. In the left eye there is a small AV shunt inferotemporal at the optic disc margin. Mesopic vision was normal.

Clinical Course

Figures 232 and 233 show the ophthalmoscopical appearance 6 months after the first examination. Fluorescein angiography confirmed the clinical diagnosis of papilledema. A neurologic examination and computed tomography were normal. The patient did not return for further follow-up examinations.

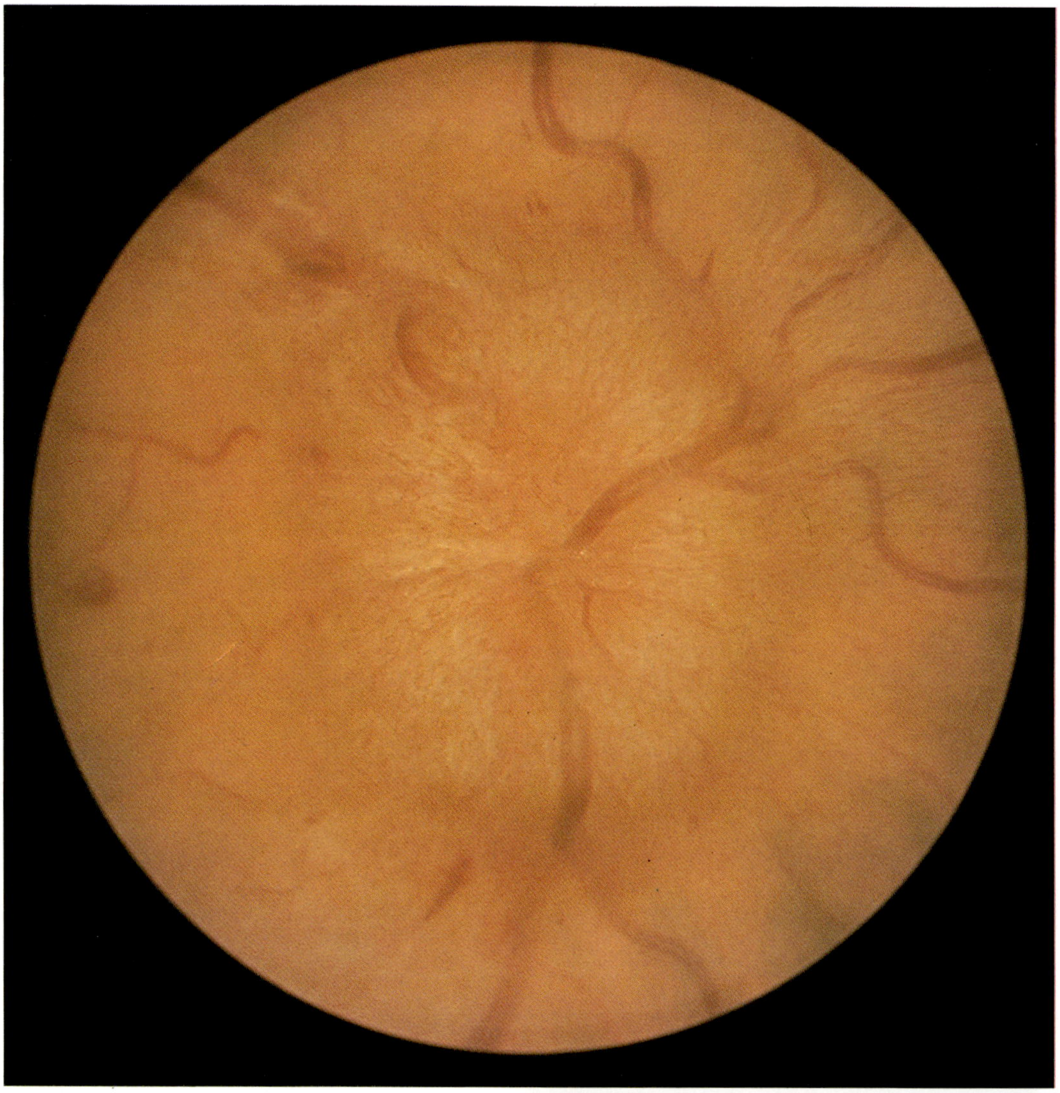

234

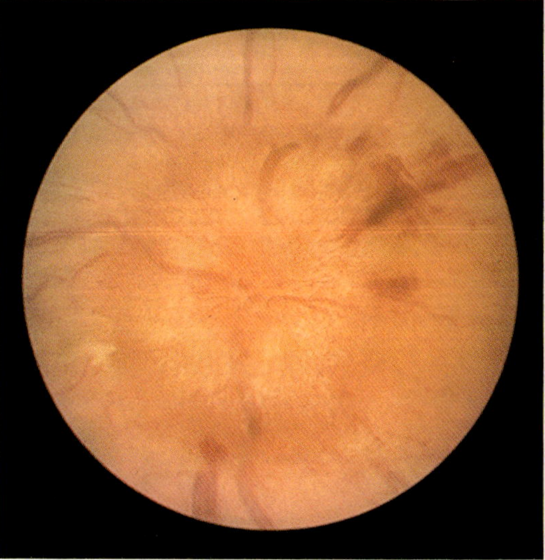

235

236 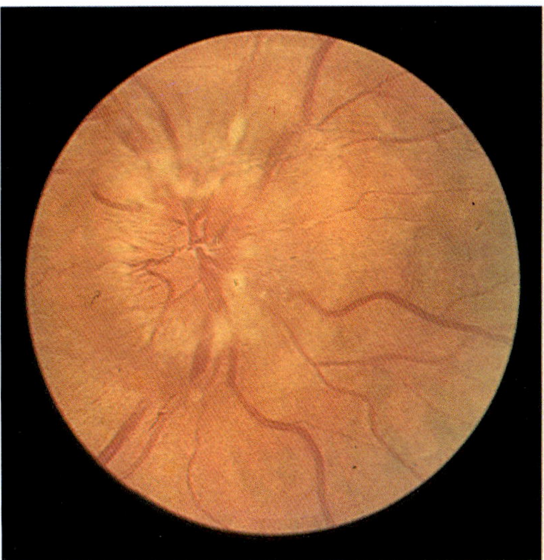

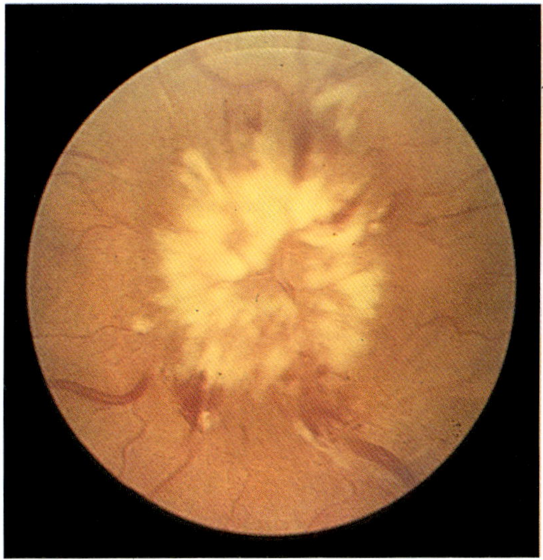 237

Figures 234 and 235. Right and left eyes of a 35-year-old male patient with papilledema associated with an astrocytoma of the left hemisphere.

Clinical Findings

Visual acuity in the right eye was 20/25, and 20/30 in the left eye. There was a bilateral papilledema and extensive visual field defects with an extinction of the supratemporal quadrant in the right visual field and extinction of three quadrants in the left eye, leaving only the inferotemporal quadrant. The most important finding of a cranial x-ray was a 1-cm right lateral dislocation of the calcified epiphyseal gland. Cranial computed tomography showed a massive tumor in the left hemisphere with a temporal parietal location. The brain ventricles were dislocated toward the right. Angiography of the carotid artery showed marked displacement of the intercerebral vessels by a left hemisphere temporal tumor. EEG findings were consistent with the tumor (delta wave focus, isolated high peaks).

Therapy

A neurosurgical operation confirmed the clinical diagnosis of a tumor measuring approximately 7 cm in diameter, located approximately 1.5 cm below the middle temporal gyrus. There was infiltration into the adjacent brain structures, and the tumor could be only partially removed. Histologic examination identified the tumor as an astrocytoma.

Figures 236 and 237. Right and left eyes of a 55-year-old male patient with bilateral papilledema associated with a brain tumor.

Clinical Findings

Six months prior to the ophthalmologic examination a glioblastoma of the left temporal lobe was removed. The patient then underwent irradiation of the tumor site with a total dose of 60 Gy. Histopathologic examination of the tumor revealed a largely necrotic glioblastoma. Visual acuity in the right eye was 20/100 and in the left eye 20/700. Intraocular pressure in the right eye was 12 mm Hg and in the left eye 16 mm Hg. There was a homonymous hemianopia to the right, and the motility of the eye was affected. The pupil dilated slowly to light. The convergent reaction could not be evaluated. An ophthalmoscopical examination showed a chronic atrophic papilledema in the right eye with an elevation of 1.5 diopters and extensive peripapillary edema. Surprisingly, the venules were not very engorged. The left eye showed a chronic atrophic papilledema with severely blurred margins and an elevation of approximately 1.5 diopters. Note the presence of inter- and preretinal venous stasis hemorrhages.

Laboratory Findings

Blood sedimentation rate was 6/22 mm. A lymphocytosis was also found. All other tests were normal. Neurologic abnormalities included a progressive cerebral edema, sensorimotor aphasia, distortions in word distinctions, and short-term memory. The patient developed an organic psychotic syndrome. Cranial computed tomography showed a glioblastoma in the parietal lobe of the left hemisphere associated with an extensive perifocal edema. The left ventricular system was compressed and the mid-brain was dislocated to the right.

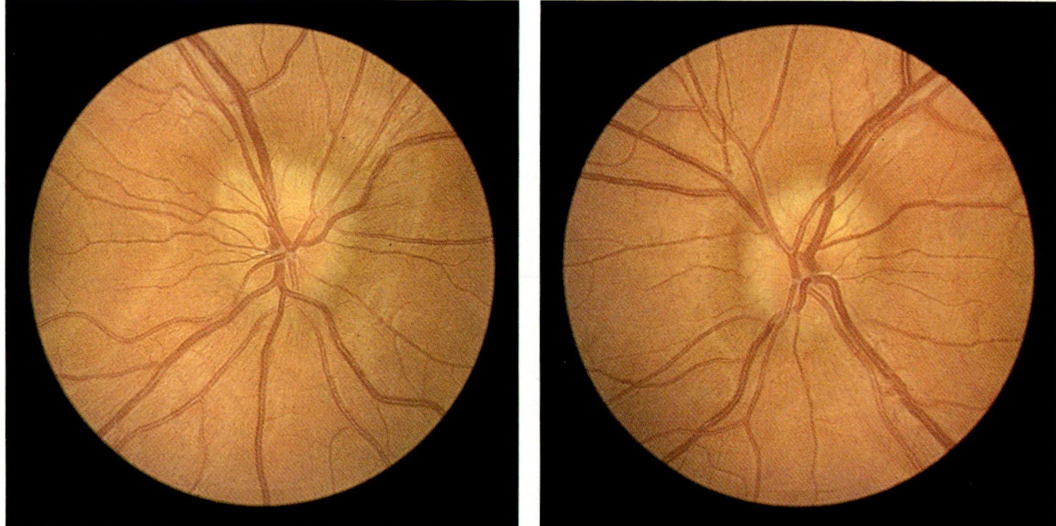

238

239

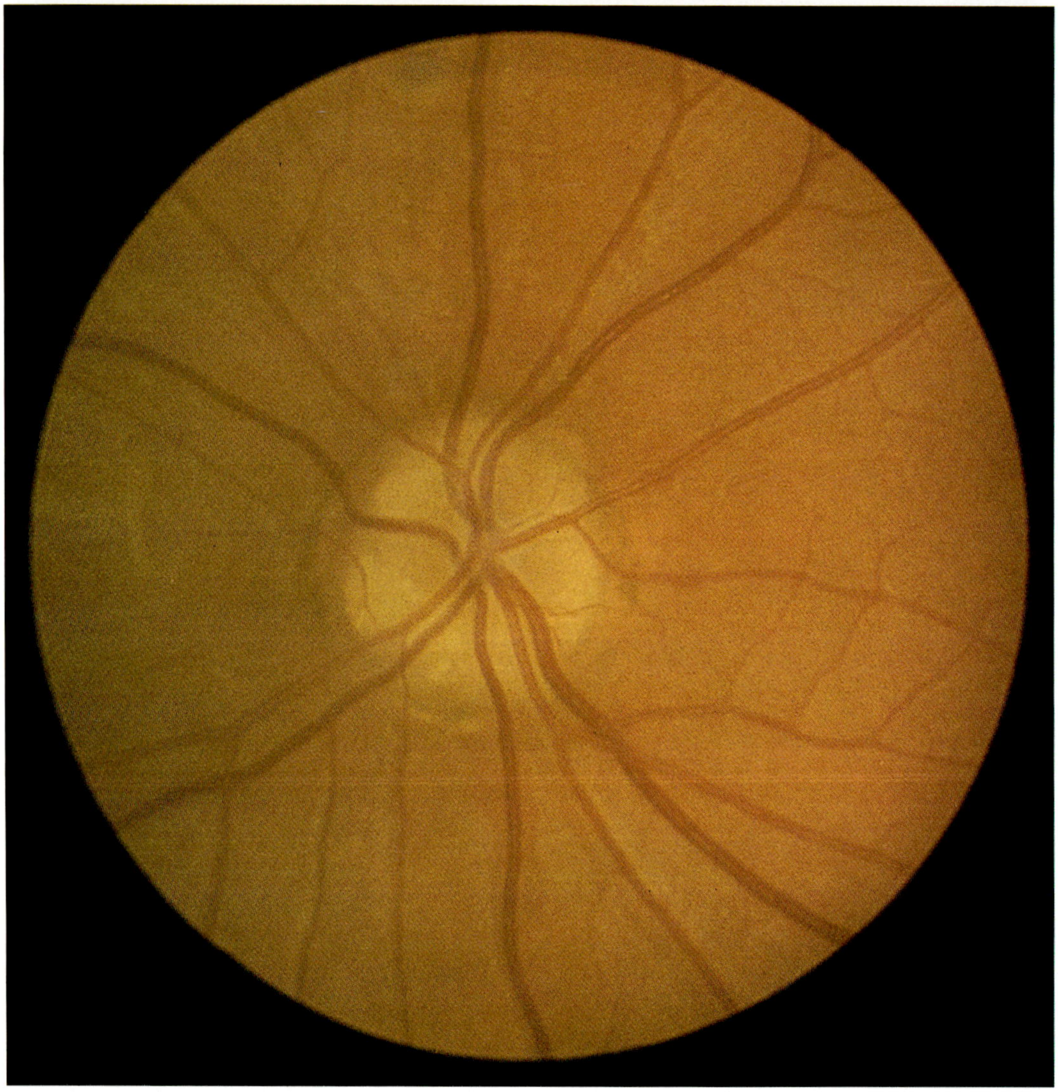

240

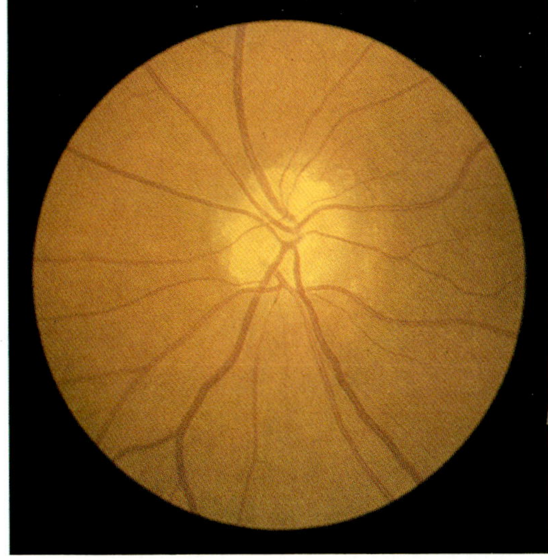

241

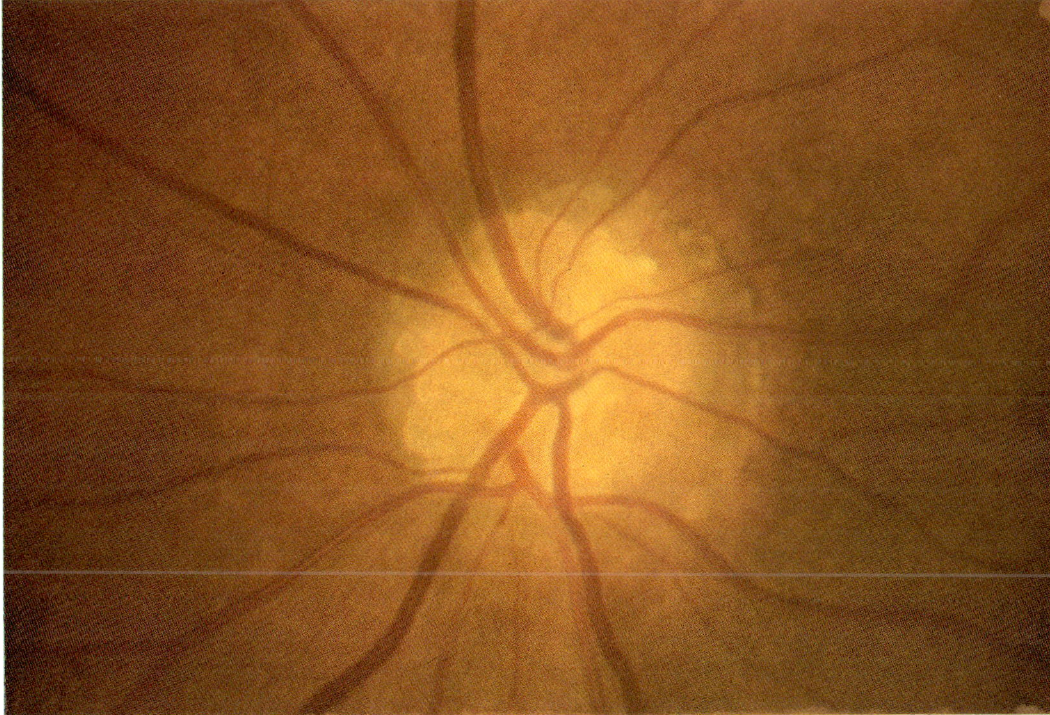

242

Figures 238 and 239. Right and left eyes of a 15-year-old female patient with optic disc drusen.

Clinical Findings

The eyes were emmetropic with a visual acuity of 20/20. The refractive media were clear and intraocular pressure in both eyes was 14 mm Hg. Visual field testing showed normal outer margins with a bilateral enlargement of the blind spot. Fluorescein angiography confirmed the diagnosis of optic disc drusen. Neurologic and internal examinations were unremarkable.

Figure 240. Right eye of a 20-year-old female patient with optic disc drusen.

Clinical Findings

With a refraction of −0.5 cylinder, axis 0°, visual acuity was 20/20. Refractive media were clear and intraocular pressure was 14 mm Hg. Visual field testing showed a moderate enlargement of the blind spot with normal outer margins. Fluorescein angiography confirmed the diagnosis of optic disc drusen. A neurolgic examination was unremarkable.

Figures 241 and 242. Left eye of a 61-year-old female patient with optic disc drusen.

Clinical Findings

With a refraction of +2.25 sphere, −1.0 cylinder, axis 10°, visual acuity was 20/40. There was a beginning age-related cataract. Intraocular pressure was 15 mm Hg. Visual field testing revealed a moderate enlargement of the blind spot with normal outer margins. Consultations by an internist and a neurologist were unremarkable except for the presence of bronchiectasia. Figure 242 is a high-power view of the optic disc.

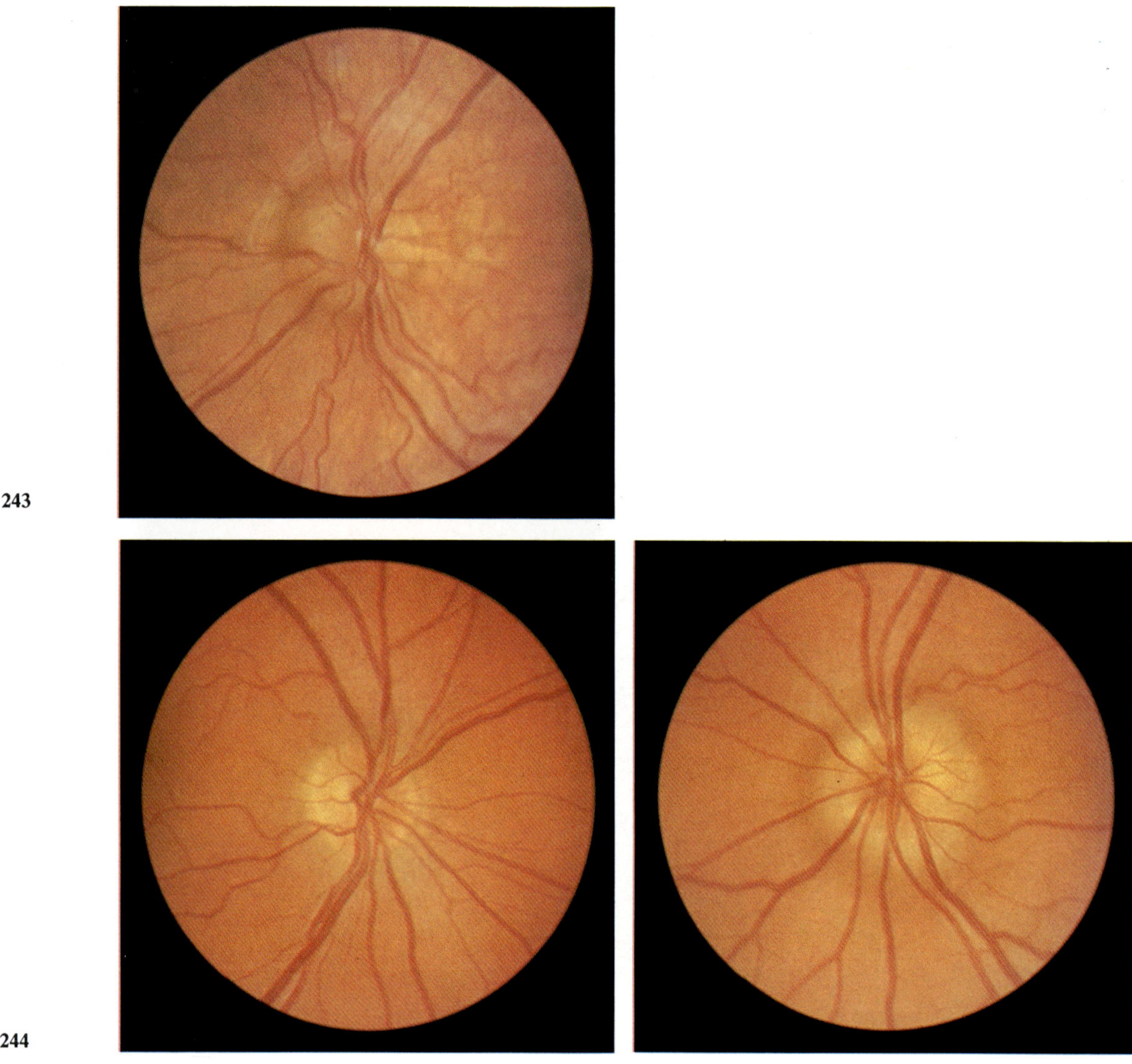

243

244

245

Figure 243. Left eye of a 7-year-old male patient with optic disc drusen.

Clinical Findings

With a refraction of −1.25 sphere, visual acuity was 20/20. Refractive media were clear and intraocular pressure was 14 mm Hg. Visual field testing revealed a moderately enlarged blind spot in the right eye with normal outer margins. The left fundus was normal. There was an anisocoria (right pupil larger than the left pupil), but the pupillary functions were normal. Fluorescein angiography confirmed a diagnosis of deep optic disc drusen. The visually evoked potential was normal. Internal and neurological examinations showed normal clinical findings.

Clinical Course

The optic disc appearance remained unchanged over a period of 3 years.

Figures 244 and 245. Right and left eyes of a 22-year-old male patient with pseudopapilledema in the left eye and a normal optic disc in the right eye.

Clinical Findings

Refraction in the right eye was +0.75 sphere, visual acuity 20/20. Refraction in the left eye was +2.5 sphere, −0.75 cylinder, axis 0°, visual acuity 20/25. Refractive media were clear and intraocular pressure was 14 mm Hg. Visual field testing was normal. Fluorescein angiography ruled out papilledema in the left eye. A consultation with a neurologist that included a computed tomography of the cranium was normal.

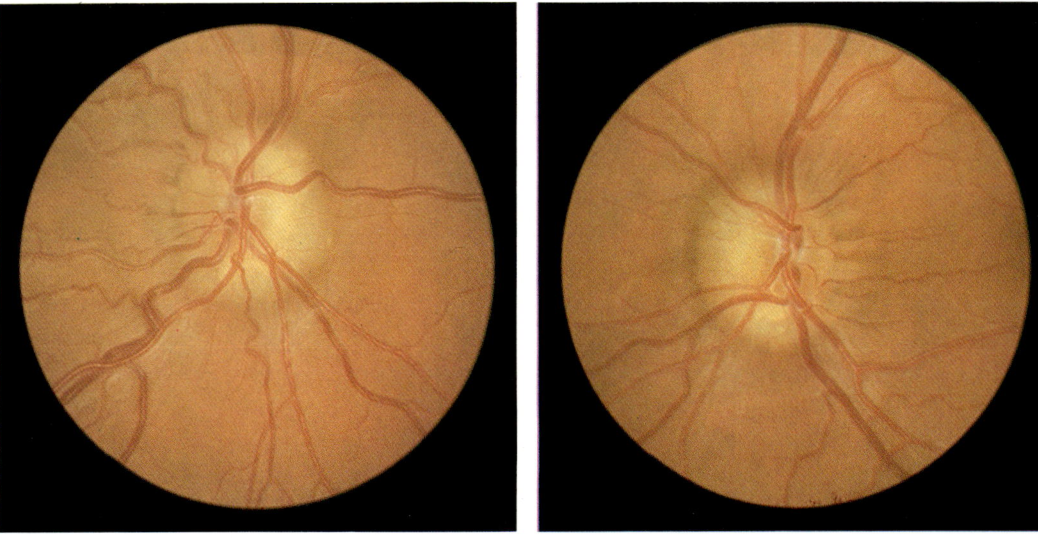

246 247

Figures 246 and 247. Right and left eyes of a 15-year-old female patient with pseudopapilledema.

Clinical Findings

Refraction in both eyes was +2.5 sphere, −0.75 cylinder, axis 90°, visual acuity 20/20. Refractive media were clear and visual fields were normal. Fluorescein angiography ruled out papilledema. Since the patient's father showed similar changes of the optic disc (elevated blurred margins), no additional neurologic tests were performed.

Clinical Course

The optic disc appearance remained unchanged over an observation period of 4 years.

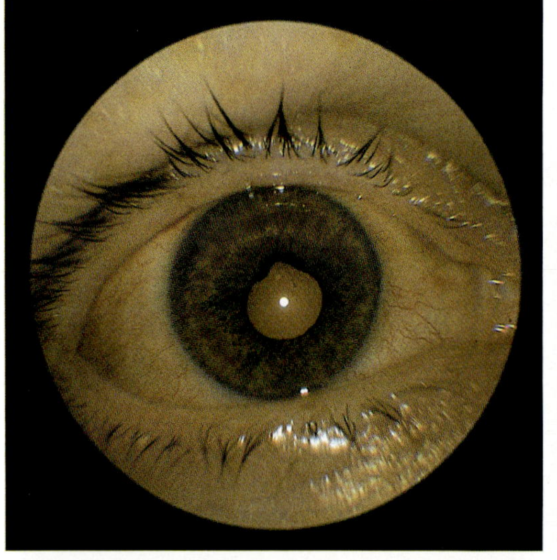

248

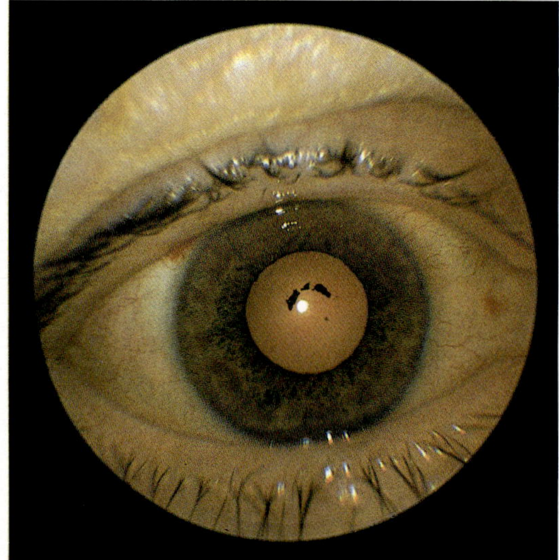

249

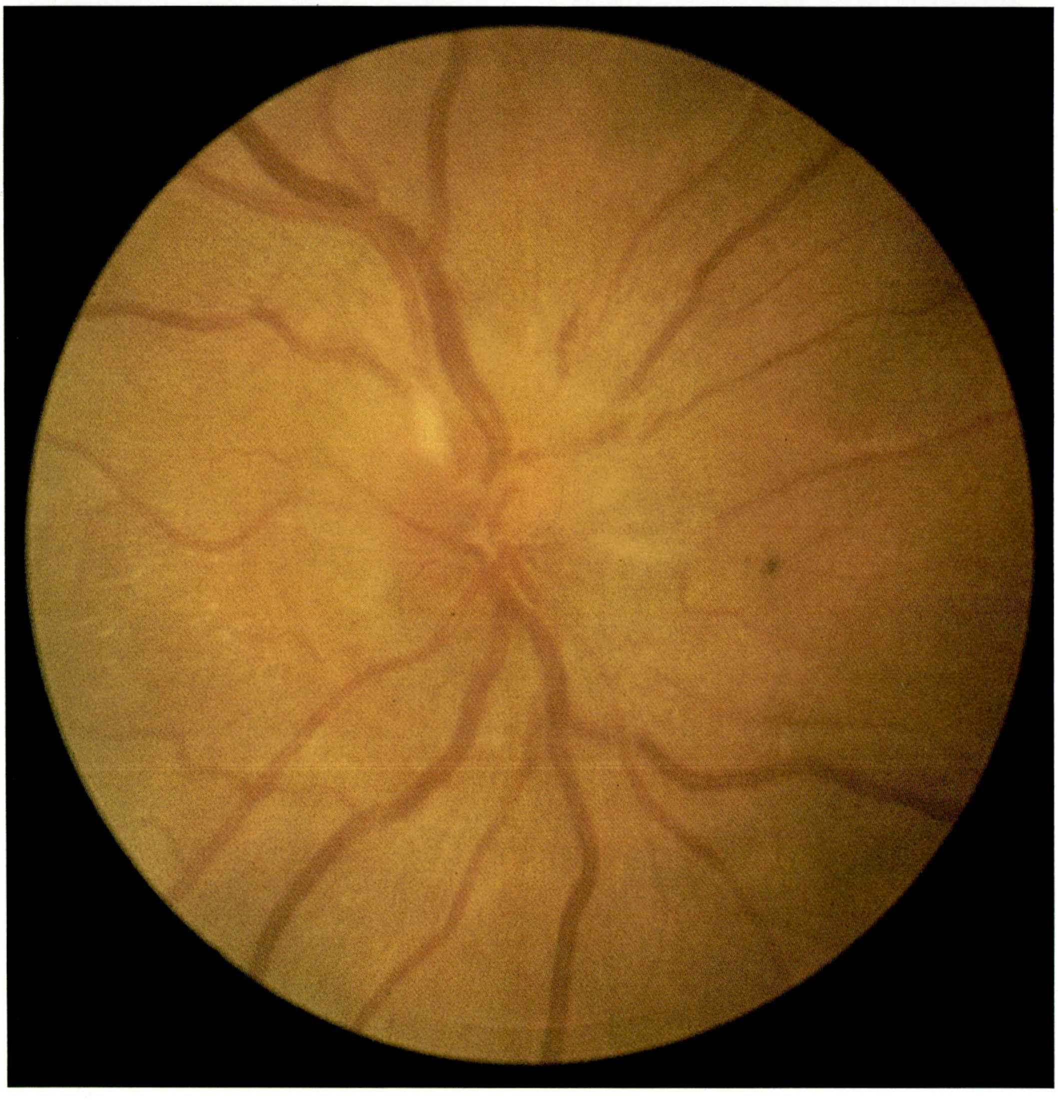

250

251 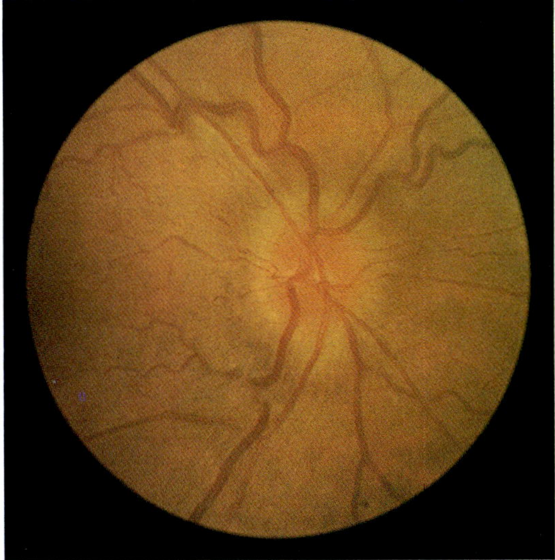

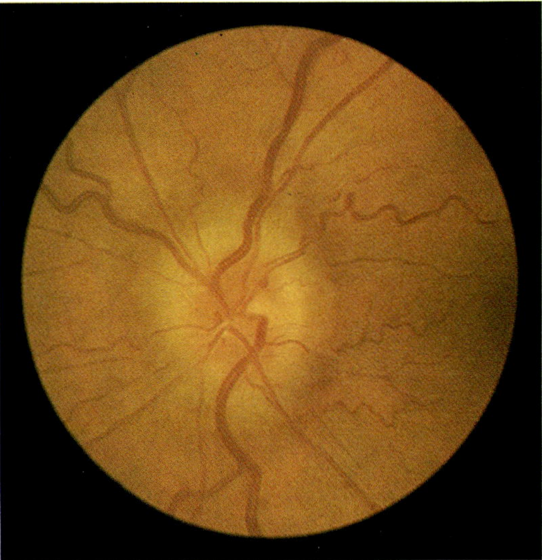 252

Figures 248–250. Right eye of a 52-year-old female patient with papilledema associated with iridocyclitis of unknown etiology.

Clinical Findings

Best visual acuity was 20/30. Intraocular pressure was 10 mm Hg. Visual field testing showed a concentric constriction of the outer margins with an enlargement of the blind spot. Slitlamp examination revealed a moderate conjunctival injection. The pupils were shaped irregularly, caused by posterior synechiae. There was an inflammation in both the anterior and posterior segments with 2+ cell and 1+ flare in the anterior chamber and 2+ cell in the vitreous. The optic disc was elevated 1.5 diopters (Fig. 250). There was a loss of normal physiological optic cupping. The capillaries were hyperemic. Note the small flame-shaped hemorrhage at the 1-o'clock position. There are age-related drusen between the optic disc and the edematous macula (*left*).

Laboratory Findings

Blood sedimentation rate 3/9 mm, erythrocytes 4.5 million, leukocytes 3800. The antistreptolysin titer was 80 units/ml. The Rose-Waaler test, latex agglutination test, and c-reaction protein test were all negative. Internal, ENT, orthopedic, and neurologic examinations were normal.

Therapy

A drug-induced synechiae lysis was performed. The patient was treated with topical corticosteroids and subconjunctival steroid injection.

Clinical Course

The inflammation subsided completely within 6 weeks.

Figures 251 and 252. Right and left eyes of a 56-year-old female patient with bilateral papilledema that may be the result of chloroquine treatment with a daily dosage of 200 mg for 2 1/2 months because of rheumatoid arthritis.

Clinical Findings

Visual acuity in both eyes was 20/30, refractive media were clear, and intraocular pressure was 14 mm Hg. Visual field testing showed normal outer margins with a mild enlargement of the blind spot. Color and mesopic vision were normal. Blood pressure was 140/85 mm Hg measured on the right arm and 130/80 mm Hg measured on the left arm. Fundus examination revealed a papilledema of 2 diopters elevation in the right eye (Fig. 251) and 3 diopters elevation in the left eye (Fig. 252). There were marked caliber irregularities of the arterioles with focal vascular spasms. In contrast, the retinal venules are engorged. The AV ratio is 1:3. A neurologic examination did not show any abnormalities except for the papilledema. Computed tomography of the cranium was unremarkable.

Clinical Course

The bilateral papilledema spontaneously resolved and blood circulation normalized after chloroquine therapy was terminated. Visual acuity in both eyes recovered to 20/20 to 20/25.

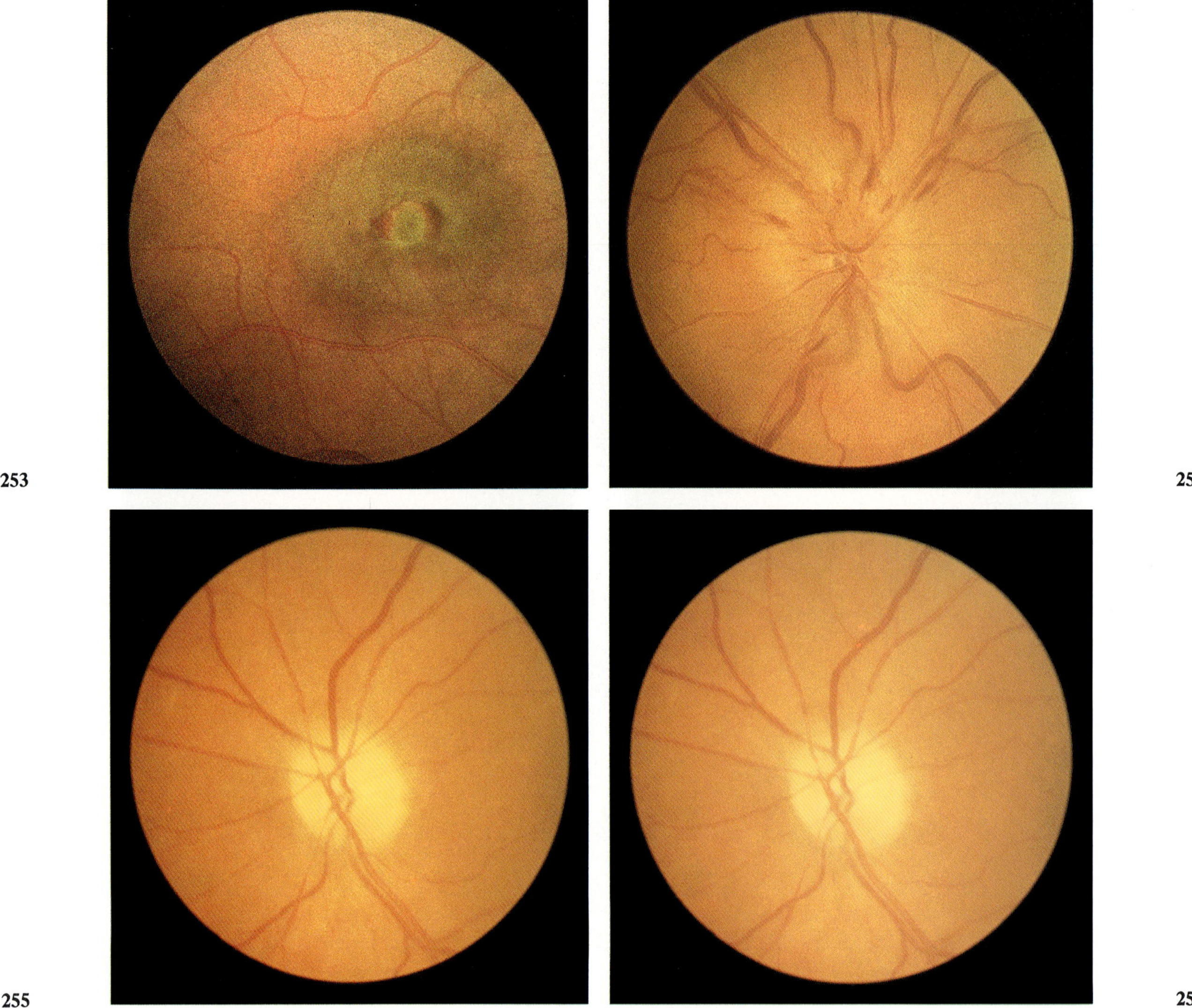

Figure 253. Left eye of a 50-year-old male patient with "bull's eye dystrophy" following chloroquine therapy over a period of several years. The drug was used to treat lupus erythematosus.

Clinical Findings

Visual acuity was 20/25 and refractive media were clear. Visual fields and mesopic and color vision were normal. Both maculae showed the same characteristic bull's-eye dystrophy.

Figures 254–256. Left eye of a 64-year-old female patient with ischemic papilledema.

Clinical Findings

In May 1980, the patient presented with visual acuity of 20/30. Intraocular pressure was 14 mm Hg. Visual field testing showed a constriction of the outer margins with a defect in the temporosuperior quadrant. Blood pressure measured on both arms was 160/95 mm Hg, and blood sedimentation rate was 14/29 mm. There were no neurologic abnormalities. Ophthalmodynamography revealed a reduced pulsation volume in the left eye. Doppler sonography showed no abnormalities of the blood flow in the internal carotid arteries. Retinal doppler sonography showed reduced peaks on the hemotachometer printout, which was confirmed by an ENT consultation. The patient suffered from a chronic sinusitis involving all the right paranasal sinuses. A temporal artery biopsy showed an unspecific fibrosis of the intima.

Therapy

The patient underwent rheologic therapy and was treated with systemic corticosteroids.

Clinical Course

In June 1980 (Fig. 255), the papilledema had resolved and there were signs of an ischemic optic disc atrophy. Visual acuity was less than 20/1000. In August 1981 (Fig. 256), the fundus appearance remained unchanged. At that time, the right eye also became affected; however, visual acuity in the right eye recovered to 20/50.

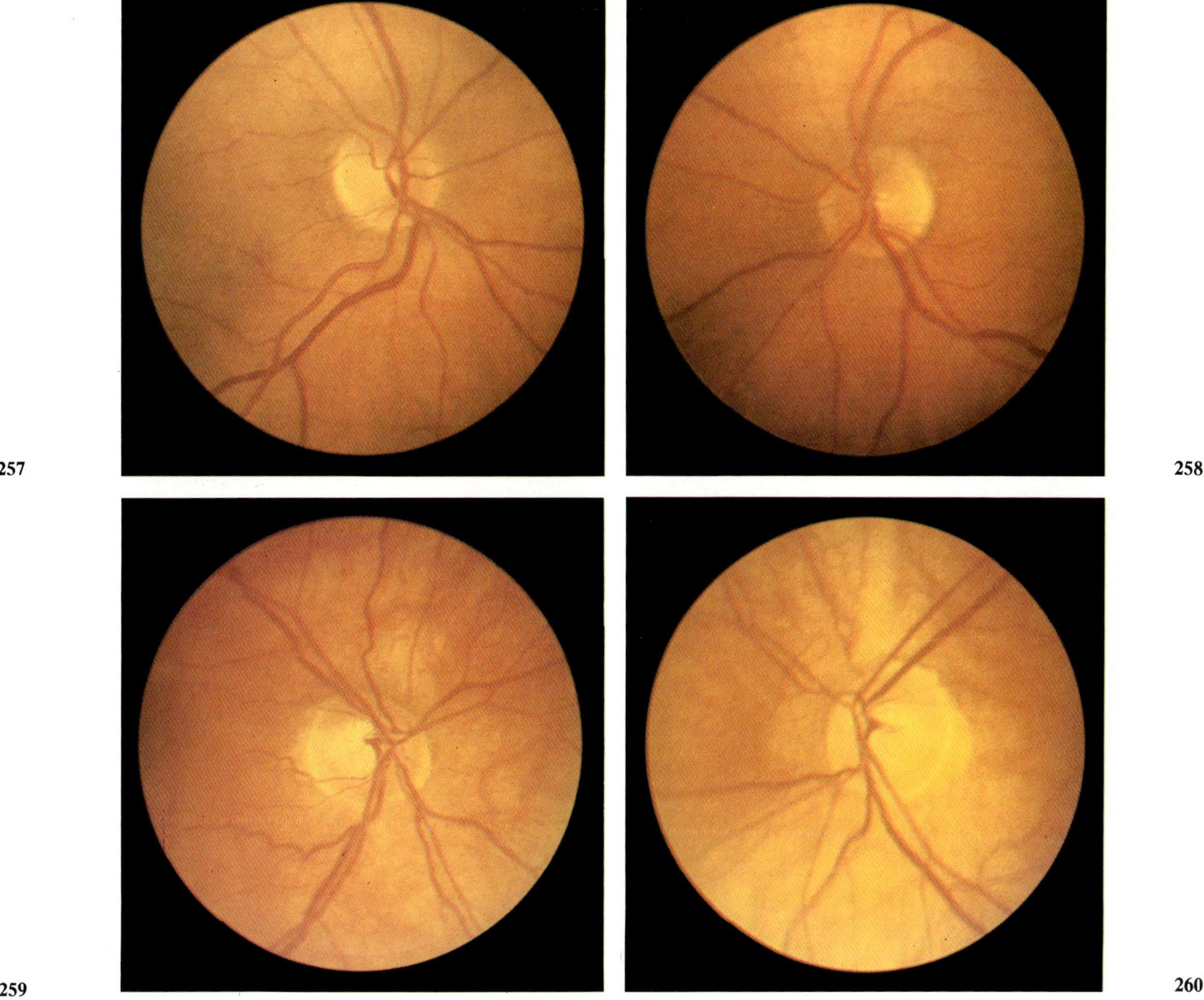

Figures 257 and 258. Right and left eyes of a 70-year-old male patient with temporal arteritis and amaurosis fugax. The patient suffered from severe temporal headache. Both temporal arteries were extremely tender to the touch with no pulsations.

Clinical Findings

Visual acuity in both eyes was 20/25. Intraocular pressure was 16 mm Hg, and there was a beginning age-related cataract. Visual field testing showed a concentric constriction of the outer margins. Blood pressure was 140/85 mm Hg measured on both arms, and blood sedimentation rate was 94/128 mm. The fundus examination was normal. A histopathologic examination of the temporal artery biopsies showed a narrow arterial lumen. The intima showed patches of thickening with areas of fibrous metaplasia. The media was partially destroyed and there were inflammatory infiltrations with lymphocytes, plasma cells, and giant cells. There were scattered chronic inflammatory infiltrates of the adventitia. A diagnosis of giant cell arteritis was confirmed by this examination.

Figures 259 and 260. Right and left eyes of a 71-year-old male patient with temporal arteritis. The patient felt very ill, suffering from nausea, vomiting, and a severe temporal headache. Both temporal arteries were extremely tender to the touch.

Clinical Findings

Visual acuity in both eyes was 20/30. Intraocular pressure in the right eye was 14 mm Hg and in the left eye 16 mm Hg. Bilateral age-related cataracts were present. Visual field testing showed an uncharacteristic concentric constriction of the outer borders. Blood pressure measured on both arms was 170/90 mm Hg and blood sedimentation rate was 70/110 mm. The fundus did not show any major pathologic changes. The diagnosis of giant cell arteritis was confirmed by a large temporal artery biopsy. The vascular lumen was extremely narrowed and there were fibrotic patches in the intima. The media was largely destroyed with granulomatous inflammation and isolated giant cells. There were chronic inflammatory cells in the adventitia of the vessel.

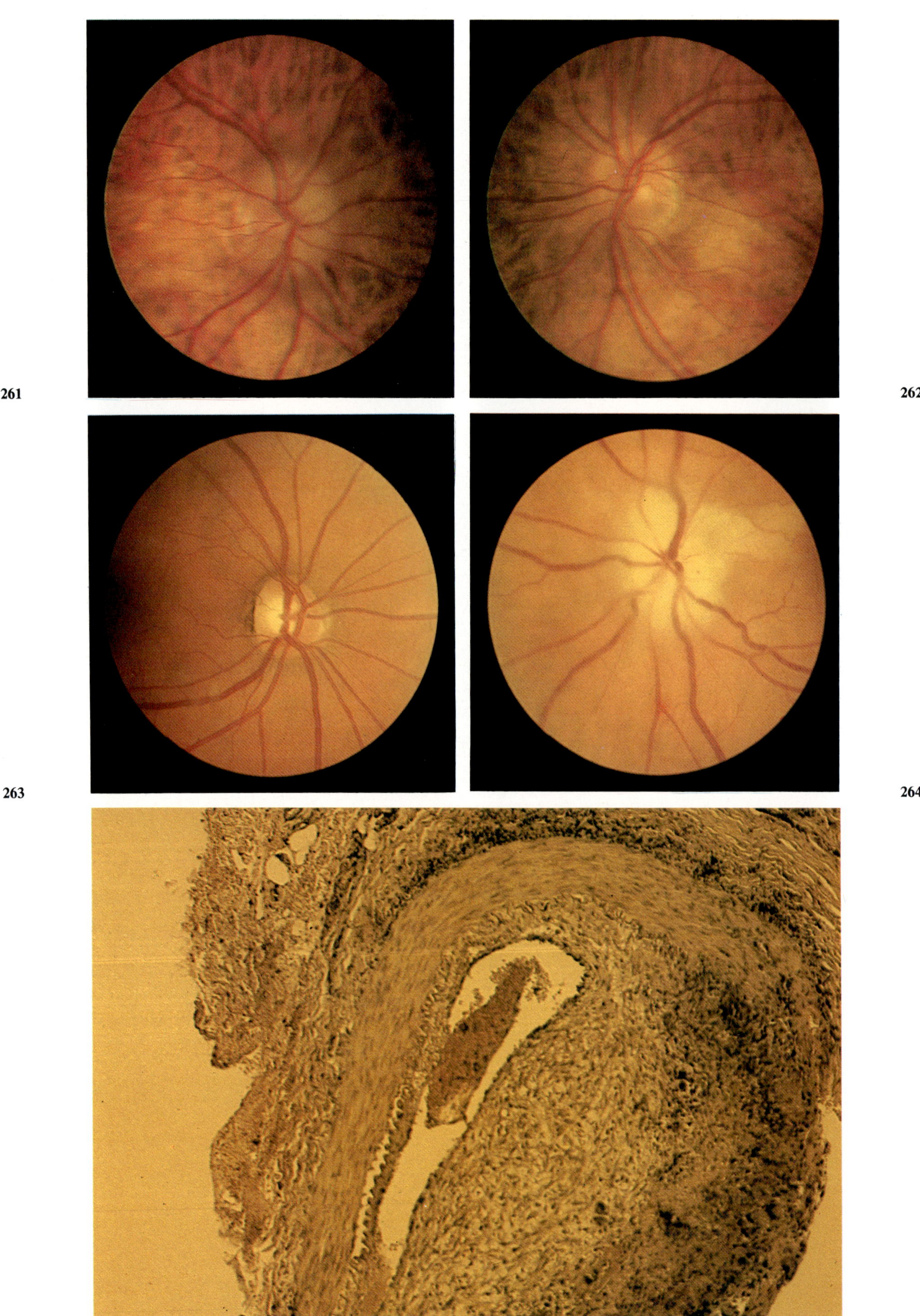

261

262

263

264

265

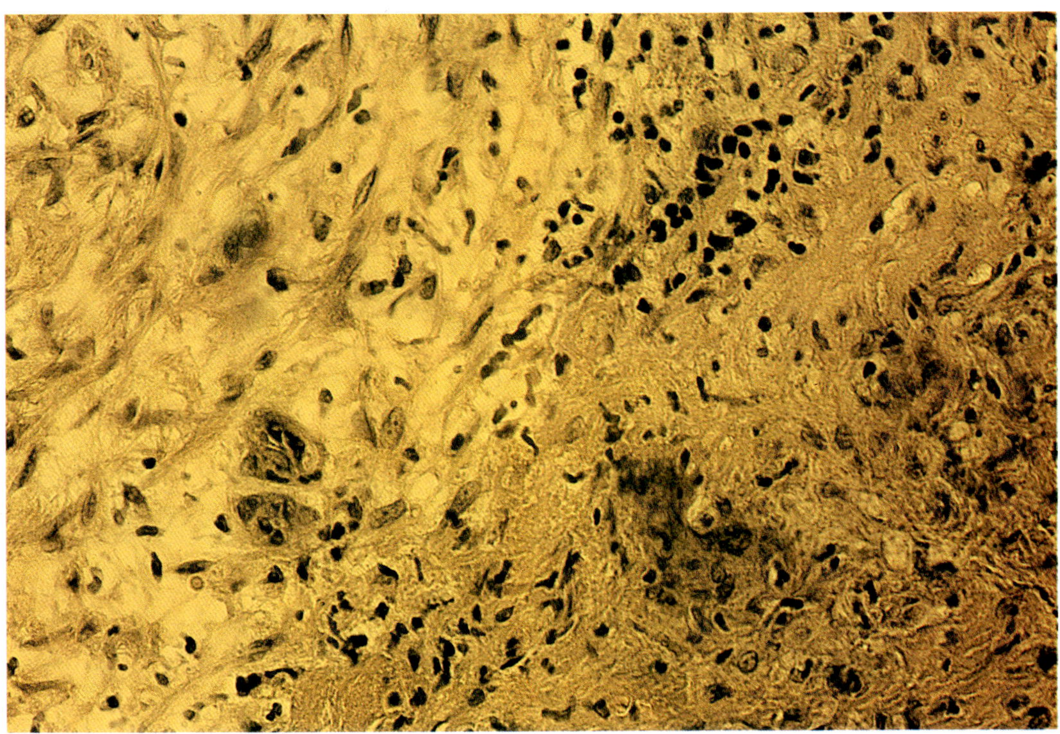

266

Figures 261 and 262. Right and left eyes of a 77-year-old female patient with temporal arteritis. The patient had blurred vision in the right eye, with a bilateral temporal headache.

Clinical Findings

Visual acuity in the right eye was 20/100, and 20/30 in the left eye. There was a beginning age-related cortical nuclear cataract in both eyes. Intraocular pressure was 16 mm Hg. Visual field testing showed a concentric constriction of the outer borders and a central scotoma in the right eye. Examination of the fundus of the right eye (Fig. 261) showed a papilledema with an elevation of 1.5 diopters. A small area between 7 and 9 o'clock was spared. There was a small peripapillary hemorrhage at the 5-o'clock position. The retinal vessels appear normal. There is a sclerosis of the choroidal vessels (senile tigroid fundus). The fundus of the left eye (Fig. 262) shows a normal optic disc. Other findings were similar to those seen in the right eye. The superficial temporal arteries were only moderately tender to the touch. There were no arterial pulsations. Blood pressure was 150/70 mm Hg measured on both arms, and blood sedimentation rate was 58/100 mm. Histologic examination of the large temporal artery biopsy showed inflammatory infiltration of the partially edematous intima layer. There were patchy areas of focal fibrinoid necrosis. There was granulomatous infection with giant cells, lymphocytes, and plasma cells. The adventitia and surrounding connective tissue were also involved. There was no thrombosis of the lumen. The diagnosis of giant cell arteritis was confirmed. As mentioned in the text, the excision of a large area of the inflamed artery is often a therapeutic tool in treating this disease.

Clinical Course

Visual acuity of the right eye could be improved to 20/25 following cataract extraction.

Figures 263–266. Left and right eyes of a 77-year-old female patient with temporal arteritis (turned 180 degrees in photographs). The patient suffered from a severe visual loss in her right eye 2 days prior to the ocular examination. She felt very ill and had a weight loss during the weeks prior to the visual loss. She also reported a severe occipital headache and neurologic symptoms.

Clinical Findings

Visual acuity in the right eye was less than 20/1000, and in the left eye 20/25. There were bilateral beginning age-related cataracts. Intraocular pressure was 18 mm Hg. The visual field could not be examined in the right eye. Visual field testing of the left eye was unremarkable. The left fundus is normal (Fig. 263). Fundus examination of the right eye (Fig. 264) showed an ischemic edema of the optic disc extending into the peripapillary retina. The arteries are narrow, and the veins are engorged. The left fundus is normal (Fig. 264). Blood pressure was 160/80 mm Hg and blood sedimentation rate was 92/123 mm.

Therapy

The indurated, tender, and pulseless temporal artery was partially removed. Histopathologic examination (Figs. 265 and 266) revealed a narrow lumen with an intact endothelial layer and fibrosis of the intima. The media layer was largely destroyed and replaced by granulomatous focal inflammation with giant cells, plasma cells, and lymphocytes. There was also lymphocytic infiltration of the adventita. These findings confirm a diagnosis of giant cell arteritis.

Clinical Outcome

Following cataract extraction, visual acuity returned to 20/25.

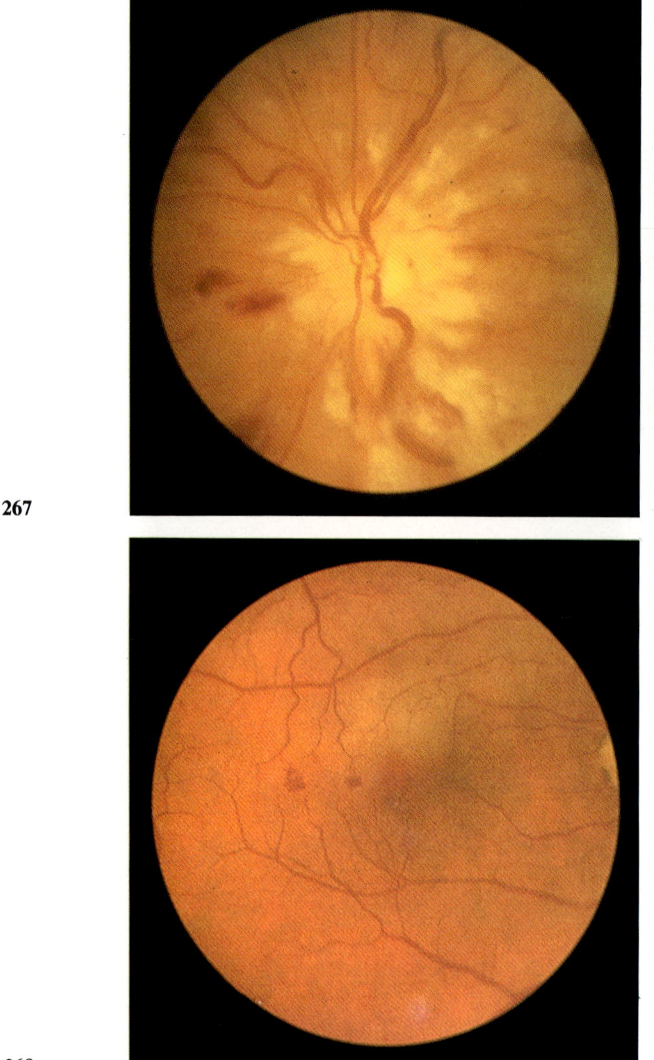

267

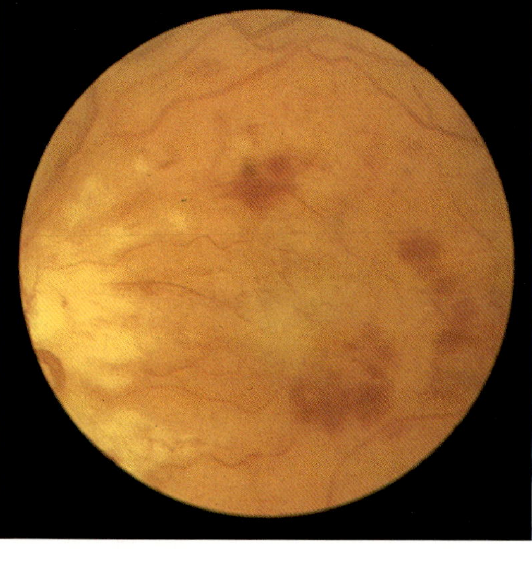

268

269

Figures 267–269. Right and left eye of a 66-year-old male patient with temporal arteritis presenting as an incomplete occlusion of the central retinal vein in the left eye, and later as a branch artery occlusion in the right eye. The patient noted a visual loss 1 week prior to the first ocular examination.

Clinical Findings

Visual acuity in the right eye was 20/20, and in the left eye 20/700. Refractive media were clear and intraocular pressure was 14 mm Hg in the right eye and 18 mm Hg in the left eye. Visual field testing was normal in the right eye. There was a central scotoma in the left eye. An ophthalmoscopic examination of the left eye (Fig. 267 and 268) showed a pale optic disc with blurred margins caused by peripapillary ischemia. The retinal arterioles are narrowed, and the retinal veins are markedly engorged and tortuous. The retinal vessels are partially masked by retinal edema. There is macular edema surrounded by dot and blot hemorrhages. Punctate hemorrhages are present on the optic disc, and peripapillary radial hemorrhages extend toward the midperiphery of the retina. Blood pressure was 160/90 mm Hg measured on both arms, and blood sedimentation rate was 20/42 mm.

Laboratory Findings

α_2-Globulin fraction was elevated. All other blood tests, including tests for rheumatoid factor and syphilis, were negative. An abdominal and thoracic computed tomography was unremarkable.

Therapy

Histopathologically, the temporal artery biopsy showed patchy thickening of the intima with narrowing of the vascular lumen. The vascular endothelium was intact. There were no inflammatory diffuse infiltrates, granulomatous inflammations, or vascular thrombosis. The patient was treated with systemic corticosteroids supplemented by rheologic therapy.

Clinical Course

The complications did not improve in the left eye and amaurosis developed. Three months later the right eye became affected and visual acuity decreased to 20/100 (Fig. 269). Blood sedimentation at that time was 129/150 mm. Doppler sonography did not show any distortion of blood perfusion in the internal carotid artery. Fundus examination of the right eye revealed a cherry-red spot of the macula with focal retinal edema superior to the macular region. There are two dot hemorrhages temporal to the macula (Fig. 269). Sludged-blood phenomenon was found in a major macular branch of the superior temporal artery. The patient was again treated with systemic corticosteroids. The branch artery occlusion resolved and visual acuity returned to 20/20 2 months after onset of symptoms in the right eye. However, the blood sedimentation rate was still 38/50 mm. Because of these very uncharacteristic findings, the diagnosis of temporal arteritis was entertained retrospectively, although the histopathologic results were atypical. However, based on the vascular symptoms, a hidden temporal arteritis seems to be the most likely explanation for the vascular changes in this patient.

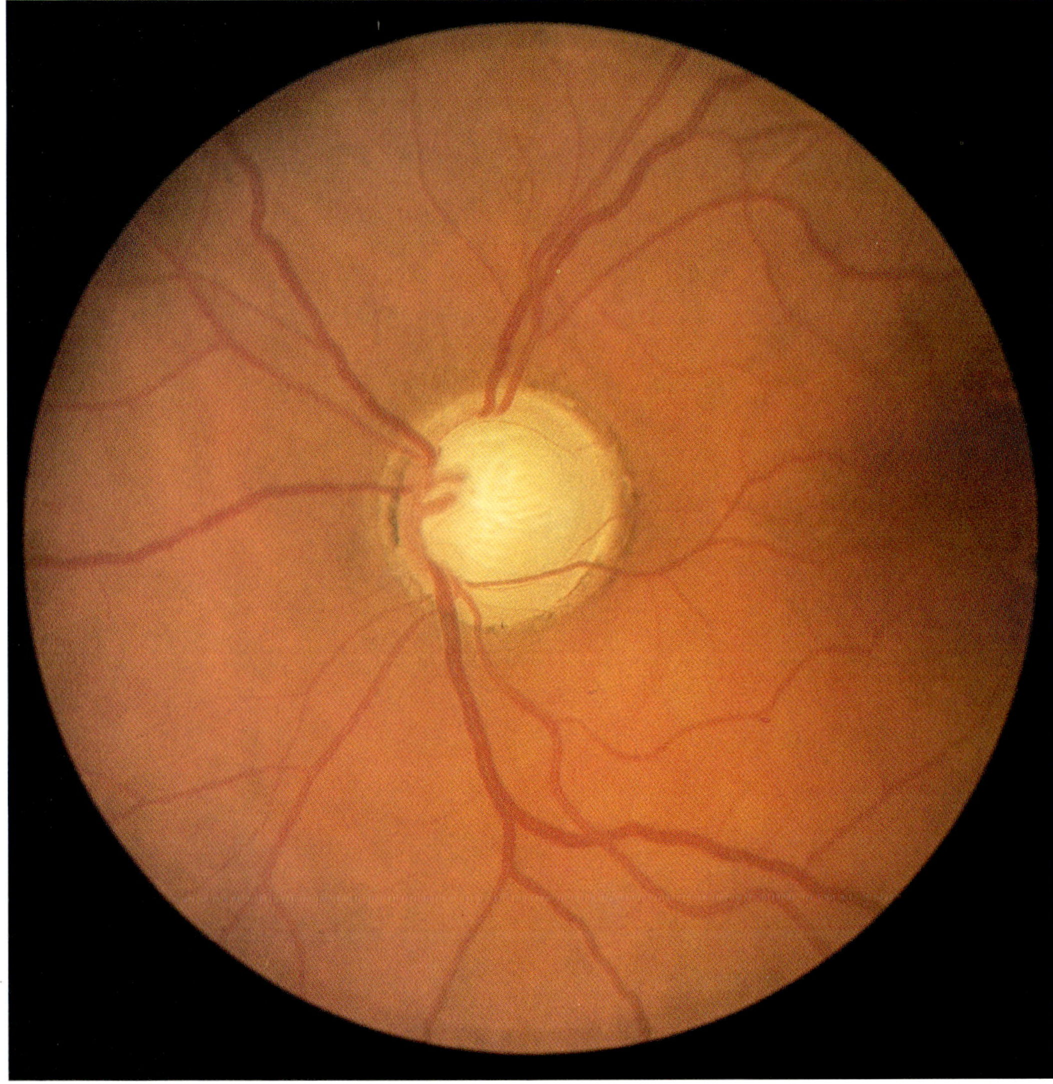

270

Figure 270. Left eye of a 47-year-old male patient with primary open-angle glaucoma and pigment dispersion (differential diagnosis: pigmentary glaucoma).

Clinical Findings

With a refraction in the right eye of −0.75 sphere, visual acuity was 20/25. Refraction in the left eye was −0.5 sphere with visual acuity of 20/40. Intraocular pressure in the right eye was 28 mm Hg, and 32 mm Hg in the left eye. Visual field testing showed a bilateral enlargement of the blind spot. Fundus examination revealed a bilateral large, deep excavation of the optic discs with a cup/disc ratio of 08:09. The lamina cribrosa is visible. Vascular trunks of the central retinal vessels are displaced nasally with typical vascular banding along the margin of the excavation. The optic discs were surrounded by a ring of irregular pigmentation (glaucomatous halo). Slitlamp examination revealed transillumination defects of the iris. Gonioscopy showed an open anterior chamber angle with dark pigmentation of the trabecular meshwork.

Therapy

Surgical intervention (Elliot's operation) was necessary.

Clinical Course

The intraocular pressure normalized after the operation.

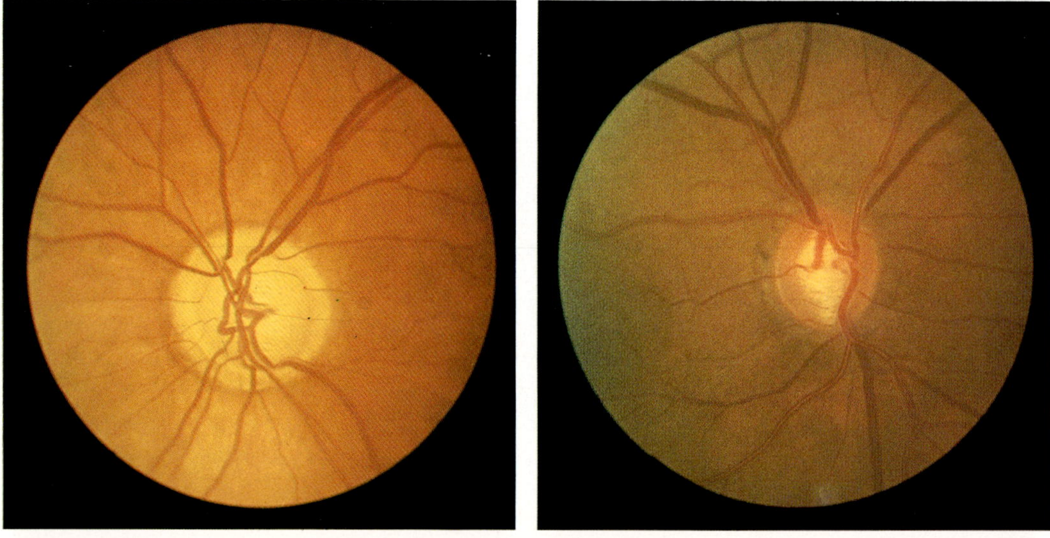

271

272

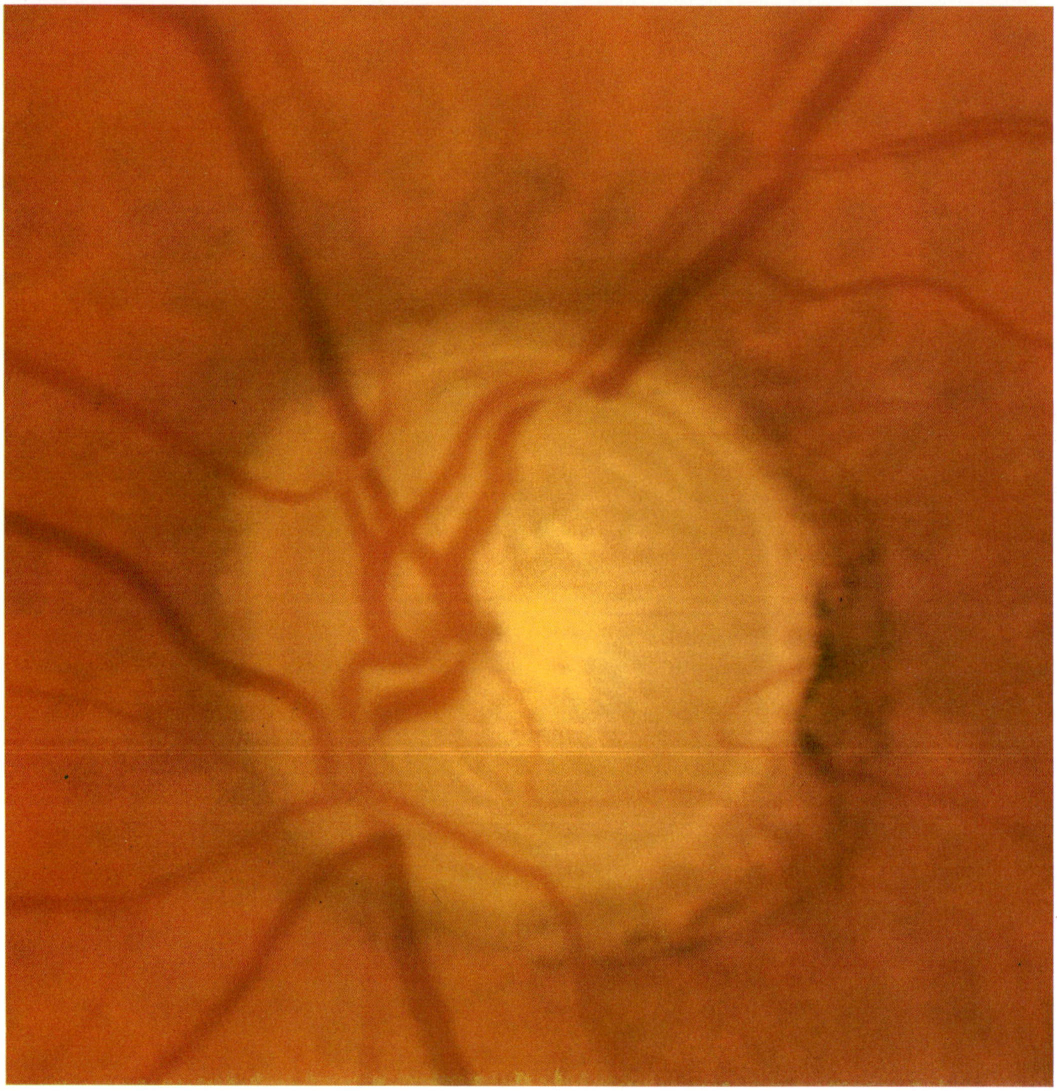

273

274 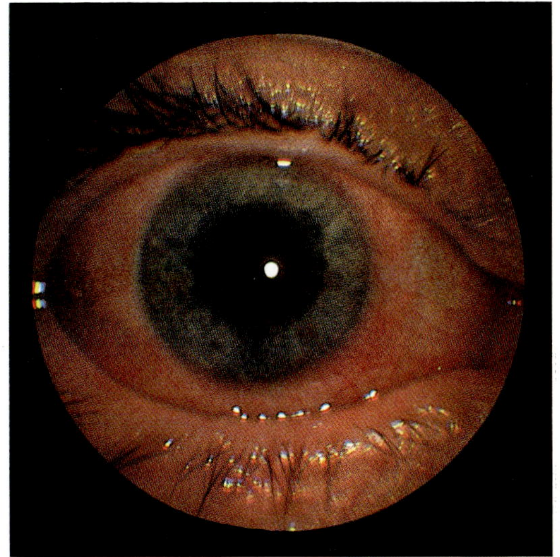

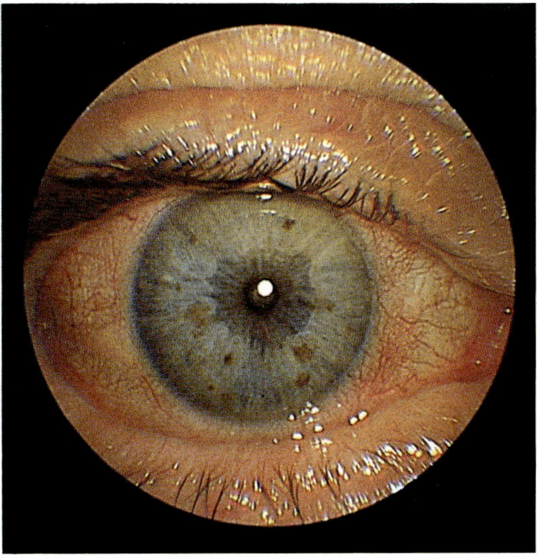 275

Figure 271. Left eye of a 70-year-old male patient with low-tension glaucoma.

Clinical Findings

Refraction in both eyes was +2.5 sphere, −0.5 cylinder, axis 90°; visual acuity in the right eye was 20/20, and in the left eye was 20/50. Intraocular pressure in the right/left eye during the day was: 7 AM, 14/15 mm Hg; 11 AM, 14/17 mm Hg; 3 PM, 16/17 mm Hg; and 7 PM, 14/16 mm Hg. Visual field testing was normal for the right eye. There was a large Bjerrum scotoma in the left eye. Fundus examination of the right eye was unremarkable. The fundus of the left eye showed a deep, large excavated optic disc with central vessels. The lamina cribrosa is visible. There were chorioretinal atrophies surrounding the optic disc (glaucomatous halo). The vessels bend over the margin of the excavated cup. Slitlamp examination revealed a bilateral transillumination defect of the iris and iris atrophy along the pupillary margin. Findings from a neurologic consultation were not significant. A cranial x-ray and computed tomography were unremarkable.

Therapy

Fistulating, filtering glaucoma surgery was performed on both eyes.

Figure 272. Right eye of a 68-year-old female patient with primary open-angle glaucoma.

Clinical Findings

Refraction in the right eye was +1.5 sphere, and in the left eye +2.5 sphere; visual acuity in both eyes was 20/25. Intraocular pressure in both the right and left eyes, measured during the day was: 7 AM, 20/22 mm Hg; 11 AM, 24/26 mm Hg; 3 PM, 24/27 mm Hg; and 7 PM, 25/23 mm Hg. Visual field testing showed a moderate enlargement of the blind spot but no paracentral scotomas. Fundus examination showed the left optic disc was centrally excavated. The central retinal vessels are nasally displaced. The excavation is oval with the longest extension in the vertical diameter, showing superior and inferior extensions toward the optic disc margin. There were bilateral beginning age-related cataracts. Gonioscopy revealed that the anterior chamber angle was open.

Therapy

The intraocular pressure was sufficiently controlled with 2% pilocarpine drops.

Figure 273. Left eye of a 70-year-old male patient with primary open-angle glaucoma.

Clinical Findings

Visual acuity in the right eye was 20/1000 with eccentric fixation, and in the left eye 20/30. Intraocular pressure in the right eye was 38 mm Hg, and in the left eye 26 mm Hg. Visual field testing showed a small temporal visual field remnant in the right eye and a Bjerrum scotoma in the left eye. Fundus examination revealed a deeply excavated optic disc in both eyes. The lamina cribrosa is visible. The central retinal vessels are displaced nasally and the vessel continuity appears interrupted at the site where the vessels curve around the margin of the excavation. There is a glaucomatous halo with irregular pigmentation surrounding the optic disc. The patient also had an advanced bilateral senile cataract. Gonioscopy showed a wide anterior chamber angle with no hyperpigmentation.

Therapy

The patient was treated with 2% pilocarpine drops.

Figures 274 and 275. Right eye of a 53-year-old male patient with acute angle-closure glaucoma.

Clinical Findings

The right eye was congested for 4 days prior to the examination and the patient suffered from headache. The eye was emmetropic and visual acuity in the right eye was 20/60, and in the left eye 20/20. Intraocular pressure in the right eye was 36 mm Hg, and in the left eye 14 mm Hg. Visual field testing revealed an enlargement of the blind spot in the right eye. Fundus examination of the right eye showed a hyperemic optic disc. Slitlamp examination revealed a mixed conjunctival injection, a moderate corneal epithelial edema, and an oval mid-sized pupil that was nonresponsive to light (Fig. 274). Gonioscopy showed a completely closed anterior chamber angle in the right eye and a narrow, but normal, anterior chamber angle without peripheral synechia, depigmentation, or neovascularization in the left eye.

Therapy

The patient was treated with an injection of 300 mg acetazolamide and strong miotics.

Clinical Course

Intraocular pressure normalized within 2 hours. The pupil constricted and the corneal epithelial edema resolved. Visual acuity recovered to 20/25 (Fig. 275).

Tumors of the Retina and Choroid

Retinoblastoma

Synonyms: Neuroepithelioma, glioma retinae, glioblastoma (all classical terms).

Retinoblastoma represents the most common malignant retinal tumor of infancy and childhood. In two-thirds of cases, it is observed within the first 3 years of life. According to the literature, bilateral occurrence is found in 25% of cases, often showing a different extension of the disease in each eye. The hereditary form of retinoblastoma is transmitted as an autosomal dominant trait with incomplete penetrance (around 80%). Bilateral cases are either hereditary or represent a mutation. In contrast, only 20% of unilateral cases represent genetic new mutations, and 80% are nonhereditary phenocopies (Höpping, 1977). However, hereditary cases cannot be differentiated either clinically or histologically from sporadically occurring tumors.

Histologically, two main forms of retinoblastoma can be identified by cell type. Poorly differentiated tumors with a high cellular density are prone to necrosis and calcification. Since the word "blastoma" means a neoplasm composed of undifferentiated immature, blast-form cells, the name retinoblastoma is appropriate for this type of tumor. Retinocytomas or neuroepitheliomas are composed of more differentiated cells that are characteristically organized around a lumen, forming the so-called "Flexner-Wintersteiner rosettes." These highly differentiated cells represent an extension of the external limiting membrane of the retina. Both forms of tumor are generically referred to as retinoblastomas.

Clinically, four different stages have been classified:

Stage 1. In this early stage there are no visible symptoms, especially in newborns, infants, and children up to 3 years. The tumor is hidden, and if discovered, it is almost always found during an early screening examination. Therefore, such examinations are indicated at regular intervals in patients with a familial occurrence of retinoblastoma. The fundus of children must be examined under general anesthesia.

Stage 2. The clinical hallmark of this stage is the leukocoria, seen as a wide pupillary reflex or amaurotic "cat's-eye reflex." The tumor protrudes well into the vitreous cavity, and the pupil is slightly dilated and shows no reaction to light. A bright chalk-white or pink-white reflex is usually present. Unilateral strabismus is often a secondary symptom. Pain caused by secondary glaucoma is rare. Most often the affected eye does not show any irritation, but a spontaneous hyphema or pseudohypopyon may develop. Occasionally, a nodular tumor growth may be seen on the iris surface.

Differential Diagnosis. The differential diagnosis includes such entities as retinal astrocytoma, pseudoglioma, (phacomatoses, i.e., tuberous sclerosis, von Hippel-Lindau disease, neurofibromatosis), congenital anomalies (persistent hyaloid artery, persistent hyperplastic primary vitreous), status after panophthalmitis, status after vitreous abscess and vitreal hemorrhages, retrolental fibroplasia, Coats' disease, and Norrie's disease (atrophia bulborum hereditaria).

Stage 3. Tumor perforation and extrabulbur extension (exophthalmus, involvement of orbital structures) are found at this stage.

Stage 4. The tumor becomes generalized with hematogenous and lymphogenous metastases. Metastases from a retinoblastoma are most commonly located in the bones and, via a direct growth along the optic tract, the brain. Less frequently, the liver, kidneys, ovaries, and lymph nodes are involved.

Ophthalmoscopical Appearance. Solitary or multiple isolated tumor nodules that are gray-white with an irregular surface are the most characteristic finding. The isolated occurrence of these tumor nodules most likely indicates multiple tumor origin rather than local metastases. The tumors are well demarcated from the nonaffected retina. In some cases the tumor is shaped like a bunch of grapes. Retinal veins show increased blood filling and tortuosity, but the arteries remain unchanged. In advanced stages, the tumor frequently causes retinal detachment.

Diagnostic Tests. Because of the age group chiefly affected by retinoblastoma, several of these tests have to be performed under general anesthesia. The diagnostic armamentarium includes slitlamp, ophthalmoscopical, and ultrasound examinations, roentgenography to verify tumor calcification, and anterior chamber paracentesis (aqueous humor cytology). A measurement of lactate dehydrogenase (LDH) should be made because elevated levels of this enzyme are frequently found in retinoblastoma patients. A difference in the ratio of LDH in blood serum compared to that in aqueous humor is an important diagnostic test.

Therapy. The ultimate goal is to save the patient's life and, secondarily, to simultaneously maintain visual function of the affected eye if possible. If the tumor completely fills the eye, it is very likely that it has already infiltrated the optic nerve. In such cases, the only therapy is enucleation of the globe together with most of the optic nerve stalk (minimum 15 mm). It is useful to thoroughly examine the optic nerve histopathologically as an isolated specimen. Such an analysis can make the judgment about optic nerve infiltration easier (Naumann, 1968). If both eyes are affected, depending on the size of the tumor, the worst-looking eye should be enucleated. Other therapeutic possibilities includes tumor coagulation (light coagulation, cryocoagulation) and tumor irradiation. In cases of recurrent retinoblastoma following enucleation or proven metastases, chemotherapy can be administered.

Complete, Spontaneous Remissions (Figs. 276–281). A complete, spontaneous remission is rare, but has been observed. Such remissions are probably related to a complete necrosis in fast growing tumors. Ophthalmoscopically, the lesion resembles a retinoblastoma after irradiation therapy. A coral-like structure surrounded by pigmented and atrophic choroid remains. Phthisis bulbi may be a late complication.

Endophytic Growth of Retinoblastoma

Synonym: Diffuse, infiltrating retinoblastoma.

In some patients, a retinoblastoma may show an endophytic growth pattern that is different than the exophytic growth previously described. In this less frequently seen form of the disease the retina has a diffuse infiltration of tumor cells without any nodular growth or tumor mass. This growth pattern, if associated with pseudohypopyon and vitreal infiltrations, may be easily misdiagnosed as uveitis.

Retinoblastoma as a Hereditary Disease

According to statistical studies, retinoblastoma patients have a higher chance of suffering from nonretinoblastoma malignancies during their life than the normal population. Malignant tumors also occur with an increased incidence in family members of retinoblastoma patients. In addition to carcinomas and sarcomas, leukemic tumors have also been reported (Stefani, 1976).

Malignant Melanoma of the Choroid

The most common primary tumor of the uvea is melanoma (melanosarcoma or melanoblastoma), which almost always occurs unilaterally. Melanomas are preponderantly found in adults. According to some authors, this tumor arises from a choroidal nevus. Pigment-containing melanomas are termed melanosarcomas, and melanomas without pigment are termed amelanotic melanomas or leukosarcomas (Fig. 282).

Histopathologically, four different types of malignant melanomas must be differentiated: (*a*) spindle A melanoma, (*b*) spindle B melanoma, (*c*) mixed tumor (spindle cell and epithelioid cells), and (*d*) epithelioid cell melanoma. This classification of cell types is ranked, according to prognosis, from the best to the poorest. Malignant melanomas metastasize via the vascular system. The liver is by far the most common uveal melanoma metastasis site. Other organs not affected as frequently are lungs, stomach, kidneys, brain, spinal cord, and bones. Metastasis is rare in the breasts, ovaries, and skin, but such growths have occurred.

Clinical Course. The development of a malignant melanoma shows four clinical stages:

Stage 1. No symptoms;
Stage 2. Retinal detachment;
Stage 3. Secondary glaucoma;
Stage 4. Tumor perforation into the orbit.

If the macula is not affected, the tumor may grow for some time without causing any clinical symptoms. Reduction in visual acuity usually indicates a tumor that has undergone extensive growth. Some patients report a slowly progressing visual field loss in the affected eye. An ophthalmoscopical examination usually shows a solid elevated tumor mass that may appear smooth or irregular and is gray to brown-black in color. At this stage, a retinal detachment is present but there is no retinal hole. After the tumor has penetrated Bruch's membrane, a mushroom-like growth protrudes into the vitreous space. A secondary intraocular pressure elevation ensues. After penetrating the sclera, the tumor may show extrabulbar growth. By the perforation stage hematogenous metastases usually have spread.

Differential Diagnosis. The differential diagnosis of malignant melanomas includes choriodal nevus, choriodal hemangioma, organized choroidal hemorrhage, choroidal detachment, senile disciform macular degeneration, granulomas of different etiologies (nematodes), or tumor metastases.

Diagnostic Procedures:

1. Ophthalmoscopy (observation of lesion over time), fundus photographic documentation.
2. Diascleral elimination (diaphanoscopic examination with subconjunctival application of light source). One of the straight ocular muscles may be temporally disinserted. If a tumor is present, neither the sclera nor a choroidal detachment appear translucent when a light is applied to the sclera adjacent to the tumor.
3. Ultrasound (A and B scan).
4. Fluorescein angiography. Typical findings are an early arterial tumor fluorescence and a late venous fluorescein diffusion.
5. Radioactive phosphorus (^{32}P) uptake test. The tumor has an increased phosphorus uptake. This test has only limited validity, especially if the melanoma is small.
6. Infrared photography. This test may be used as a differential diagnostic method, particularly in the early stages.

Therapy. Previously, enucleation of a uveal malignant melanoma was the only therapy. Now more conservative radiation therapy is used more frequently (^{106}Ru application). If the tumor has invaded the sclera, an orbital exenteration with subsequent irradiation (6000 rad) is the usual treatment.

Benign Choroidal Tumors

Benign choroidal tumors include choroidal nevi and, less frequently, angiomas, fibromas, neurofibromas (often associated with phacomatoses, i.e., tuberous sclerosis, von Hippel-Lindau disease, and neurofibromatosis).

Metastatic Choroidal Tumors

Most choroidal metastases appear approximately 6 months after the primary tumor. Metastases are associated most often with breast cancer and, less frequently, with lung or stomach cancer. Metastases also may arise from malignant intestinal carcinomas, renal carcinomas, epirenal carcinomas, thyroid carcinomas, and carcinomas originating in the thymus, liver, pancreas, prostate, testicles, and uterus.

Arteriovenous Hemangiomas in the Elderly

In contrast to von Hippel-Lindau disease, angiomatoses in the elderly do not show any changes in the afferent feeder arteriole and the efferent draining venule (Pau, 1974a). The vessels show neither an increased diameter nor any tortuosity. They appear hemogenously dark, with no changes in coloration. Therefore, differentiation between an arteriole and a venule is possible only by fluorescein angiography (Figs. 284 and 285).

The vascular tumor has a reddish brown appearance. It may be nodular or cystic (angioma cysticum) and, only rarely, measures up to 1 optic disc diameter. In the proximity of the lesion, other arteriovenous (AV) shunts can be found. The lesion may show a slight progressivity (Fig. 283).

Since a retinal hemangioma may be associated with an extracranial (orbital) or intracranial hemangioma or other vascular abnormalities (von Hippel-Lindau disease, Wyburn-Mason syndrome), a neurologic or neuroradiologic examination is always indicated. Secondary retinal changes may be present in the form of a circinate retinopathy. Complications include retinal and vitreous hemorrhages, retinal detachment, and secondary glaucoma.

Differential Diagnosis. Differential diagnosis includes choroidal hemangiomas, glial hamartomas (Fig. 286), vascular proliferations following retinal vascular occlusions, Leber's miliary aneurysms, or Coats' disease.

Therapy. The tumor may be coagulated using diathermy, laser or xenon light coagulation or cryocoagulation. If a retinal detachment occurs, it must be repaired surgically.

Wyburn-Mason Syndrome

Synonyms: Bonnet-Dechaume-Blanc syndrome, neuroretinoangiomatosis.

This entity represents a mostly unilateral occurring, congenital angiomatous malformation.

Ophthalmoscopical Appearance. Wyburn-Mason syndrome is an association of intracranial angiomatous malformations with similar racemose angiomas of the hemolateral retina. The intracranial lesions are located mostly within the diencephalon and mesencephalon. Radiologic examination may reveal a dilated optic foramen on the affected side, indicating an ateriovenous anastomosis surrounding the optic nerve. The skin and mucous membranes may be affected, and unilateral telangiectasias and hemangiomas may be found. Neurologic symptoms such as contralateral pyramidal sign, cranial nerve palsies (III, IV, and VII nerves), and symptomatic epilepsy may be present. Other ocular symptoms include reduced visual acuity, visual field defects (homonymous hemianopsia) and, rarely, a pulsating exophthalmos.

Diagnosis. The diagnosis is based on the characteristic fundus changes of racemose, serpentine, plexiform, or cavernous hemangiomas, and cirsoid aneurysms. The neurologic symptoms, as well as typical skin and mucous membrane lesions, may be absent. A neuroradiologic examination and carotid angiography may help to ascertain the diagnosis.

Differential Diagnosis. The differential diagnosis basically includes other angiomatous phacomatoses such as von Hippel-Lindau syndrome, Klippel-Trenaunay-Weber syndrome, and Sturge-Weber syndrome.

Therapy. Ocular treatment is indicated if the angiomas hemorrhage, e.g., light coagulation of the tumor. Secondary glaucoma is almost never a part of this disease. The tumor generally has a very mild, benign course. The intracranial lesion may require neurosurgical treatment. If the tumor is inoperable, a partial artificial thrombosis may be induced via the internal carotid artery to reduce the intracranial hemangiomatous tumor mass (Schlieter and coauthors, 1976).

Choroidal Metastases

Reports about choroidal metastases of malignant, extraocular tumors are found only sporadically in the ophthalmic literature. Because most of the publications are case reports, it may be misleading to conclude that choroidal metastases are a rare entity. The lack of opportunities to examine tumor patients ophthalmologically at a time when a tumor has become generalized may explain a lack of information about metastatic ophthalmic tumors. Cases with painful secondary glaucoma are quite rare.

Some physiologic-anatomic vascular findings may explain why the left eye is affected more often than the right eye. This may be partially because the left internal carotid artery originates from the aortic arch, whereas the internal carotid artery and the arteria supraclavia dextra originate at the brachiocephalic trunk.

Ophthalmoscopical Appearance. Intraocular metastases appear as an isolated (rarely multiple) gray to yellow-gray lesion that measures up to several optic disc diameters. Breast cancer metastases often show flat, barely elevated growth; whereas metastases of intestinal carcinomas are more prone to elevated, prominent growth. The latter metastases rarely reach the size of a malignant melanoma. The surface of the tumor may show slight pigment irregularities with pigment granules that are gold to brown. The tumor may be surrounded by small hemorrhages and/or whitish degenerative areas. Characteristically, a secondary exudative retinal detachment, which is usually flat, can be found at an early stage. When a retinal detachment occurs, the choroidal metastasis (the underlying reason for the detachment), may be masked (differential diagnosis: inflammatory processes) (Figs. 287 and 288).

Diagnosis. The diagnosis is based on the photographically documented opthalmoscopical findings that show any progressive growth of the tumor. Other diagnostic tools are chromatoophthalmoscopy (infrared), ultrasound (A and B scan), and fluorescein angiography. A thorough general examination by an internist, including radiologic and hormonal screening, are also indicated. Other medical specialists may be consulted depending on each case.

Clinical Appearance. The patients may be free of any ocular symptoms for a long period of time. Often a metastasis is discovered incidentally during an ophthalmoscopical examination. This is especially true for early metastasizing pulmonary, intestinal and thyroidal tumors, and hypernephromas. Visual acuity may be affected if the metastasis is located at the posterior pole. Inflammatory changes may be present, but secondary glaucoma is not often an early symptom.

Therapy. Ophthalmologically, the first therapy includes irradiation. Enucleation of the affected eye should only be performed as a last therapeutic option. Generally, the ocular therapy is adjusted to fit the treatment of the primary tumor. An endocrinological approach may be chosen with tumor metastases from the endocrine system (ovarectomy, adrenalectomy, hypophysectomy). Other tumors may be treated by using only chemotherapy or irradiation.

Breast cancer metastases are usually seen an average of 3.5 years after the primary tumor was diagnosed. Quite often such metastases occur 5–10 years or later after discovery of the primary tumor. According to the literature, the average life expectancy after a choroidal metastasis has been diagnosed is approximately 9 months.

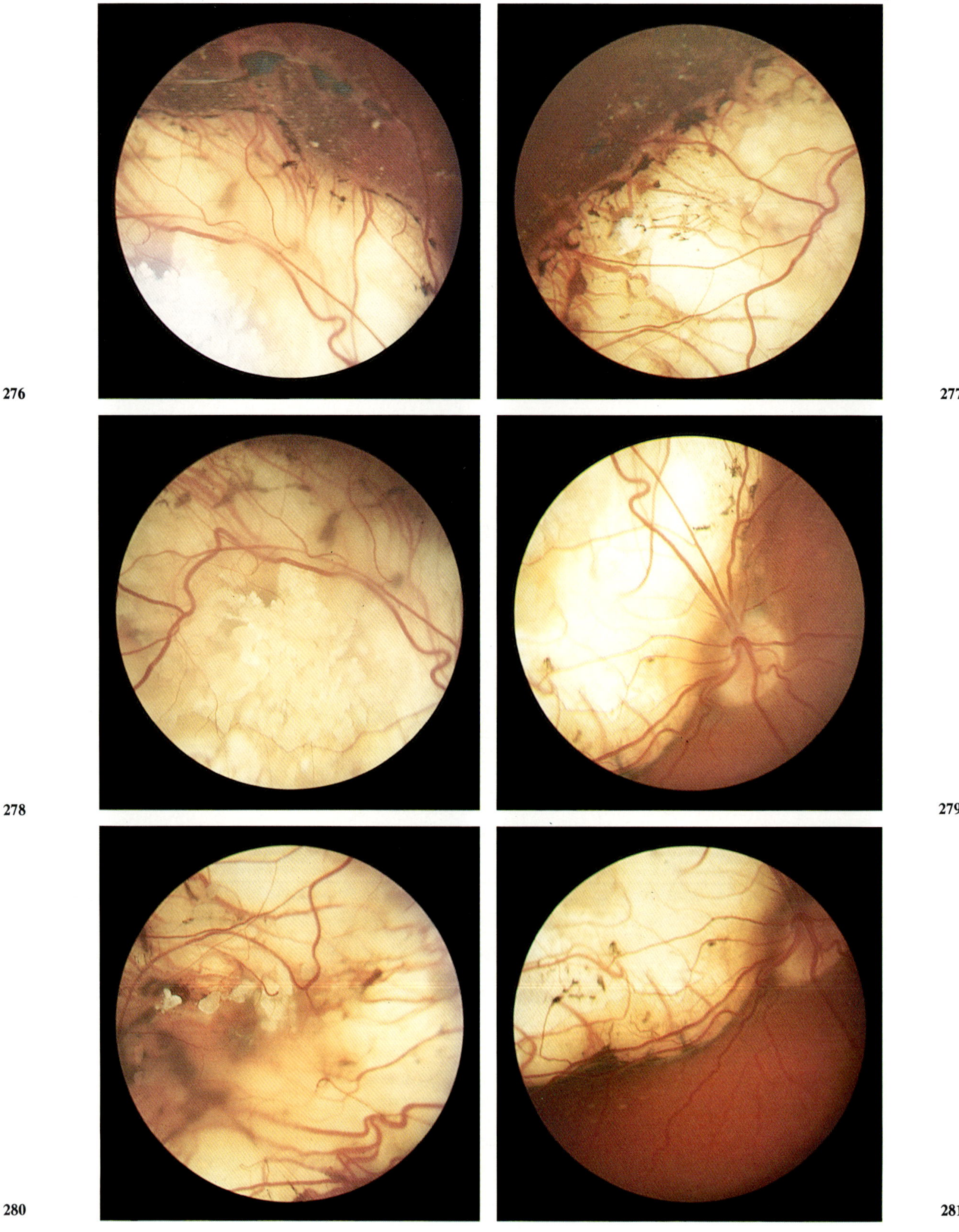

276 277

278 279

280 281

282 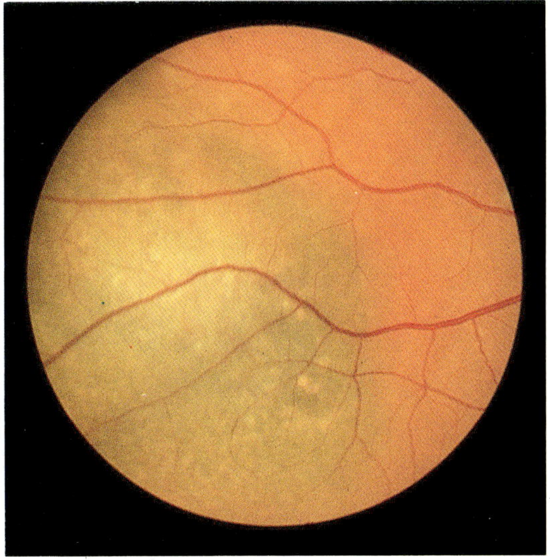

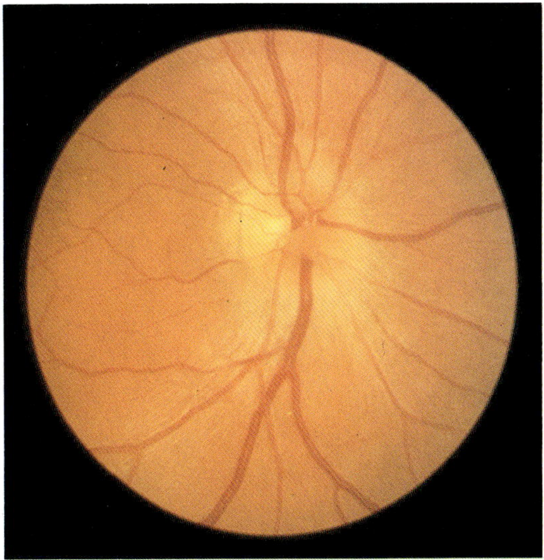 283

Figures 276–281. Right eye of a 9-year-old female patient with spontaneous remission of a retinoblastoma.

Clinical Findings

Visual acuity was 20/1000. Refractive media were clear and intraocular pressure was 14 mm Hg. There was secondary exotropia. Fundus examination showed the entire posterior pole was covered with a large scar with coral-like irregular deposits in the center of the lesion. The margins of the lesion were not elevated and show marked choroidal atrophy. There was enhanced pigmentation along the margins. The family history was unremarkable regarding retinoblastoma or other tumors.

Figure 282. Right eye of a 58-year-old female patient with malignant melanoma of the choroid.

Clinical Findings

The refraction in this eye was +1.0 sphere, visual acuity 20/25. Refractive media were clear and intraocular pressure was 18 mm Hg. Fundus examination showed an elevated, pigmented tumor measuring 4 optic disc diameters superotemporally from the macula. Fluorescein angiography showed a highly suspicious vascular pattern for malignant melanoma of the choroid. The eye was enucleated and histopathologic examination confirmed the clinical diagnosis. The tumor had not infiltrated the optic nerve.

Clinical Course

Ten years after the enucleation no metastases had occurred.

Figure 283. Right eye of a 47-year-old female patient (turned 180° in photograph) with papilledema associated with meningioma of one wing of the sphenoid bone that extended into the orbital apex.

Clinical Findings

At the time of examination, visual acuity had decreased over 1 week to 20/100. The refractive error was +2.5 sphere, −1.0 cylinder, axis 45°. Refractive media were clear, and intraocular pressure was 16 mm Hg. There was a central scotoma and temporal hemianopia in the right eye. Visual fields in the left eye were normal. Fundus examination of the right eye revealed papilledema involving nearly the entire optic disc, which was most evident nasally. There was a peripapillary retinal edema extending from 5 to 1 o'clock. The retinal veins were engorged, indicating a decreased venous outflow. Exophthalmometer readings were 18-85-19 mm. A neurologic examination was unremarkable. An EEG, echoencephalography, and brain centigram were unremarkable. An x-ray in Rheese's position showed a narrowed optic channel with blurred margins. Cranial computed tomography helped confirm a diagnosis of meningioma of the sphenoidal wing.

Clinical Course

The patient refused neurosurgical intervention and did not return for follow-up examination.

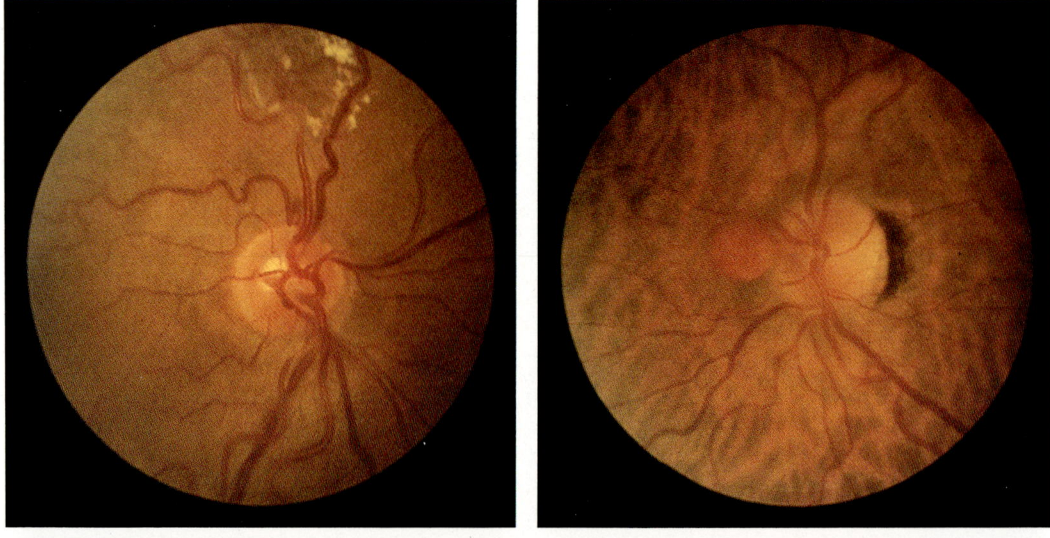

284

285

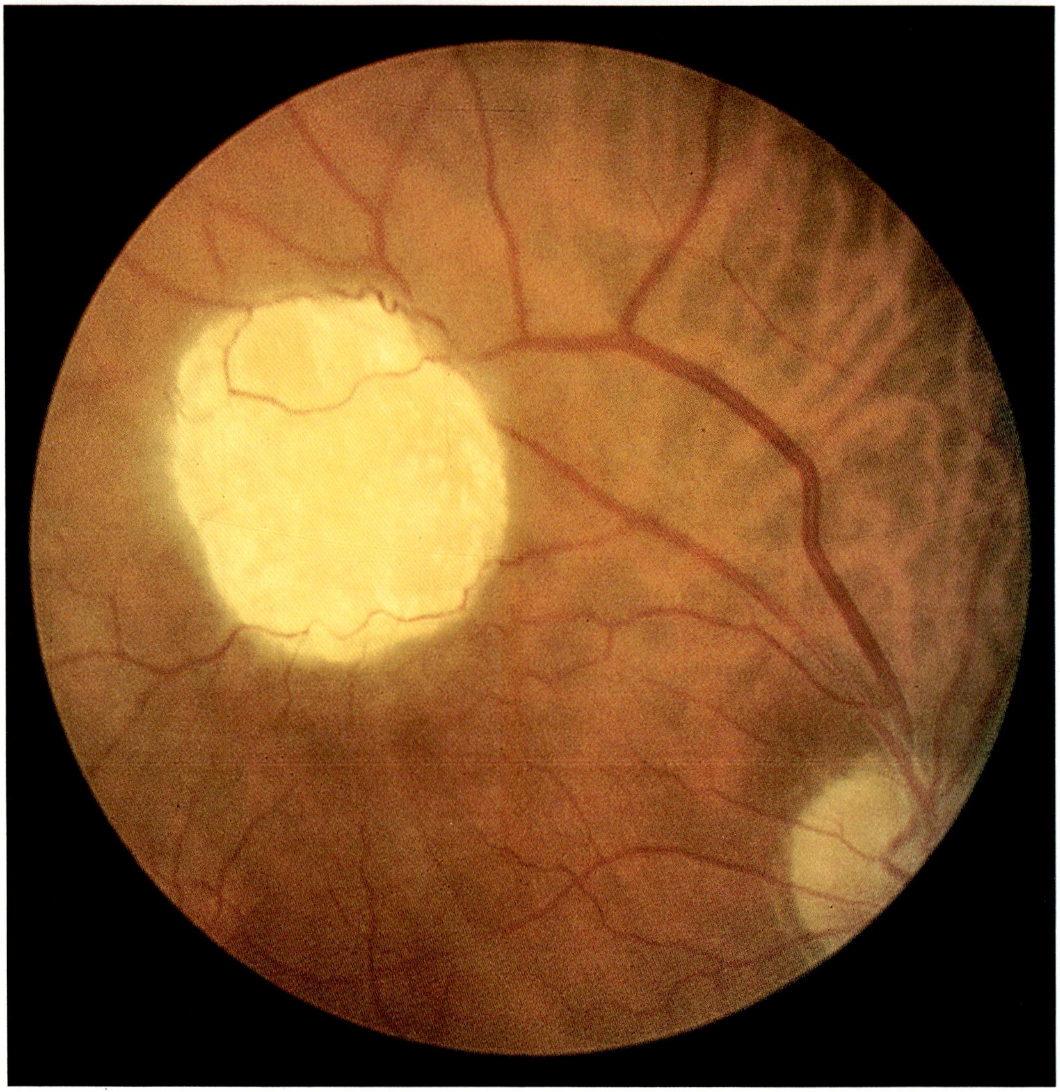

286

287 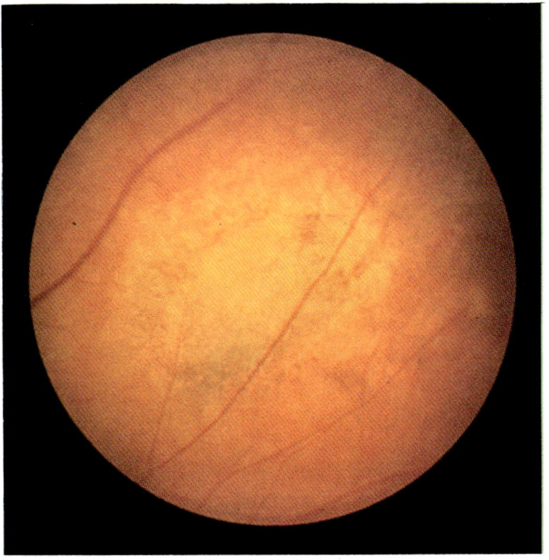

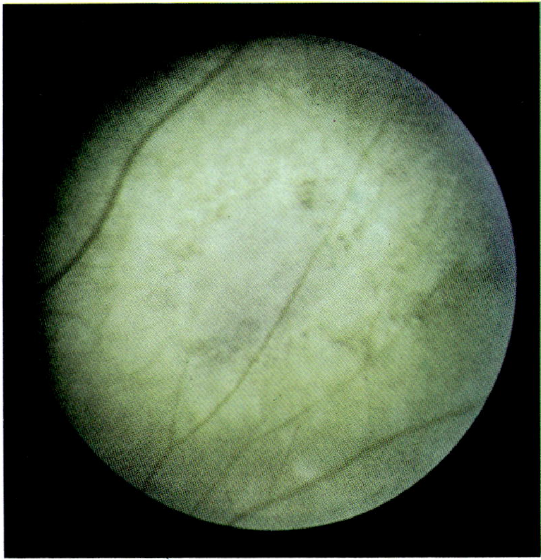 288

Figure 284. Right eye of a 68-year-old male patient with ateriovenous hemangioma of the retina (*top*) and late stage hypertensive retinopathy.

Clinical Findings

The patient was first seen following a cerebral stroke associated with left hemiparesis. There was a history of arterial hypertension (blood pressure 220/120 mm Hg measured on both arms). Visual acuity was 20/60, and there was an age-related cataract.

Clinical Course

The patient died 4 weeks later.

Figure 285. Left eye of a 62-year-old male patient with capillary hemangioma.

Clinical Findings

With a correction of −2.0 sphere, −0.5 cylinder, axis 155°, visual acuity was 20/20. Visual fields were normal. Fluorescein angiography confirmed the diagnosis of a capillary hemangioma immediately adjacent to the optic disc.

Clinical Course

The hemangioma was photographed and followed at regular intervals.

Figure 286. Right eye of a 56-year-old male patient with glial hamartoma.

Clinical Findings

The eye was emmetropic and visual acuity was 20/30. Refractive media were clear and intraocular pressure was 16 mm Hg. Visual field testing showed the defect shown in this photograph. Neurologic and radiologic consultations ruled out symptoms usually asssociated with von Hippel-Lindau syndrome, Bourneville-Pringle disease, or von Recklinghausen's disease.

Clinical Course

The ophthalmoscopic appearance of the lesion remained unchanged over an observation period of 10 years.

Figures 287 and 288. Left eye of a 38-year-old female patient with choroidal lesion that appeared to be a metastasized primary tumor of unknown origin.

Clinical Findings

Refraction in both eyes was +1.0 sphere, and visual acuity was 20/20. Refractive media were clear and intraocular pressure was 14 mm Hg in the right eye and 15 mm Hg in the left eye. Visual fields were normal. The right fundus was normal. The fundus in the left eye (Fig. 287) showed a flat yellow-brown lesion measuring approximately 1 optic disc diameter located in the midperiphery of the retina with irregular pigmentations along the edges and surrounding choroidal atrophy. However, there was no exudative retinal detachment. Infrared photography was positive for melanocytic pigment (Fig. 288). In the late venous stage of fluorescein angiography, the tumor stained in irregular patches. The fluorescein leakage can be seen. A general medical workup of the patient, including a mammography, thermography of the breast, x-ray of the colon, endoscopy of the gastrointestinal system, and x-ray of the paranasal sinuses, was negative for a primary tumor. All laboratory findings were within normal limits. A gynecologic workup was also negative.

Clinical Course

The lesion remained unchanged.

Fundus Changes Associated with Pregnancy

The first report regarding fundus changes associated with pregnancy was given by von Graefe. In 1855, he reported the case of a woman who suffered from Bright's disease during the puerperal period: "Besides very broad, wide retinal exudates, there was an extensive retinal detachment inferiorly. I was quite astonished to see this patient several months later with a completely attached retina."

Not only can a retinal detachment be observed during a subsequent pregnancy that is associated with gestosis and preexisting renal disorders, but it can also be found during a severe gestosis in a unipara or multipara, independent of the month of gestation. According to Schiötz (1919), unilateral retinal detachment seems to be exceptional; most often both eyes are affected. However, development of a retinal detachment in the fellow eye may be delayed (see Table 25 for nomenclature).

Hollwich (1960) studied retinal vessels in 500 healthy pregnant women by using Lobeck measuring oculars, which are based on the heliometer principle. The vessels were evaluated by using the normal values of the physiological thickness of the central retinal artery (0.090–0.112 mm). These normal values were established using the same method introduced by Badtke in 1937. In his series, Hollwich (1960) found measurable abnormalities of the arterial thickness in 206 cases (41.2%) during the last 3 months of gestation. Either some isolated branches of the central retinal arteries showed thinning when curving from the optic disc onto the retina, or all the retinal branches showed a decreased caliber (generalized spasm). The nasal arterial branches were affected most often and also showed these changes earlier than the temporal branches. According to Hollwich (1961), a vasoconstriction exceeding 40%, combined with a blood pressure elevation of approximately 25%, marked the average transition from a physiological to a pathological condition.

Table 25. Nomenclature of Gestosis (Disorder of Pregnancy)

EPH	Edema, proteinuria, hypertension.
IE	Imminent eclampsia (monosymptomatic or polysymptomatic gestosis without cerebral convulsions during pregnancy, birth, or as a puerperal gestosis), precursor of eclampsia with cerebral convulsions. *Synonyms:* preeclampsia, retinopathia gravidarum. In preeclampsia, all retinal changes may resolve completely after birth.
CE	Convulsive eclampsia. *Synonyms:* eclampsia, retinopathia eclamptica. After birth, a complete resolution of all retinal changes is possible.
Gestosis superimposed on preexisting, chronic vascular disorders such as arterial hypertension and renal disorders (German, "Pfropfgestosis": "to graft" to gestosis).	*Synomyms:* symptomatic gestosis, retinopathia albuminurica gravidarum, gravidic or toxemic retinopathy. Gestosis causes progression of preexisting retinovascular and retinoparenchymatous changes, which do not resolve completely afer birth.

Ophthalmoscopical Appearance. Gestosis edema, proteinuria (preeclampsia), and hypertension may be associated with the following ophthalmoscopical changes (all of which may resolve completely after the birth):

1. Retinal arteries develop spasms, especially nasal arterial branches. As the vasospasm increases, arteries may change appearance and appear spindle- or bead-shaped. These constrictions may simulate a peristalsis.
2. The retinal parenchyma reveals hemorrhages, cotton wool exudates, and a milk-white edema that may involve the optic disc.
3. In contrast to a gestosis superimposed on a preexisting renal disease, typical vascular changes associated with renal disorders affecting the retinal vasculature and parenchyma are missing (Figs. 289–294).

Eclamptic Amaurosis

According to pathologic and anatomic studies (von Baunmühl, 1928; Benoit, 1931; Bodechtel, 1934), eclamptic amaurosis is caused by arterial spasms and functional circulatory distortions in the visual cortex. This entity is characterized by an acute bilateral visual loss with a normal fundus appearance and normal pupillary motions. After several hours or days, vision spontaneously recuperates. Eclamptic amaurosis may precede an eclamptic attack or immediately ensue. The incidence of this condition ranges from 5 to 9.8% (Mönckeberg, 1931).

Differential Diagnosis. The differential diagnosis includes such complications of pregnancy as icterus gravis, uremic amaurosis, optic neuritis associated with pregnancy, or hysteria.

Retinal Detachment during Pregnancy

As mentioned, a unilateral or bilateral retinal detachment may occur in a unipara or multipara patient at any time during gestation. Spontaneous reattachments have been reported by von Graefe (1855), Schiötz (1919), and Verderame (1911). However, most authors (Velhagen, 1940; Gasteiger, 1953; Heydenrieich, 1955; Legerlotz, 1971; Mewe, 1981) agree that the pregnancy should be interrupted, by cesarean section if necessary, for renal complications if, despite optimal therapy, the mother's life is severely endangered. Depending on when the retinal detachment occurs, the birth of a healthy child is very unlikely, but this depends on the severity of the underlying disease (Velhagen, 1940).

Retinal detachments caused by other than renal complications are not an indication for interruption of the pregnancy or for a cesarean section at full term. To abbreviate the labor, a vacuum extraction may be performed. A cesarean section is indicated only if additional complications are present.

Optic Neuritis during Pregnancy

Clinical Appearance. The clinical appearance of optic neuritis during pregnancy is similar to that of optic neuritis not associated with pregnancy. This condition is most often observed between the 4th and 7th month of gestation. All stages and types (intrabulbar and retrobulbar) of optic neuritis can be observed. A wide range of manifestations may be observed from mildly distorted visual acuity to the most severe form of neuritis that leads to optic nerve atrophy and blindness. Unilateral and bilateral involvement is possible. If both eyes are affected, each one may show a varied degree of inflammation. The clinical course is often prolonged, and neuritis can recur during the same pregnancy or with subsequent pregnancies.

According to Weigelin (1908), there is an etiologic connection between pregnancy and optic neuritis. Weigelin based this conclusion on an extensive literature search and on his own findings. He noted that after spontaneous or iatrogenically induced birth the ocular inflammation subsides. However, recurrent inflammation was observed in subsequent pregnancies. He also ruled out other possible causes (in particular, nephritis) by careful examination.

Mewe (1981) speculated that occurrence of optic neuritis during pregnancy is simply coincidental. Therefore, he objected to interruption of the gestation. Also, during the puerperal period, the occurrence of optic neuritis (lactation neuritis) has been observed. In this instance, the mother should stop nursing the baby.

Differential Diagnosis. The differential diagnosis includes inherited diseases (Leber's optic atrophy), optic neuritis caused by intoxication (quinine abuse), amaurosis associated with icterus gravis, uremia, eclampsia, hysteria (which does not proceed into optic atrophy), or hypophyseal tumors.

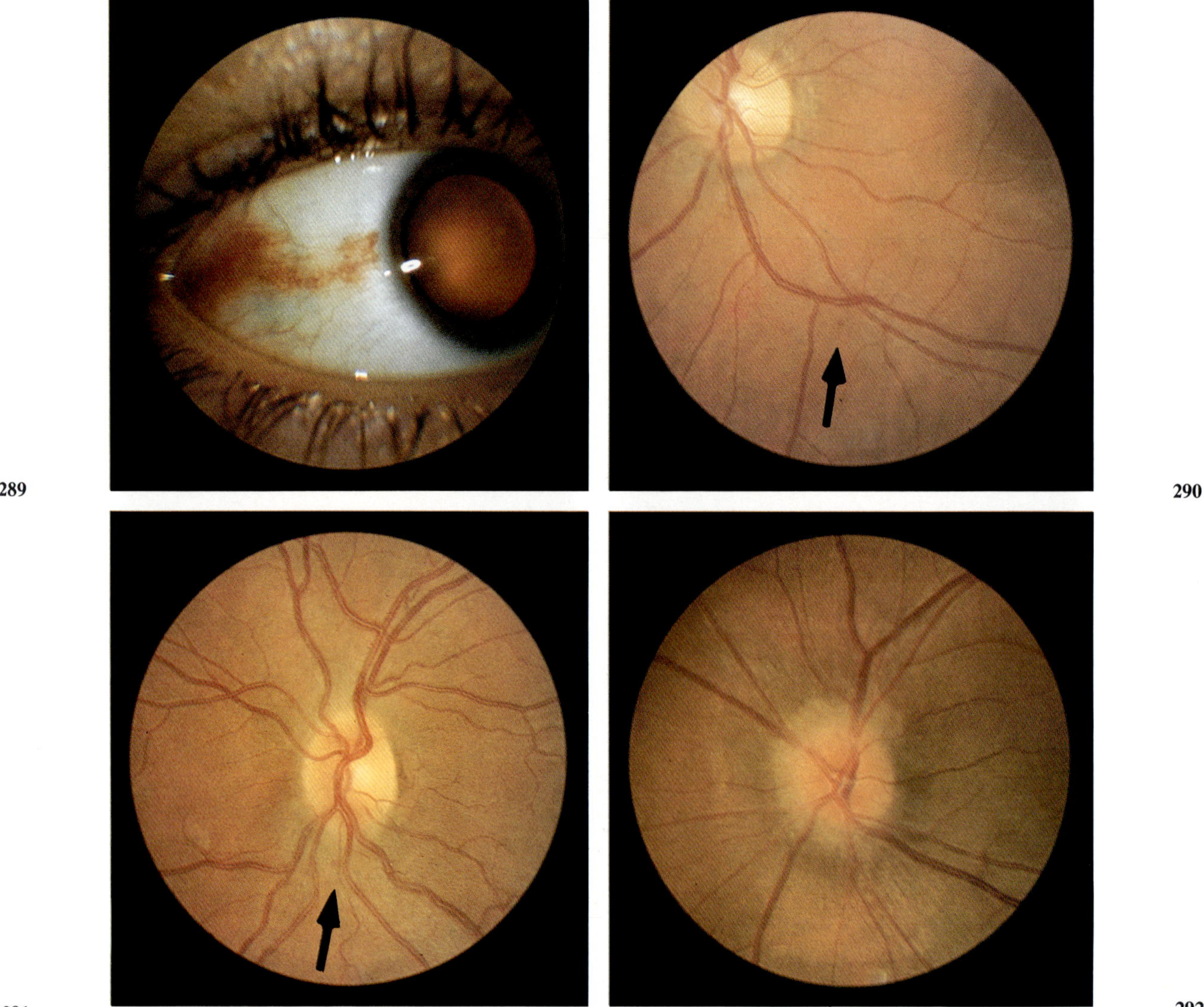

Figure 289. Right eye of a 35-year-old female patient with subconjunctival hemorrhage following normal delivery.

Clinical Findings

The patient gave birth to her third child 2 days earlier. A subconjunctival hemorrhage was found, extending temporally from the insertion of the lateral rectus muscle. Visual acuity in both eyes was 20/20. The fundus was normal and blood pressure was 130/85 mm Hg.

Figure 290. Left eye of a 28-year-old female patient with proteinuria (preeclampsia) during delivery of a second child.

Clinical Findings

The eyes were examined after birth. Visual acuity in both eyes was 20/20. Blood pressure measured on both arms was 170/110 mm Hg. There is an isolated punctate hemorrhage located away from the optic disc (*arrow*). Differential diagnosis for this lesion includes microaneurysm. The patient did not want to undergo fluorescein angiography because of the renal involvement.

Clinical Course

Three weeks after the first examination, the hemorrhage had resolved. Note: In 10 cases of clinically confirmed toxemia, identical hemorrhages (most unilateral and always inferiorly located) were found (Huismans, 1984b). Such retinal hemorrhages may possibly represent a specific finding in cases of preeclampsia or eclampsia. Other characteristic findings are generalized arterial vascular spasms.

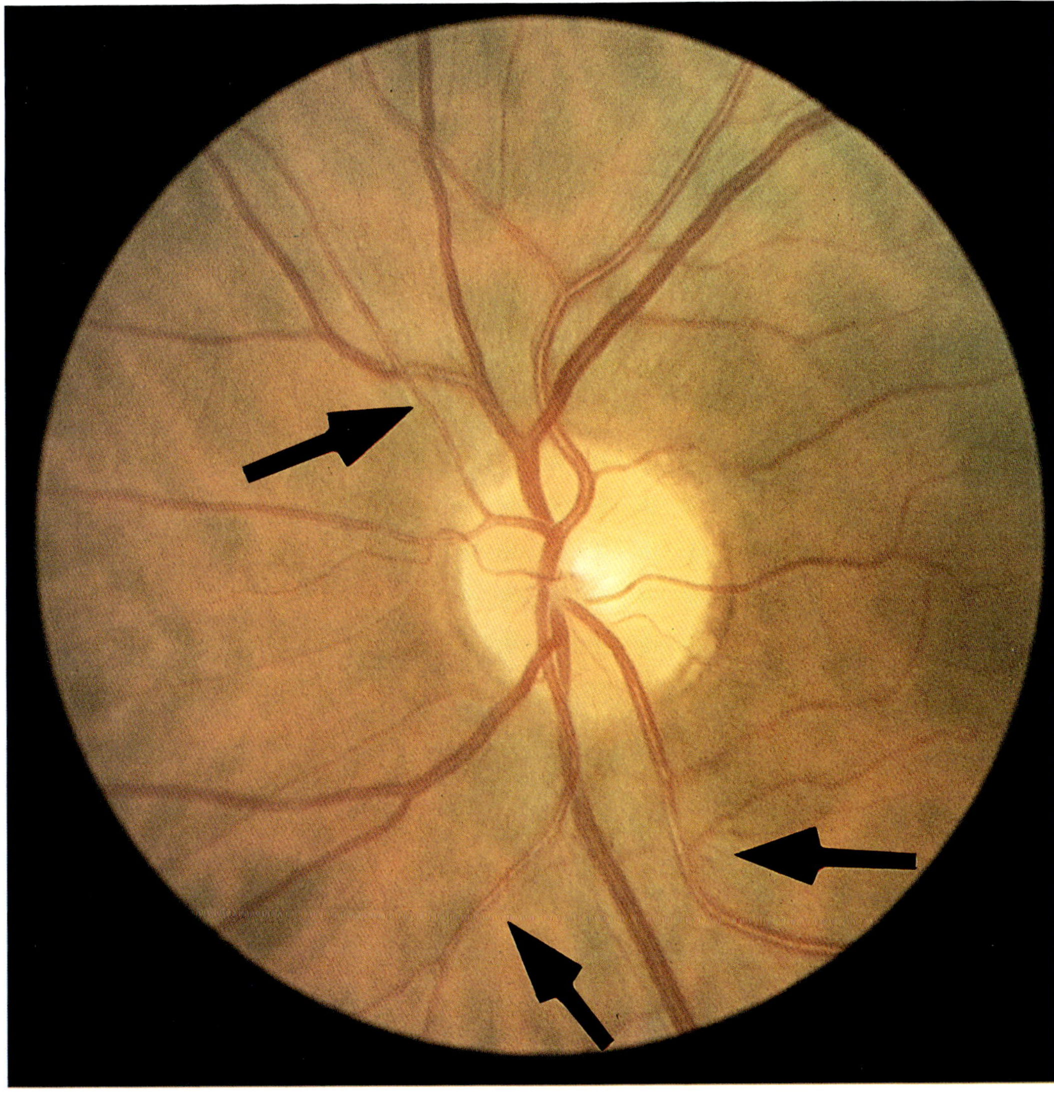

293

Figure 291. Left eye of a 25-year-old primipara patient with toxemia during the 8th month of gestation.

Clinical Findings

Peripapillary retinal edema and a small perivascular punctate hemorrhage (*arrow*) inferior to the optic disc (compare with Fig. 290) are seen. Arterial spasms are present, especially nasally. Blood pressure measured on both arms was 145/95 mm Hg.

Clinical Course

After a spontaneous delivery, the punctate retinal hemorrhage resolved.

Figure 292. Left eye of a 25-year-old primipara patient with toxemia during the 9th month of gestation.

Clinical Findings

Papilledema and disseminated arterial spasms with blood pressure of 155/95 mm Hg measured on both arms.

Figure 293. Left eye of a 30-year-old primipara patient with preeclampsia 4 days after delivery.

Clinical Findings

Visual acuity in both eyes was 20/25. Arterial spasms (*arrows*) are visible. Visual fields and color, mesopic, and scotopic vision were normal. Delivery was complicated by a forceps extraction. Blood pressure during delivery varied from 180/120 to 200/120 mm Hg but normalized after the birth.

294

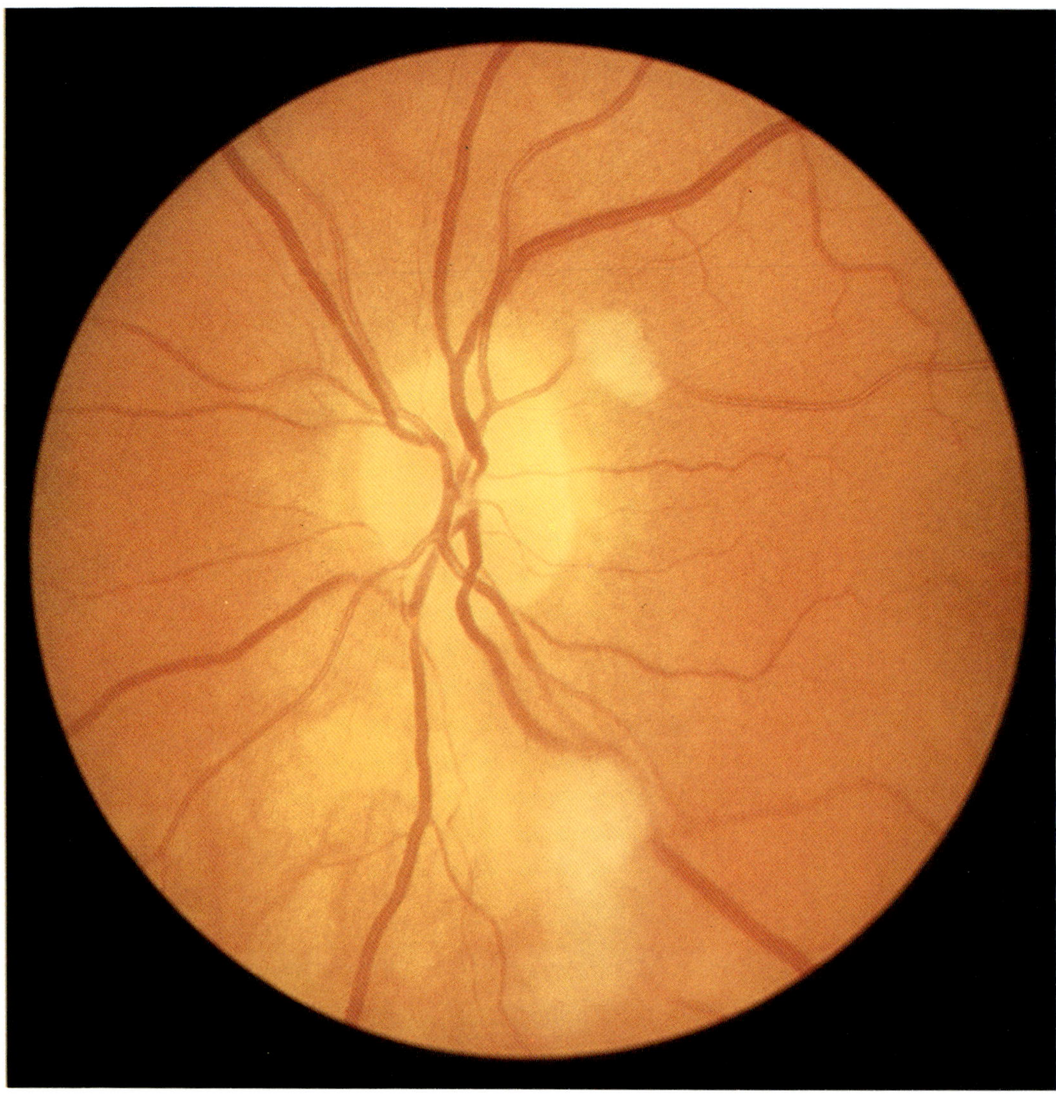

Figure 294. Left eye of a 35-year-old female patient with toxemia superimposed on essential hypertension. A hypertensive crisis occurred during the birth of this patient's second child.

Clinical Findings

One week before delivery, the patient had hyperlipidemia, uremia, and a fatty hepatomegaly. The patient presented at the hospital with generalized edema, coughing, and blood pressure of 230/140 mm Hg on the scheduled date for delivery. A cesarean section was performed. During the operation, blood pressure raised to 300/140 mm Hg but slowly stabilized after delivery. Visual acuity was 20/30. The fundus showed extreme narrowing of the arterioles and several cotton wool spots.

Fundus of Infants and Childrens

Fundus of the Premature Newborn

An ophthalmoscopical examination of a premature infant is difficult because the pupil does not dilate very well (maximum dilatation is 3 mm). Tropicamide can be used to achieve pupil dilatation. In addition, a Barraquer lid speculum is useful during the examination.

Indirect ophthalmoscopy provides superior results compared with direct ophthalmoscopy. Direct ophthalmoscopy using a hand-held ophthalmoscope is only possible with the addition of a −20 diopter lens, which can usually be added by switching the ophthalmoscope into that position. Honegger (1969) explained this phenomenon by citing the extreme myopia of the newborn within the first 4–6 weeks of life. However, Gernet (1964) found, by ultrasound examination of 36 newborns between the ages of 1–5 days, that a hyperopia averaging 2.8 diopters was present. Two of 21 male newborns in his group had a myopia of 3 and 4 diopters. None of the other eyes showed any myopia. The difficulties of ophthalmoscopically examining the newborn eye therefore can not be explained only by refractive anomalies. A physiological corneal edema within the first days of life is probably the reason for these varying difficulties. Other problems may include peripheral vitreous infiltrates, hyaloid artery remnants, the tunica vasculosa lentis, and the pupillary membrane.

Ophthalmoscopical Appearance. The entire fundus appears pale due to a lack of pigment. The retina shows a yellowish white discoloration, and the bright gray of the retinal periphery may resemble a retinal detachment (pseudoretinal detachment) (Honneger, 1969). Large choroidal vessels are visible. The central foveal reflex is absent. The optic disc appears gray-white with blurred margins. The arterioles are very thin and barely visible. The caliber of the veins is larger. Vascular branching is seen at the superior or inferior optic disc margins. Congenital retinal hemorrhages can be found in an average of 13% of premature infants.

Fundus of the Full-Term Newborn

Normal retinal pigmentation develops after the first 6 months of life. Therefore, the fundus of a mature newborn initially shows a generalized lack of pigment. The choroidal vessels are easily visible during the first phase of life, and the intervascular spaces have only a small amount of pigmentation. The irregularity of this pigmentation resembles the "salt and pepper" fundus that is usually associated with congenital syphilis. The optic disc appears gray to gray-white and, in the majority of cases, has sharply demarcated margins. An excavation is often present. Retinal vessels and vascular branching are unremarkable. Initially, the central foveal reflex is missing or only barely visible because the central fovea is not completely developed before the 4th month of life. More normal, vital disc coloration can be seen around the 5th month of life.

Congenital retinal hemorrhages can be observed in an average of 20–25% of full-term infants. Such hemorrhages are found more often after complicated deliveries (vacuum extractions). They are found less frequently following a cesearean section. Such retinal hemorrhages may have a punctate or dot and blot shape. Band- or flame-shaped hemorrhages may also be observed. In some cases, massive hemorrhage can be found, which may resemble a central retinal vein thrombosis.

Fundus of Children

In general, the fundus of a child resembles that of an adult except a child's fundus commonly has extremely bright reflexes. The retinal reflexes reveal a kaleidoscope of blue tones (interference colors) (Brückner, 1966). This finding is most pronounced in the macular area. The background color of the infantile central macula appears grayer than the peripheral macula when brightly illuminated.

Retinopathy of Prematurity

Synonyms: Retrolental fibroplasia, Terry's retrolental fibroplasia.

This entity was first reported in 1942 by Terry, who described the condition as a "fibroplastic overgrowth of persistent vascular tissue behind each crystalline lens," stating that what is now termed "retinopathy of prematurity" was simply a persistent embryonic tunica vasculosa lentis. The mechanisms of oxygen toxicity were discovered more than a decade later. This pathological condition is most frequently found in infants with a birth weight between 800 and 1500 grams, born prematurely between the 26th and 32nd week of gestation. Typically, these newborns were treated with a hyperbaric oxygen therapy in an incubator.

During the 1950s, retrolental fibroplasia was one of the most common causes of blindness in newborns in several countries of the world. Today, blindness caused by this condition is seen much less frequently. Generally, milder, less progessive, "abortive" forms of this condition are observed (Lemmingson, 1959).

In these abortive forms, typically the neovascularization does not extend beyond the retina. No preretinal or vitreal neovascularization occurs. The temporal arterioles show severe tortuosity, and the veins are extremely dilated. More peripherally, the retina is partially thickened and may have folds. These retinal changes can resolve spontaneously, resulting in clumped pigment irregularities and atrophic areas. Sometimes the diagnosis of retinopathy of prematurity is made retrospectively when peripheral retinal folds surrounded by irregular pigmentation are present, and the patient's history of oxygen therapy supports the diagnosis.

Prophylaxis. The arterial oxygen tension (pO_2) has to be monitored several times daily in the at-risk premature infant who is undergoing incubator therapy. Also, precautions and strict controls must be observed if artificial ventilation is necessary. Repeated ophthalmoscopical examinations are indicated, initially daily.

Differential Diagnosis. The differential diagnosis includes congenital findings such as persistent tunica vasculosa lentis, persistent hyaloid artery, congenital falciform retinal folds, Coats' disease, Norrie's disease, "shaken-baby" syndrome, birth trauma, epiretinal membrane, retinoblastoma, or toxoplasmosis.

Therapy. Corticosteroids are recommended when a progression of the early retinal complications is observed.

Histopathologically, the retinopathy of prematurity represents a proliferation of the capillaries and glial tissue. Normally the most peripheral areas of the sensory retina are incompletely vascularized before birth. Physiologically, between the 6th and 7th month of gestation the retinal capillarization takes place. During normal embryogenesis the vascular buds emanate from the disc and reach the nasal ora serrata by the 8th gestational month. The temporal ora serrata is not fully vascularized until several weeks after birth. When oxygen is administered to a premature infant, the still developing angioblastic tissue of the peripheral retina is stimulated toward vasoconstriction and later neovascularization. This phenomenon is observed if the arteriole oxygen tension exceeds values of 50–55 mm Hg (Heydenreich, 1979).

Clinical manifestation of the retinopathy of prematurity is differentiated into an active, proliferative stage and a cicatricial stage. Both the active and cicatricial stages can be subdivided into five grades:

Active Stage

Grade 1. Between 2 and 10 weeks after birth, the still developing angioblastic tissue of the retinal periphery is stimulated toward an initial primary stage of vasoconstriction. This is followed by a dilatation of the arteries and veins combined with severe vascular tortuosity.

Grade 2. Neovascularization, retinal hemorrhages, and temporal and peripheral gray retinal edema ensue.

Grade 3. A peripheral retinal detachment and vitreal capillary neovascularization develop.

Grade 4. The retinal detachment extends to involve the posterior pole and neovascularization progresses and vitreous hemorrhages occur.

Grade 5. Eventually, the retina becomes detached completely.

Cicatricial Stage

Grade 1. The cicatricial phase of the retinopathy of prematurity develops between the 3rd and 5th months after birth. Initially, a temporally located infiltration and cloudiness of the retinal periphery can be seen.

Grade 2. The retinal infiltrates become more dense and cause a localized peripheral retinal detachment.

Grade 3. At this point the fundus changes resemble congenital falciform retinal folds that extend into the retrolental space. White-gray glial proliferations that exert a temporal traction on the pale disc are characteristic findings.

Grade 4. Vascularized retrolental membranes are present and the retina is largely detached.

Grade 5. The entire pupillary area is filled with a gray-white retrolental membrane. No normal fundus reflexes can be seen.

Ophthalmoscopical Appearance. As the retinopathy of prematurity progresses, additional ocular complications may be observed such as anterior and posterior synechiae, corneal opacities, cataract, secondary glaucoma, and phthisis bulbi. However, spontaneous remissions have been observed up to Grade 3 of the active stage.

Contraceptive Drugs

There are numerous case reports regarding ocular disorders associated with oral contraceptives. A connection between a contraceptive drug and pathologic retinal findings can be assumed if the patient has no history of preexisting disease and other etiologies can be ruled out. Often, the symptoms resolve once the contraceptive drug is discontinued.

There seems to be a connection between the amount of estrogen in a contraceptive drug and the risk of a thromboembolic disorder. Therefore, the estrogen concentration of most contraceptive drugs has been lowered so that most such preparations today have a concentration of only 0.03 mm.

Ocular Complications Associated with Contraceptive Drugs

Conjunctiva: hemorrhages
Cornea: edema
Lens: anterior and posterior cortical cataract (cataractogeneous effect of steroids)
Vitreous: hemorrhages
Retina: hemorrhages, edema
Retinal vessels: central retinal artery occlusion, branch arteriole occlusion, prethrombosis, central retinal branch vein occlusion (Figs. 295–302).
Optic disc: intra- and retrobulbar optic neuritis, optic atrophy
Ocular muscles: paresis
Refraction: manifestation or worsening of myopia, astigmatism, contact lens intolerance

Extraocular Complications Associated with Contraceptive Drugs

Arterial hypertension: thrombosis (brain vessels, cavernous sinus, lung, peripheral thrombosis)
Coagulation effect: decreased glucose tolerance
Migraine: increased susceptibility, increased duration and severity of migraine attacks
Cerebral pseudotumors: associated with ocular muscle paresis, hemianopia, and Parinaud's syndrome
Other complications: nausea, gastrointestinal disorders, increased body weight, coagulation disorders, breast pain.

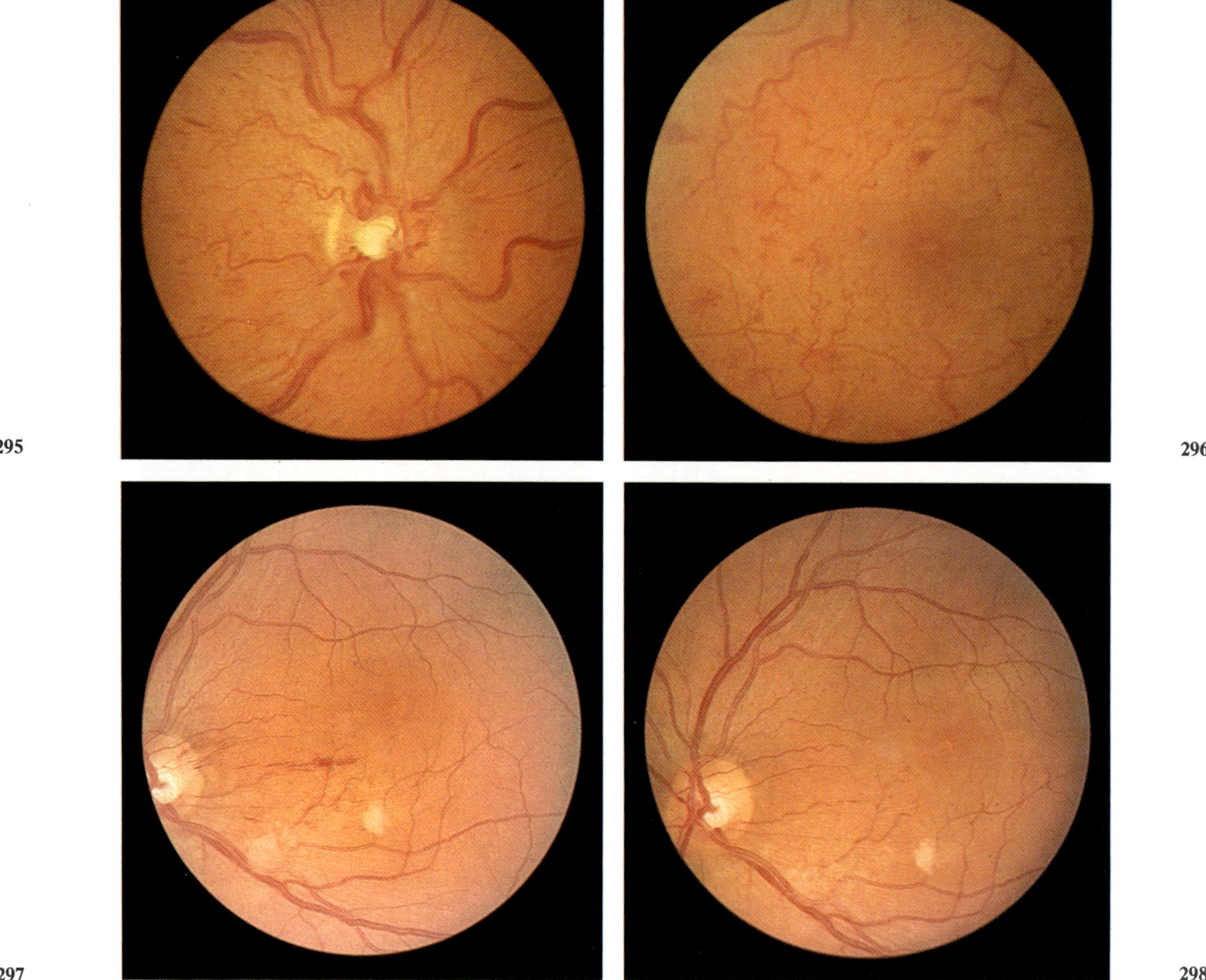

Figures 295 and 296. Right eye of a 35-year-old female patient with an incomplete central retinal vein occlusion.

Clinical Findings

The patient took an oral contraceptive drug for 2 years that was a combination of progesterone and estrogen. Visual acuity was 20/50. Visual field testing showed an enlargement of the blind spot, concentric constriction of the outer margins, and a relative central scotoma. Blood pressure was 160/100 mm Hg and blood sedimentation rate was 2/3 mm. Bleeding time was 4 minutes, 55 seconds. The coagulation parameters were normal.

Laboratory Findings

Blood cell counts and electrophoresis showed normal values. Cholesterol, 216 mg/100 ml; triglycerides, 142 mg/100 ml; β-lipoproteins, 400 mg/100 ml; urea, 24 mg/100 ml; serum creatinine, 1.02 mg/100 ml.

Therapy

Use of the contraceptive drug was terminated. The patient was treated with a regimen of prednisolone and an anticoagulant.

Clinical Course

Visual acuity completely recovered to 20/20.

Figures 297 and 298. Left eye of a 37-year-old female patient with isolated vascular retinal ischemia of unknown etiology.

Clinical Findings

The patient had taken various contraceptive drugs. Visual acuity was 20/400. There was a central scotoma. Fundus examination revealed radial and some punctate hemorrhages extending between the optic disc and the macula (Fig. 297). Several small cotton wool spots are visible along the inferotemporal artery. Blood pressure was 150/90 mm Hg measured on both arms.

Laboratory Findings

All laboratory findings were unremarkable.

Therapy and Clinical Course

Contraceptive drug use was terminated. Figure 298 shows the fundus 8 days later, and in another 8 days visual acuity had fully recovered and the retinal changes had resolved. The patient was treated with an anticoagulant regimen.

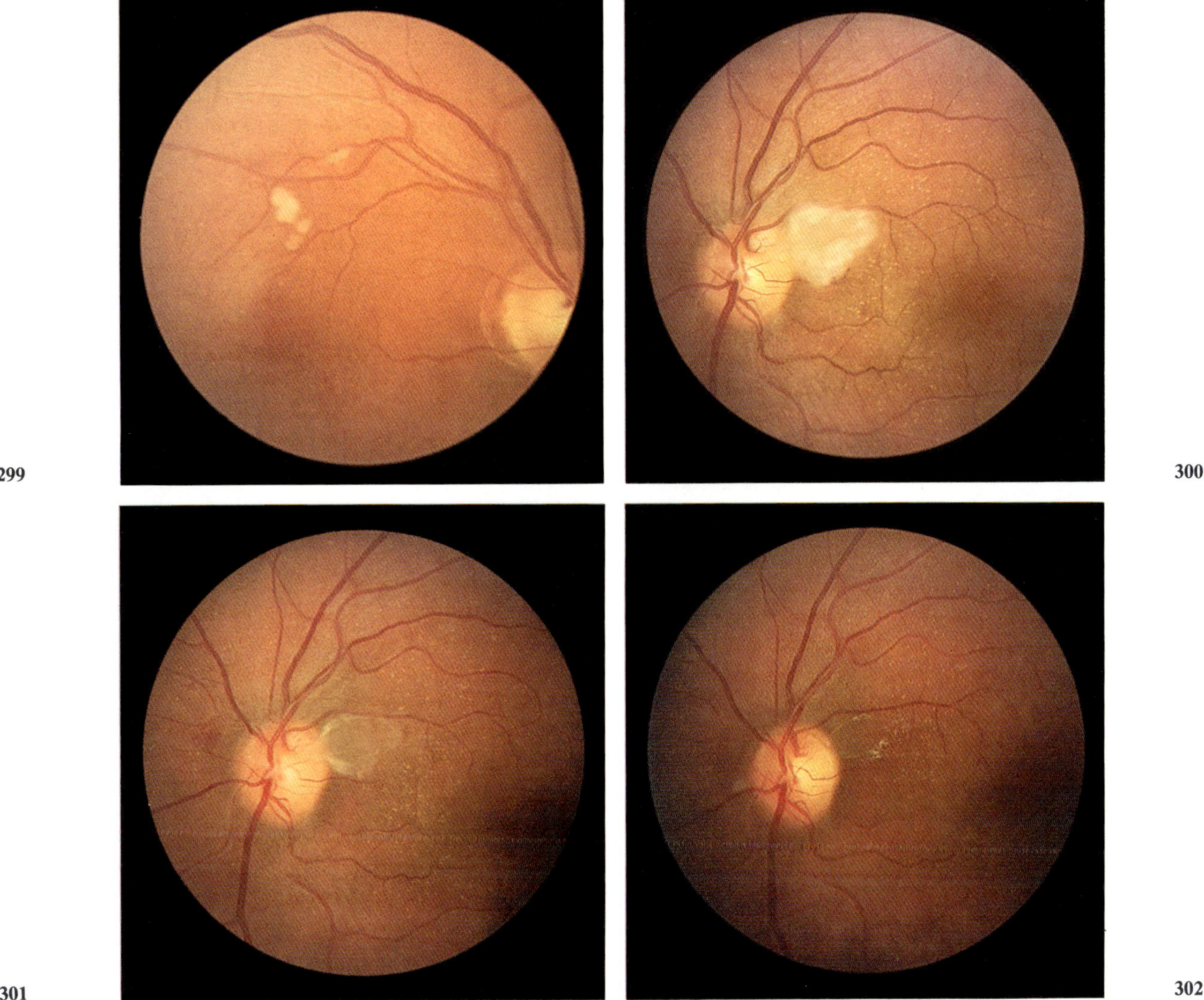

Figure 299. Right eye of a 35-year-old female patient with retinal ischemia caused by isolated arterial spasm.

Clinical Findings

The patient had taken two different contraceptive drugs for a total of 7 years. Visual acuity was 20/50. There was an absolute sector-shaped scotoma corresponding to the ischemic retinal areas (superotemporal artery). Fundus examination showed several cotton wool spots along the superotemporal artery. Extensive retinal edema was present superotemporally, extending toward the macula. Ophthalmoscopically, this lesion also corresponded to an embolic occlusion of the central retinal artery. Note the similarity of the findings in Figures 297 and 298. Blood pressure measured on both arms was 140/85 mm Hg. Laboratory findings were unremarkable.

Therapy

The contraceptive drug was discontinued. The patient was treated with an anticoagulant regimen.

Clinical Course

There was full visual rehabilitation within 2 weeks.

Figures 300–302. Left eye of a 38-year-old female patient with embolic occlusion of a cilioretinal artery and an albipunctate dystrophic fundus.

Clinical Findings

The patient had taken various contraceptive drugs for a period of 8 years. She suffered from a transient hypertension and varicosis. Visual acuity was 20/400. There was a centrocecal scotoma present and the outer margins of the visual field were concentrically constricted. Fundus examination shows a localized ischemic zone that extends from the optic disc (between 1 and 3 o'clock) toward the periphery (Fig. 300). This area was supplied by a cilioretinal artery originating at the 1 o'clock position from the optic disc. Blood pressure measured on both arms was 240/140 mm Hg. Blood cell count and differential blood cell counts were unremarkable.

Therapy

The contraceptive drug was discontinued. The patient was treated with an anticoagulant regimen.

Clinical Course

Blood pressure normalized and the retinal edema resolved. Visual acuity recovered to 20/20 (Figs. 301 and 302). Note the presence of an albipunctate dystrophic fundus.

Traumatic Fundus Changes

Birth Trauma

Congenital Retinal Hemorrhages

Congenital hemorrhages are observed in approximately 13% of all premature newborns and in 20-25% of all mature newborns. Congenital retinal hemorrhages may result from extravasation of erythrocytes or from rupture of the vessel. These conditions are caused by a venous pressure elevation during birth.

Depending on the infant's age when the ophthalmological examination was performed and on the technique used, the incidence percentage varies widely in case reports of congenital retinal hemorrhage. A prolonged delivery (primipara, narrow pelvis), vacuum extraction, or a forceps delivery increase the incidence of retinal hemorrhage. In contrast, the incidence of such hemorrhages after a cesarean section is much lower.

A possible connection is mentioned in the literature between congenital retinal hemorrhages, especially macular hemorrhages, and late amblyopia in patients who have no refractive anomalies or strabismus.

Ophthalmoscopical Appearance. All types of monocular or binocular retinal hemorrhage can be observed, including punctate or dot and blot hemorrhages (located with the nuclear layers), radial band- or flame-shaped hemorrhages (within the nerve fiber layer), and extensive preretinal hemorrhages. Clinically, the fundus sometimes resembles that seen with central retinal vein occlusion. In general, vitreous hemorrhages are rare.

The extravasated blood cells are usually resorbed within the 1st to 3rd week after birth. An exception are cases of vitreal hemorrhage in which the blood may not be resorped for several months.

Congenital Papilledema

Congenital papilledema is rare, but when present it may progress into an optic atrophy (differential diagnosis: congenital hereditary optic atrophy). It is difficult to determine whether head injuries during the delivery cause this condition.

Commotio Retinae

Synonym: Berlin's edema.

Within the first hour following a blunt ocular trauma (contusio bulbi), a contrecoup effect may cause a posterior retinal edema. The white appearance of the retina is caused by a localized ischemia related to arteriole spasms. Mild retinal hemorrhages may also occur. If the posterior pole is directly affected, a so-called cherry-red spot may result. This spot occurs when the normal choriocapillaris becomes visible within the edematous region because the central retina and macular area are not affected by the edema due to a lack of axons (Fig. 306). In most cases, the edema resolves spontaneously within a few days. Persistent defects are an exception.

Contusio Retinae

In contrast to commotio retinae, the retinal damage associated with contusio retinae does not completely resolve. A blunt trauma causes Berlin's edema and associated retinal hemorrhages, and after these hemorrhages are resorbed, pigment irregularities (contusion scars) remain (Figs. 303-305 and 307-308). Depending on their location, these lesions may cause persistent visual acuity and visual field alterations. Complications of this condition are traumatic macular hole development and retinal detachment.

Traumatic Retinopathy

Synonyms: Purtscher's disease, angiopathia retinae traumatica Purtscher, traumatic retinal angiopathy.

The fundus changes in this condition are observed following skull trauma or compression injuries of the body. These changes are therefore secondary effects of thoracic, abdominal, or cranial injuries without direct ocular involvement.

According to Seitz (1968), traumatic retinopathy represents primarily a choroidal disorder caused by microembolic occlusion within the choroidal vascular system via the short posterior ciliary arteries. In addition, retinal vessels may be affected. Seitz based his conclusion on the subretinal location of exudates that are observed in connection with this retinal trauma. Fatty inclusions develop in the vascular lumen. These changes can be proven histologically by special fat stains.

Ophthalmoscopical Appearance. After a few hours, multiple, bright white patches can be seen, which vary in size and may partially accrue. This finding is in contrast to true fat emboli, which do not appear for 1 to several days. The lesions are usually found in groups surrounding the optic disc and involve the posterior pole. The margins are not well demarcated. Often the lesions are observed in retinal veins. Preretinal and intraretinal hemorrhages and cotton wool exudates are usually present. Retinal vessels are affected, particularly when the thorax was the site of the underlying trauma. The veins are engorged, and the arteries have a narrow lumen and appear tortuous. The peripheral retina at the equator is not affected. The lesions are always observed bilaterally except in some cases of cranial trauma.

Fluorescein angiography immediately following the trauma reveals capillary dilatations on the optic disc with vascular leakage and nonperfusive areas. Tenner and coauthors (1972) also found segmental constrictions and dilatations of the peripapillary arteries (major branches) during follow-up examinations. These bead-shaped vascular abnormalities were typically associated with otherwise completely normal vessels, including the retinal veins. The optic disc barely shows any fluorescence, and the papillary capillaries were rarified, indicating atrophy of several vessels in this region.

Functional losses depend on the extent of macular involvement. The visual acuity may be reduced, and central or pericentral scotomas may be present. This condition is transient; however, only an occasional full and complete recovery is reported. Partial or total optic atrophy may be a late complication.

Therapy. The therapy for this condition is limited to treatment of the underlying trauma. There is no specific therapy for the retinal changes.

Retinopathia Sclopetaria

Synonyms: Retinitis sclopetaria, pseudoretinitis, chorioretinitis sclopetaria.

This condition was named because it was often observed in association with war injuries. It is caused by severe blunt traumas of the orbit and globe, which are often caused by projectiles that may have directly touched the sclera.

Ophthalmoscopical Appearance. Retinopathia sclopetaria may closely resemble retinitis pigmentosa and therefore is one of the conditions often diagnosed as pseudoretinitis pigmentosa (Fig. 309). At an early stage, extensive preretinal and intraretinal hemorrhages, as well as choroidal hemorrhages, can be found. Once the hemorrhages are resorbed, extensive, irregularly pigmented brown-black chorioretinal scars remain. If the optic nerve is affected, an optic nerve atrophy with partial or total optic disc pallor may be seen. Strand-like scars and membranes are found quite often (Figs. 310–312). Functional loss depends on the location of the chorioretinal involvement.

Therapy. Therapy consists of treatment for the underlying trauma and has to be adjusted to the ocular symptoms.

Choroidal Rupture

A rupture within the choroidal tunic may be caused by a severe blunt ocular trauma. These ruptures are found either at the site of the direct impact (direct rupture) or at the site where the contrecoup effect is involved (indirect rupture).

Ophthalmoscopical Appearance. Initially, edema and hemorrhages may overlie the site of choroidal damage. Retinal hemorrhages usually appear light red to beefy red. Choroidal hemorrhages may appear washed-out and gray. After resorption of the hemorrhages, a single isolated or several arcuate or sickle-shaped white scleral areas may become visible. Quite often these choroidal lesions are arranged concentrically around the optic disc. Sometimes the injured choroid shows a few, isolated choroidal vessels crossing the area of the rupture. The secondary pigmentation may vary in color or it may be totally absent (Fig. 313). Functional loss depends on whether the macular region is affected.

Therapy. No reparative therapy is known.

Choroidal Detachment

Synonyms: Spongiosis chorioidea, ciliochoroidal detachment.

The first pathologic, anatomic description of a choroidal detachment (hydrops chorioidae externus) was given by von Zinn in 1755. In 1858, von Graefe provided the first clinical observation of a choroidal detachment. The etiology of this condition is unknown.

A choroidal detachment may occur in the following conditions:

1. Postoperative: following cataract extraction (Figs. 314–316) or glaucoma surgery (iridectomy, sclerectomy, cyclodialysis, iridencleisis (Holth's operation), trephining of the globe (Elliot's operation)).
2. Posttraumatic: following direct or indirect injury, perforating ocular injuries, or secondary to perforation of a corneal ulcer.
3. Exudative: inflammatory (associated with iridocyclitis, chorioretinitis, including chorioretinitis caused by the Vogt-Koyanagi syndrome or the Harada syndrome, tenonitis, scleritis); vascular (nephritis, arterial hypertension, uremia, polyarteritis nodosa, leukemia, syphilis); congestive (intrabulbar or extrabulbar tumor, including orbital or lacrimal gland tumors).
4. Hemorrhagic: limited explusive hemorrhage.
5. Purulent: purulent choroiditis.
6. Secondary to traction: phthisis bulbi.
7. Spontaneous serous choroidal detachment: cyclitis anularis exudativa pseudotumorosa.

Ophthalmoscopical Appearance. There are three morphological types of choroidal detachment: anular, globular, and planar. A choroidal detachment shows a green to brown-pink coloration, appears solid, and does not fluctuate. The retinal vessels deviate from their normal course at the base of the tumor and then ascend onto the elevated tumor. Choroidal vessels never become visible. The detachment is often largest where it extends toward the temporal or nasal quadrant. Sometimes four isolated segmental lesions can be found depending on the location of the vortex veins. In other cases, the choroidal detachment becomes so severe that the elevated areas show a tunnel-like appearance, leaving only a very small portion of the posterior pole visible. A planar, slightly elevated choroidal detachment may form parallel, horizontal folds. A retinal detachment can also complicate this condition, even without development of a retinal hole.

A postoperative choroidal detachment usually reaches the maximum size after 5–6 days and spontaneously resolves within 2–3 weeks. In some cases, however, it may persist over months or years. Complications such as iridocyclitis or secondary glaucoma often ensue in such cases. The retina often becomes involved when choroidal detachment is present for a long time. The retinal pigment epithelium develops a spotty atrophy. Often, pigmentary clumps and lines, which may be hook-shaped or arcuate, can be found. The pigmentary lines are usually slightly broader than the diameter of the retinal veins.

The most commonly observed functional losses affect visual acuity and visual fields. A complete amaurosis may develop in cases in which the choroidal detachment persists for years.

Other ocular abnormalities may be present, depending on the underlying reason for the choroidal detachment. A detachment in an eye with a shallow anterior chamber must be differentiated from a detachment associated with a normal anterior chamber. Except for cases of serous choroidal detachment, pressure of the globe is reduced. The diagnosis is based on diascleral transillumination and echography. Transillumination reveals an interruption of the normal ring shadow caused by the ciliary body. When the light source is supplied to the sclera immediately adjacent to the detachment, the sclera shows an increased translucency, causing a very bright pupillary reflex.

Differential Diagnosis. The differential diagnosis includes such conditions as retinal detachment, choroidal ring melanoma, choroidal hemorrhage, or angioma of the choroid.

Therapy. The therapy must be adjusted according to the underlying disease. Atropine drops may be used to prophylactically avoid synechia formation. Corticosteroids are recommended. Surgical intervention is believed to worsen the course of the disease. Sautter and coauthors (1972) recommended a "mini-keratoplasty" in special cases if a postoperative choroidal detachment does not resolve spontaneously. Leakage of aqueous humor and/or fistula formation may be determined by applying the Seidel test.

Light or Radiation Trauma of the Macula

The classic example for this type of trauma is solar retinopathy (solar retinitis or eclipse retinopathy). This type of radiation injury usually occurs following solar eclipses as a result of direct observation of the sun without an adequate filter. In essence, this sun-gazing produces a thermal burn of the macula by infrared light.

Other retinal and macular radiation injuries include lesions caused by ionizing rays (atom bomb explosion) and following intensive roentgen therapy (tumor irradiation).

Ophthalmoscopical Appearance. Initially, a central retinal edema can be found. The foveal reflex is absent. Brown-black granular hyperpigmentation and scar formation ensues. The symptoms associated with this condition resemble a macular hole.

Therapy. No efficacious therapy is known.

Optic Nerve Trauma

Traumatic Optic Atrophy

A traumatic optic atrophy may be caused by a cranial bone fracture. Optic nerve damage is frequently found if the injuring force comes from the frontal or frontoparietal direction. This type of trauma is quite rare statistically and can be found in only 0.8–1.0% of all head injuries (Huber, 1966). Other possible causes of traumatic optic atrophy are stab, gunshot, and impaling wounds. Traumatic optic atrophy may also be observed following severe blunt ocular traumas.

Diagnosis. If the patient is unconscious, the diagnosis of an optic nerve trauma may be based on the presence of an amaurotic or amblyopic pupil. In the latter case, the pupil of the affected eye does not show any light reaction at all, or reacts in an extremely attenuated manner when directly illuminated. When the other eye is exposed to light, the affected eye reacts normally. A partial or total optic atrophy with sharply demarcated margins develops 3 weeks after a head trauma in 97% of cases with injury to the optic nerve. This optic atrophy is caused by the postinjury edema and/or damage to the optic nerve's nutritional source, i.e., the optic nerve vessels (Huber, 1966). This type of damage plays a much more important role than a direct injury of the nerve by a bone fracture, e.g., a fracture of the lesser wing of the sphenoidal bone, which only rarely extends into the optic foramen. Furthermore, not every fracture in this area causes a direct optic nerve lesion (Fig. 317). The radiographic proof of dislocated bone fragments (roentgenoscopy of Rheese-Goalwin and tomography of the optic foramen) are rather rare findings despite their mention in the older literature.

Ophthalmoscopical Appearance. Ophthalmoscopical changes can only be found in approximately 2% of patients with acute head trauma who do not suffer from a direct lesion of the globe and orbit (Huber, 1966). Usually papilledema appears in a more attenuated form in cases of epidural, subdural, or intracerebral hematoma. It is often limited to a part of the optic disc. Sometimes only a hyperemia of the optic disc with dilated veins and distinct nasal juxtapapillary retinal hemorrhages can be found. In cases of optic nerve trauma, it is rare to find papilledema, but if present, it seldoms exceeds an elevation of 2 diopters. Often within 3 weeks, the optic nerve head proceeds to optic atrophy with blurred margins. Initially, the optic lesion does not cause any ophthalmoscopically evident symptoms in most cases. Without any preceding papilledema, the atrophic optic disc appears bright white.

The rarification of capillaries and nerve fibers may lead to a cupping of the optic disc, depending on the extent of glial proliferation. The retinal vessels are not affected in every case. If affected, the arteries appear markedly narrow, linear, and show a whitish-gray ensheathing. The veins usually remain unchanged (Figs. 318 and 319).

Depending on the extent of the optic nerve damage, different visual functional losses can be found. The spectrum of losses may cover all types of visual disabilities from simple reduction of visual acuity up to complete amaurosis. Other symptoms include peripheral visual field defects, pericentral or central scotomas, and distortions in color vision.

Therapy. Because an injury of the optic nerve is only rarely caused by a fracture of the bony structures of the optic foramen and optic nerve channel, a neurosurgical decompression is only rarely indicated. This is especially true when considering the poor prognosis for successful treatment of a primary optic nerve lesion. However, secondary amaurosis of the undamaged eye may be prevented by this type of surgical intervention. In some cases of optic nerve concussion, high doses of corticosteroids for a limited time may relieve edema and improve the visual prognosis.

Hematoma of the Optic Nerve Sheath

This condition is caused by a direct hemorrhage into the optic nerve sheath and may be associated with cranial bone fractures or cerebral contusions.

Ophthalmoscopical Appearance. According to Huber (1966), a hematoma of the optic nerve sheath does not normally cause papilledema. Therefore, this entity becomes manifest clinically only because of functional disturbances. Immediately following the injury, the pupil may appear amaurotic. No red blood cells are seen in the aqueous humor. Initially, the optic disc does not show any pathological alterations, but after several weeks a sharply demarcated optic atrophy develops. In some cases the hematoma-related papilledema closely resembles papilledema caused by other diseases. The optic disc margins appear blurred, elevated, and white. Radial folds develop in the surrounding retina, and retinal veins are engorged and tortuous. Radial peripapillary hemorrhages, which may be ring-shaped, may also be present.

Without immediate neurosurgical therapy the eye may undergo a partial or complete visual loss (see "Traumatic Optic Atrophy"). In cases of bilateral injury, both eyes may become amaurotic.

Traumatic Disruption of the Optic Nerve

Synonyms: Evulsio nervi optici, evulsio fasciculi optici.

Penetrating or impaling injuries, an acute and extensive pressure rise within the orbit, and frontobasal head trauma may cause a total or partial luxation of the globe anteriorly, i.e., luxation of the eye anterior to the lids or into the nasal sinuses. Such extreme globe dislocation may cause rupture of the optic nerve, most often at the site where the nerve penetrates the sclera.

Ophthalmoscopical Appearance. In the acute stage, the optic nerve may not be seen at all because of extensive vitreous hemorrhage. There is an extreme peripapillary retinal ischemia. Later, a deep hole develops at the original site of the optic nerve head. No vessels are present, and proliferating glial and connective tissue may later cover the defect. The clinical appearance may be supplemented by radial retinal scars and choroidal ruptures that vary in size.

Therapy. No therapy is possible.

Foreign Body Embedded in the Optic Disc

As with other intraocular foreign bodies, the prognosis following foreign body penetration of optic disc tissues depends on the size and material of the foreign body and whether it was contaminated with pathogenetic microorganisms. A direct injury of the central retinal vessels usually causes total visual loss. Aluminum, lead, glass, or small stone fragments may not cause any inflammation. Iron-containing foreign bodies may cause siderosis bulbi. Copper and copper-containing foreign bodies may cause chalcosis bulbi.

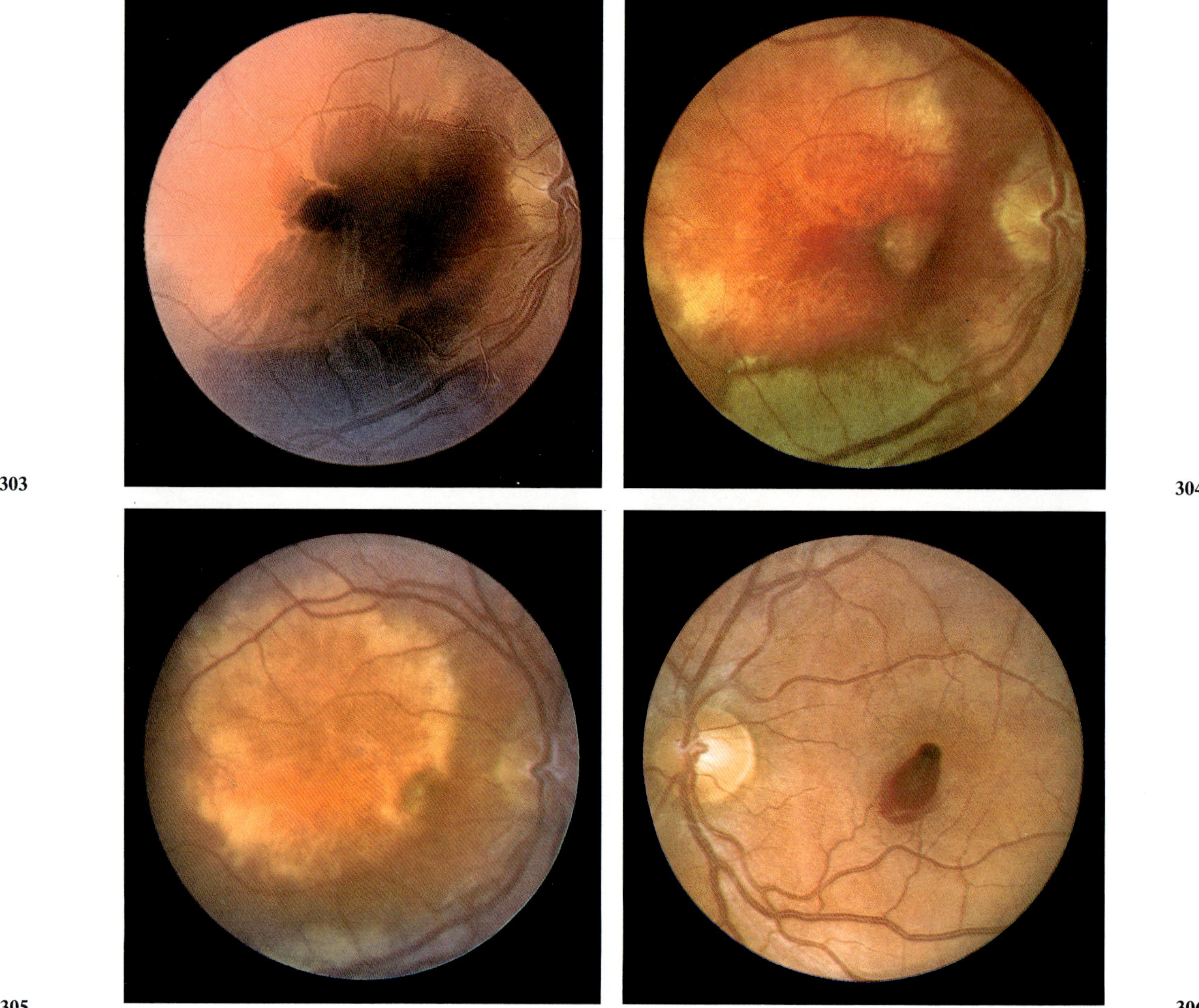

Figures 303–305. Right eye of a 15-year-old male patient with severe retinal contusion caused by blunt trauma. The patient was hit in the eye by his own goggles while jumping into water.

Clinical Findings

Figure 303 shows the fundus of the right eye during the first examination 3 days after the injury. Visual acuity was 20/400. Refractive media were clear. There was a large central scotoma. It is remarkable that the anterior segment was completely normal, whereas the fundus had large hemorrhages extending from the optic disc toward the macular region and inferiorly. The hemorrhages were located both subretinally and intraretinally. The flame-shaped hemorrhages surrounding the macula are located in Henle's nerve fiber layer.

Therapy

The patient was treated with radiation and rheologic therapy.

Clinical Course

Figure 304 shows the fundus 2 1/2 weeks after the trauma. Visual acuity at this time was 20/60. Figure 305 shows the fundus 6 weeks after the trauma, and visual acuity then was 20/30. The hemorrhages had almost completely resolved. A large contusion scar developed on the posterior pole.

Figure 306. Left eye of a 16-year-old male patient with retinal contusion caused by blunt trauma. He was hit in the left temporal region by a fist.

Clinical Findings

Visual acuity was 20/200. Refractive media were clear. There was a central scotoma. The anterior segment was unremarkable. There is a drop-shaped retinal hemorrhage involving all retinal layers that extends from the macula inferiorly.

Therapy

The patient was treated with radiation and rheologic therapy.

Clinical Course

The hemorrhage quickly resolved, leaving a small central scar. The final visual acuity was 20/30.

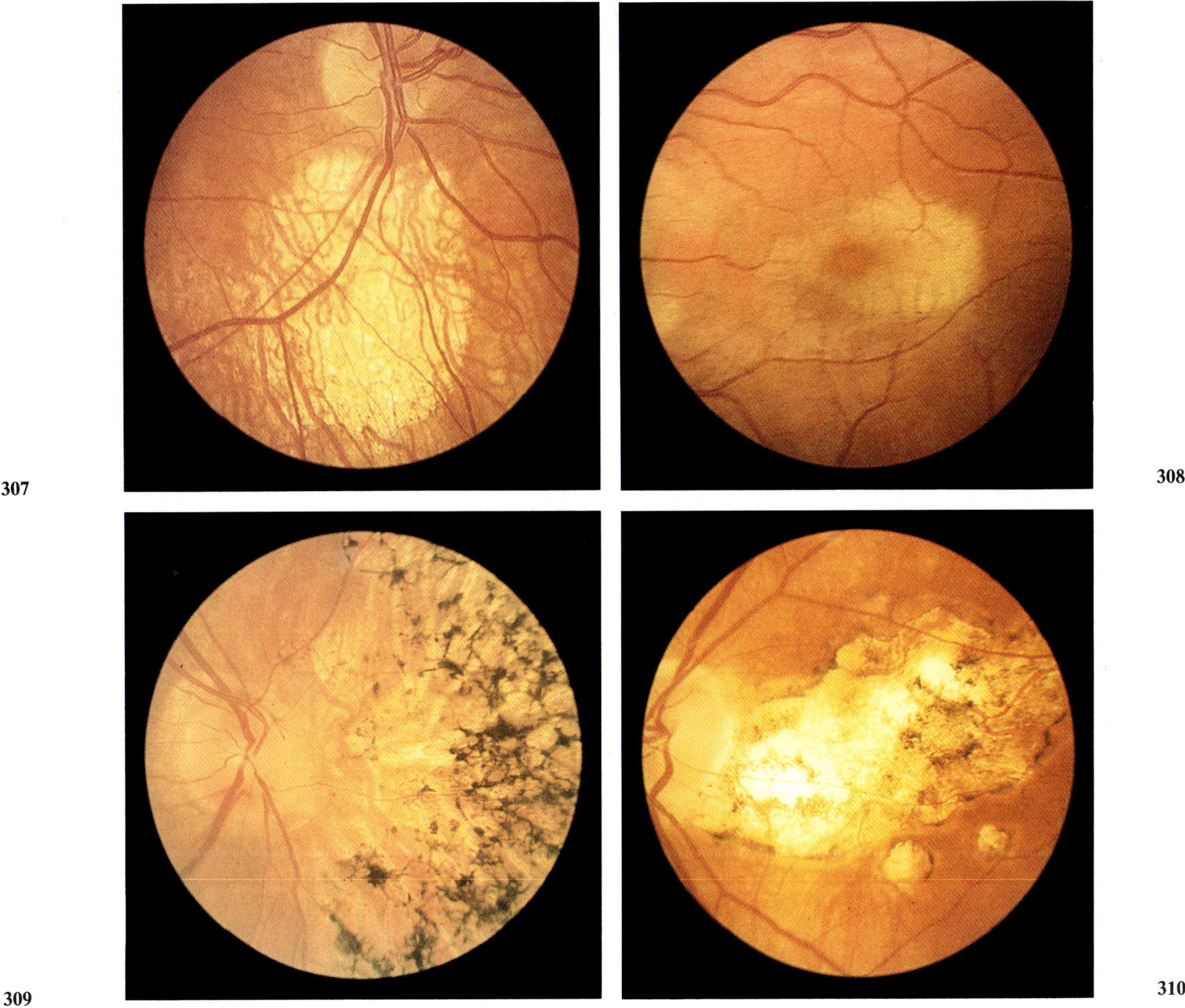

Figure 307. Right eye of a 12-year-old female patient with retinal contusion scars 2 months after a blunt ocular trauma that occurred during a volleyball game.

Clinical Findings

Refraction was 0.25 sphere, −0.5 cylinder, axis 130°, visual acuity 20/20. Refractive media were clear and intraocular pressure was 14 mm Hg. There was anisocoria. The visual field had a large corresponding defect in the superior half.

Figure 308. Left eye of a 20-year-old male patient with retinal edema (Berlin's edema) caused by blunt ocular trauma, due to an exploding bottle, which occurred 8 hours prior to the examination.

Clinical Findings

Visual acuity was 20/200. Refractive media were clear and intraocular pressure was 10 mm Hg. There was a central scotoma, a pseudoptosis, moderate conjunctival injection, traumatic mydriasis, and Berlin's edema. Gonioscopy revealed there was no angle recession.

Figure 309. Left eye of a 59-year-old female patient with pseudoretinitis pigmentosa caused by a severe blunt trauma 15 years earlier. The patient was hit in the eye by a cow's tail.

Clinical Findings

Refraction was +1.5 sphere, visual acuity 20/50. There was an incomplete contusion rosette of the crystalline lens. Intraocular pressure was 16 mm Hg. Visual field testing showed a large temporal defect.

Figure 310. Left eye of a 56-year-old male patient with traumatic retinopathy following an injury by a bullet, (retinopathia sclopetaria).

Clinical Findings

Visual acuity was 20/1000. Refractive media were clear and intraocular pressure was 15 mm Hg. There was a large central scotoma and a concentric constriction of the outer margins of the visual field. The fundus showed extensive scarring of the posterior pole.

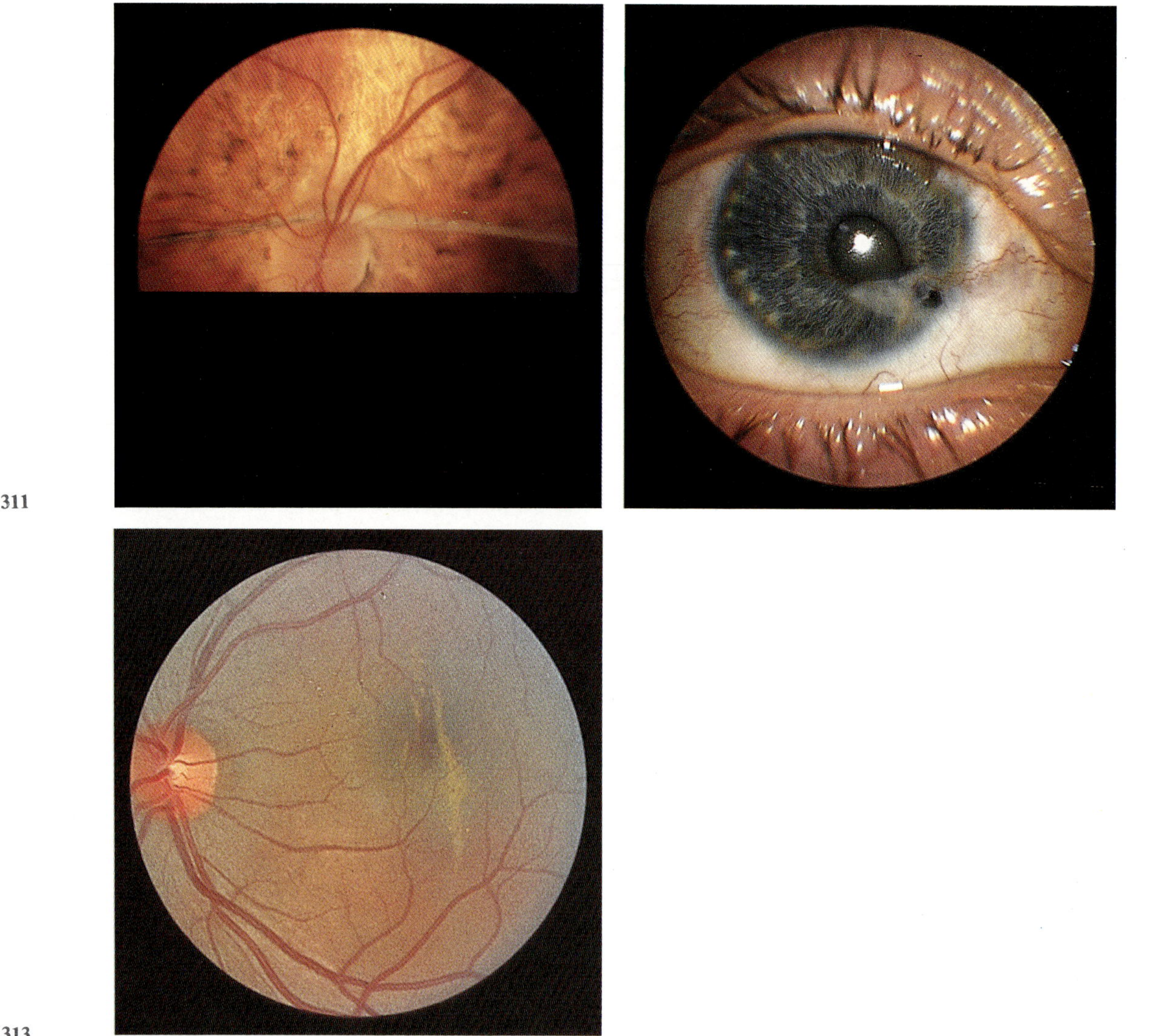

311

312

313

Figures 311 and 312. (Note: Figures 311 and 312 are reversed.) Right eye of a 28-year-old male patient showing status following perforating trauma 10 years earlier with corneal and lenticular injury. A descemetocele is now present.

Clinical Findings

After a small keratoplasty and removal of the secondary cataract, extensive chorioretinal scarring and proliferation strands became visible. The best corrected visual acuity achieved in this eye with a correction of +13.5 sphere, −2.0 cylinder, axis 35° was 20/400. A secondary exotropia had developed.

Figure 313. Left eye of a 25-year-old male patient showing fundus status after blunt injury caused by a kick in the eye 4 years earlier.

Clinical Findings

With a refractive correction of +1.0 sphere, visual acuity was 20/30. Refractive media were clear. There was metamorphopsia as documented by an Amsler grid. Note the longitudinal choriodal ruptures at the posterior pole.

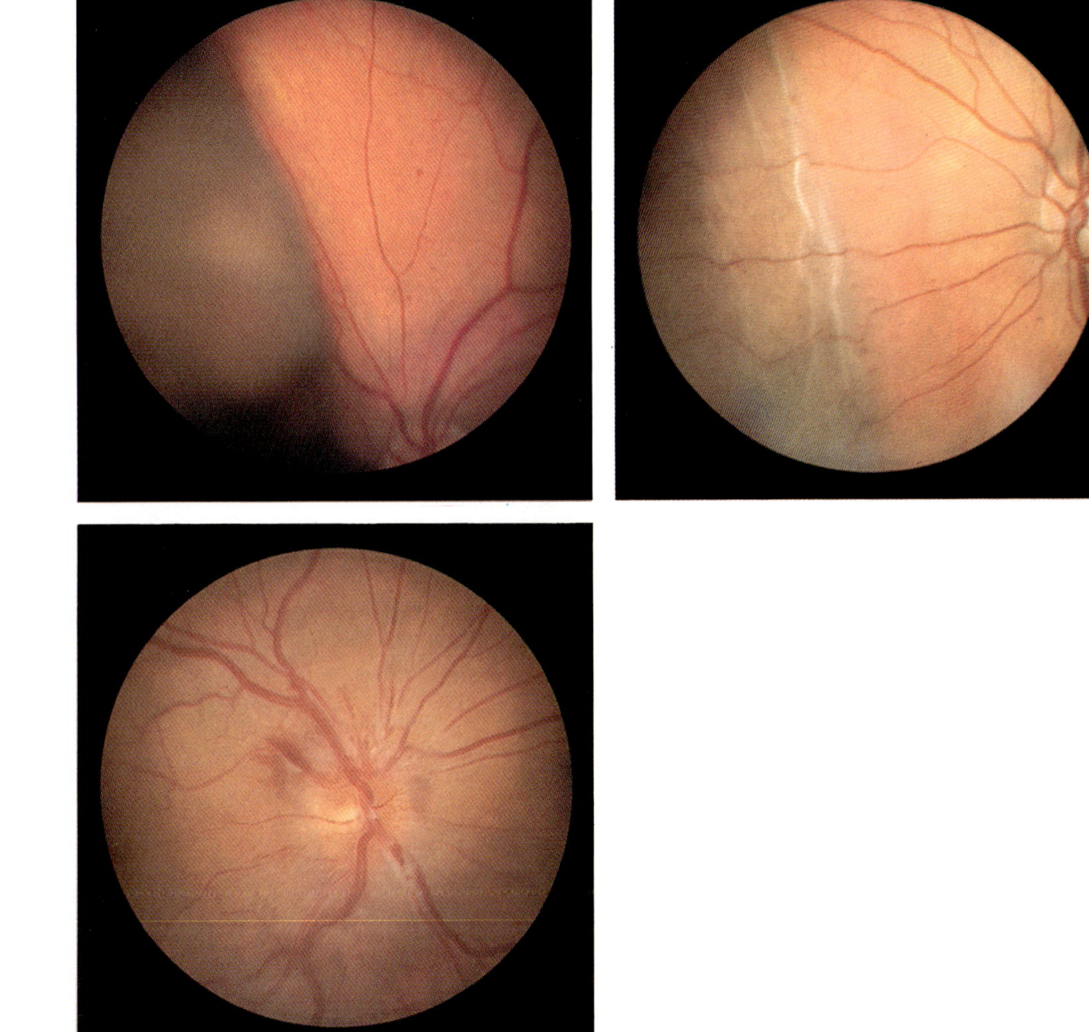

Figures 314 and 315. Left eye of a 68-year-old female patient with late choroidal detachment following cataract extraction. The right eye was amaurotic following central retinal artery occlusion.

Clinical Findings

There are signs of early hypertensive retinal changes. Stage 1 diabetic retinopathy is evident by the punctate hemorrhage and/or microaneurysm. Eighty days following an uncomplicated intercapsular cataract extraction, the patient presented with photopsia and a constriction of the nasal visual field. With a correction of +14.0 sphere, −1.25 cylinder, axis 110°, visual acuity was 20/20. Intraocular pressure in the right eye was 17 mm Hg and in the left eye was 15 mm Hg. Gonioscopy showed a nasally flat anterior chamber, an open peripheral iridectomy at 12 o'clock, and an intact anterior hyaloid face. The fundus showed a translucent choroidal detachment seen with transillumination. The typical dark-brown staining characteristic of a choroidal detachment is seen in Figure 314.

Therapy

The patient was treated with corticosteroids, topical 1% atropine, and radiation therapy. Figure 315 shows the fundus 5 days later. Note the vertical dune-like folds.

Figure 316. Right eye of a 68-year-old male patient with ocular hypotension and showing status of the eye following intracapsular cataract extraction.

Clinical Findings

With a correction of +12.5 sphere, −1.0 cylinder, axis 95°, visual acuity was 20/20! Intraocular pressure was 8 mm Hg. The anterior chamber was narrow. There is a small filtration bleb of the conjunctiva at 12 o'clock.

Clinical Course

Fourteen days later the retinal changes and hemorrhages spontaneously resolved. Visual acuity remained 20/20 and intraocular pressure was 16 mm Hg. At that time the optic disc was also normal. The filtering bleb had disappeared.

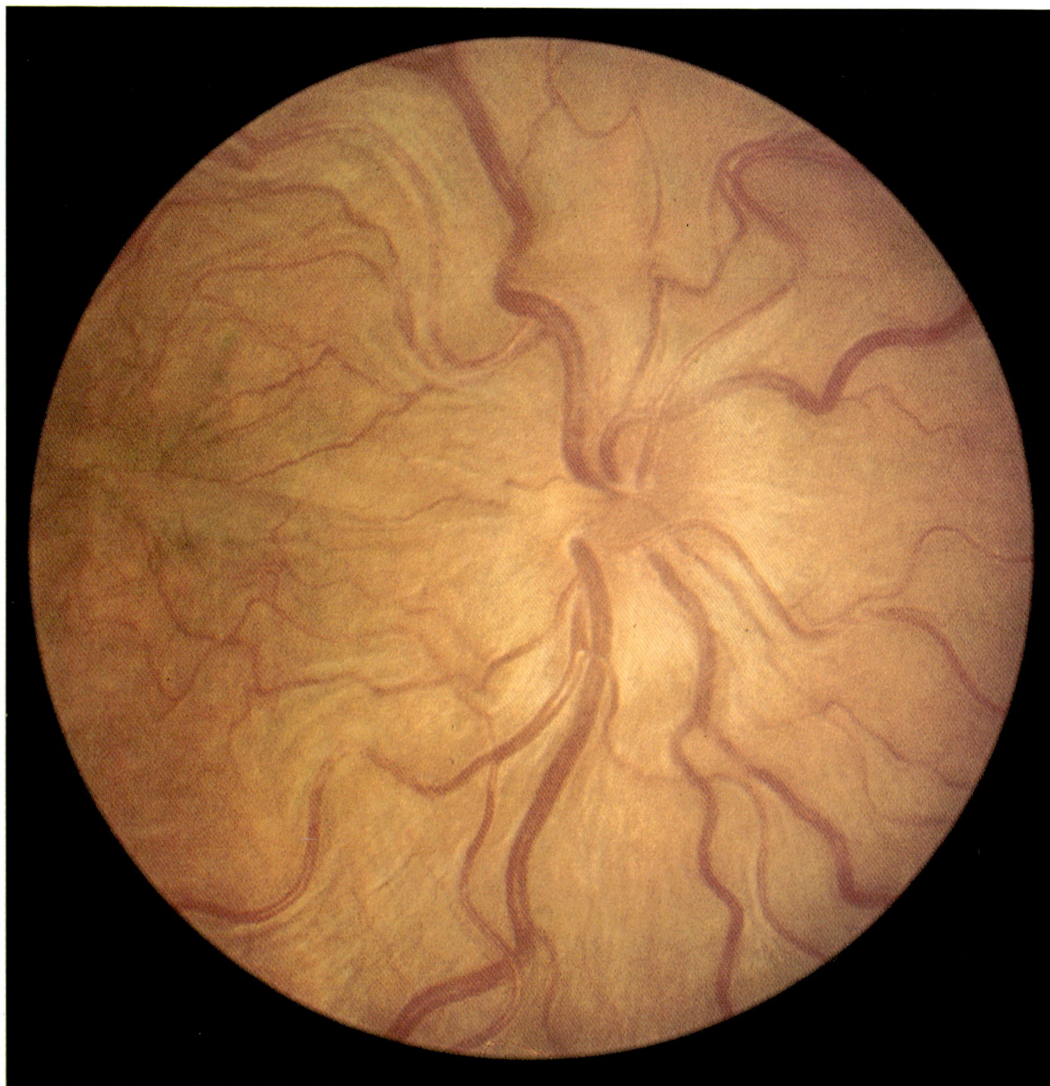

317

Figure 317. Right eye of a 38-year-old male patient with chronic ocular hypotension following severe ocular contusion caused by a snowball hitting the eye when he was 7.

Clinical Findings

Refraction was +6.0 sphere, −2.0 cylinder, axis 0°, visual acuity 20/50. There is an incomplete anterior contusion rosette of the lens and iris sphincter ruptures at 11, 2, and 5 o'clock. Intraocular pressure was 10 mm Hg. The blind spot was enlarged and the outer margins of the visual field were concentrically constricted moderately. The optic disc was elevated 1.5 diopters. There are retinal folds along the posterior pole. The retinal vessels appear tortuous. Gonioscopy showed a wide anterior chamber angle with increased pigmentation of the trabecular meshwork. There were no peripheral synechiae or pathological vessels in the anterior chamber angle. The exophthalmometer measurements were 14-97-14 mm. Ophthalmodynamography showed a pulsation volume of 58.3 ml in the right eye and 72.6 ml in the left eye. Neurologic consultations and computed tomography were normal.

Figure 318. Right eye of an 18-year-old male patient with traumatic optic atrophy caused by a motorbike accident 3 years prior to the examination. There was a secondary exotropia.

Clinical Findings

The eye was amaurotic. Refractive media were clear and intraocular pressure was 12 mm Hg. The fundus showed a bright white optic disc. There was a complete lack of optic disc capillaries, extremely narrow retinal arterioles, but normal retinal venules.

Figure 319. Right eye of a 37-year-old male patient with traumatic optic atrophy caused by a car accident 5 years earlier. A secondary exotropia developed.

Clinical Findings

The eye was amaurotic. Refractive media were clear and intraocular pressure was 13 mm Hg. The fundus showed a white-yellow optic disc with narrow, partially ensheathed retinal arterioles, and slightly engorged retinal venules.

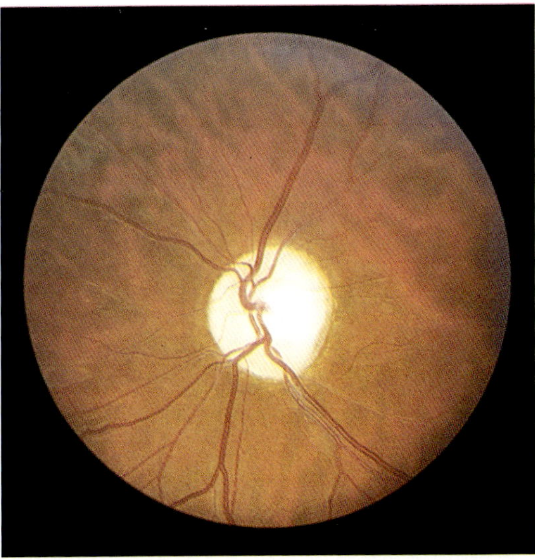

318

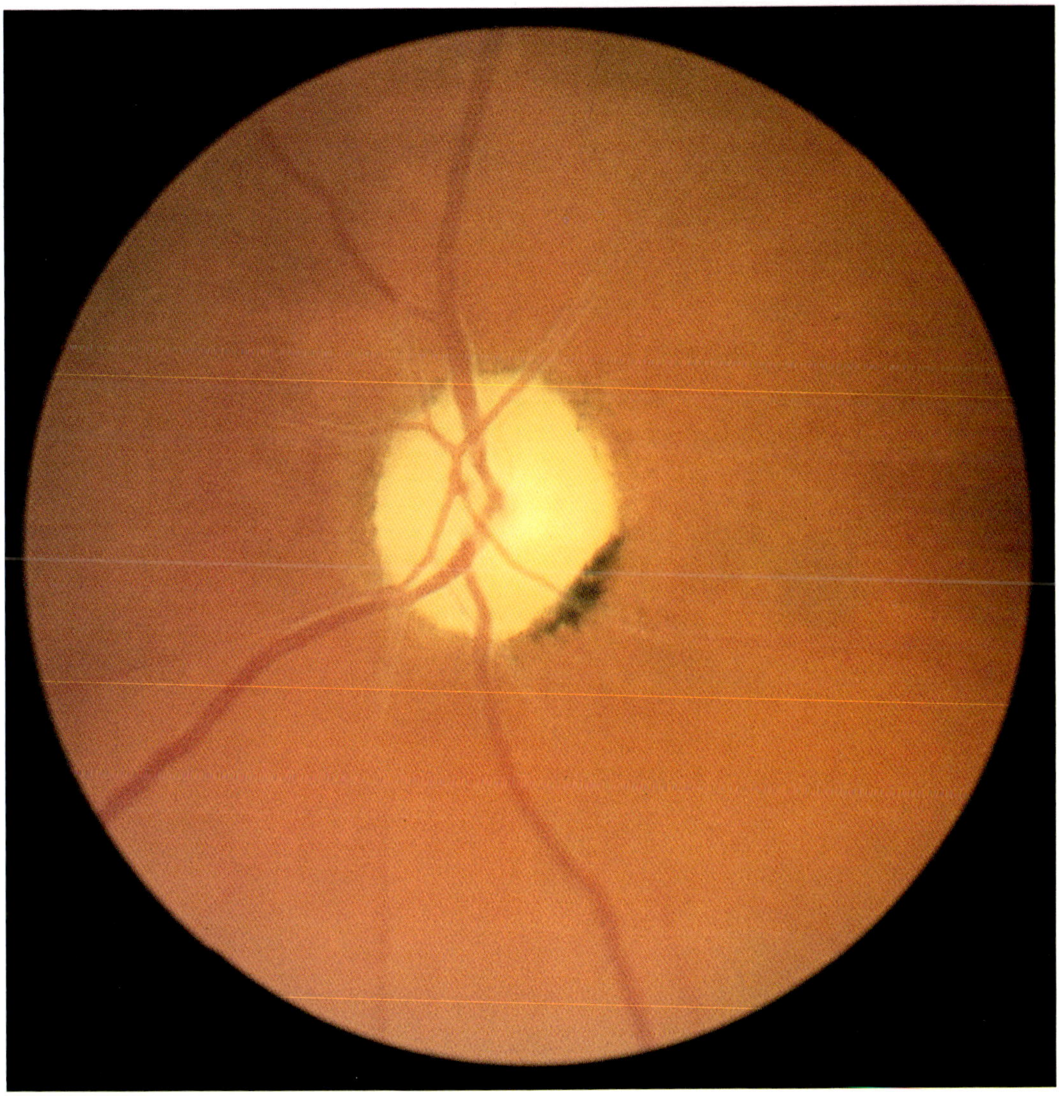

319

Retinal Detachment

Synonyms: Amotio retinae, ablatio retinae.

Two types of retinal detachments must be differentiated: (*a*) a primary, idiopathic type, and (*b*) a secondary type.

Primary Retinal Detachment

Predisposing factors for the development of a retinal detachment (Figs. 320–326) are degenerative changes of the retina and vitreous (Fig. 327), associated with a moderate myopia in older patients in the 5th to 6th decades of life and often associated with arteriosclerosis and aphakia, especially after loss of vitreous. The retinal detachment may be induced by a direct or indirect trauma.

The term "retinal degeneration" denotes a deteriorative atrophy of retinal tissue, resulting from acquired processes such as aging, vascular diseases, exudative or inflammatory insults, mechanical forces, trauma, or toxicity. Some retinal changes predispose to retinal detachments. One of the major degenerative sclerotic areas found ophthalmoscopically, "snail track degeneration" or "lattice degeneration," is seen frequently with pigment irregularities (Pau, 1977). Depending on their location between the ora serrata and the equatorial region of the globe, the lesions are defined as peripheral or equatorial detachments. Small thread-like connections between retina and vitreous (vitreoretinal attachments) are often seen with this condition.

The vitreous also shows degenerative changes, losing its normal gel-like consistency. A decrease in the hyaluronic acid contents of the vitreous destablizes the fibrillar-collagenous network and reduces normal vitreous pressure. Ring-shaped posterior (rarely anterior) vitreous detachments can be found. Such condensed vitreous material is deformed during head movements and may exert stretch and stress on degenerative, sclerotic retinal areas. Retinal detachment may be complicated by development of a retinal hole.

The following are types of retinal holes:

1. Horseshoe-shaped retinal tears occur in 60% of cases and are located primarily in the temporal or superior quadrants. The opening of the horseshoe most often points toward the peripheral retina.
2. Round, circular tears are found in 30% of cases. Often a series of holes, which line up like pearls on a circular necklace, are found within the degenerative retina area.
3. Tears at the ora serrata are found in 10% of cases and are located primarily within the temporoinferior quadrant. In contrast to the temporal or superior horseshoe holes, these tears usually cause very late symptoms. A decrease in visual acuity and enlargement of visual field defects are quite rare observations, and the prognosis is generally good.

The presence of a retinal break does not necessarily mean that the retina will detach immediately. The most important factor for development of a retinal detachment is the degeneration or detachment of the vitreous overlying the break. Smaller vitreous strands may exert traction on the retinal tissue adjacent to the break, and liquified vitreous may then protrude through the retinal hole into the subretinal space, eventually leading to retinal detachment.

The retinal detachment may be preceeded by certain prodromi that include the observation of muscae volitantes (French: Mouches volantes) and the perception of flashing lights or stars. Sometimes patients report seeing a rain of dust particles. This symptom may indicate a small vitreous hemorrhage has already occurred. An advanced retinal detachment becomes clinically manifest as a visual field loss that progresses like a curtain into the visual field. Once the retinal detachment involves the posterior pole, permanent, severe visual loss ensues. Pain is not normally associated with a retinal detachment.

Ophthalmoscopical Appearance. Initially, the detached retina appears translucent; as this condition persists, it becomes more and more opaque and the retina appears gray or gray-green to gray-red. No choroidal structures can be seen underneath the area of retinal detachment. Arteries and veins appear prominent and tortuous and may have a very dark color. The vessels ascend onto the elevated level of the detached retina and follow the contours of the detachment. A wave-like formation of multiple folds (sand dune phenomenon) or a fluctuating flap may be seen.

Quite frequently, the retinal tear is located at the most elevated site of the detachment. The retinal hole appears bright red because the underlying choroid is now visible through the hole. Sometimes retinal vessels cross the retinal break like a bridge. If these vessels rupture, a massive vitreal hemorrhage may ensue. In patients in which the cause of the retinal detachment—one or more retinal holes—is not detected in time, a complete retinal detachment may result. In such cases, the retina appears gray-white and rigid and may show multiple folds.

In rare cases in which there is only a partial retinal detachment, spontaneous remission or reattachment may occur. When examined ophthalmoscopically after a reattachment, these eyes simply show hyperpigmentation and depigmentation that demarcate the margin of the former retinal detachment. The lines are created by pigment clumps that indicate the site to which the detachment progressed before it healed spontaneously (Figs. 320-326).

Therapy. The therapeutic goal in cases of rhegmatogenous retinal detachment is occlusion of the retinal tear. Once this hole is sealed, the subretinal fluid will resolve and the retina may reattach. There are several means for surgically occluding the retinal hole or reattaching the retina at the area where the formation of the retinal break occurred. Part of the sclera may simply be excised or inverted. The sclera can also be pressed toward the inside by affixing a silicone scleral buckle (cerclage) 360° around the sclera to form a circumferential, equatorial band. Other means of reattaching the retina include diathermy, cryopexy, and light and xenon laser coagulation.

Secondary Retinal Detachment

As the term indicates, a secondary retinal detachment is always associated with or caused by other systemic or ocular diseases, including retinal or choroidal tumors, ocular parasites, as a symptom of the Vogt-Koyanagi syndrome and Harada's syndrome, following severe blunt injuries (severe vitreous hemorrhages), or severe perforating injuries (with vitreous loss and intraocular foreign body injuries). Secondary retinal detachment may also be seen in late stages of hypertensive retinopathy, with gestosis (extremely altered vascular permeability), and proliferative retinopathy, Coat's disease, von Hippel-Lindau disease, and Eales' disease.

Therapy. Therapy consists of treatment for the underlying disease or trauma.

Macular Holes

Macular holes represent the final stage of a variety of different diseases. With the exception of an acute traumatic hole, macular hole formation involves the complete thickness of the retina and is always caused by long-standing macular edema that has progressed into cystoid macular degeneration with subsequent hole formation. A macular hole usually causes severe deterioration of the central visual acuity (central scotoma).

The most common causes of macular hole formation are:

Trauma
- Blunt trauma (contusio retinae)
- Perforating trauma
- Severe and abrupt changes in atmospheric pressure (acute decrease of atmospheric pressure, explosion)
- Light or radiation injuries (solar retinitis)

Inflammation
- Iritis, iridocyclitis
- Extraocular localized infections

Cardiovascular system
- Arteriosclerosis, central retinal artery occlusion, arterial branch occlusion, central retinal vein occlusion, venous branch occlusion, periarteritis, Eales' disease, periphlebitis retinae, hypertensive retinopathy, diabetic retinopathy

Refractive anomalies
- High myopia

Retinal detachment
- Degenerative lesions (disciform macular dystrophy)

Hereditary degenerative diseases
- Retinal pigment dystrophies
- Stargardt's disease

Spontaneous macular holes

Ophthalmoscopical Appearance. Typically, a circular dark-red central lesion, measuring 1/6–1/3 optic disc diameter (rarely larger), can be found within the macula. Morphologically, the lesion looks like a circular piece of retina has been cut out. The bottom of the hole is 0.5 to 1.0 diopters deeper than its margins. The surrounding retina may be edematous, and in later stages traction on the retina can cause radial folds. Small granules and, in some eyes, small shimmering crystalline deposits can be seen at the bottom of the hole. The hole shows a white discoloration if the choroid becomes atrophic. Secondary macular holes, in particular, may have partially jagged or irregular margins.

The diagnosis of a macular hole is confirmed by applying the Goldmann lens on the cornea. When examining the macula with a slit image, the slit is interrupted at the site of the hole. A macular hole is a rare cause of retinal detachments, occurring most commonly in association with pathological myopia.

Therapy. Therapy depends largely on the underlying disease. One possible surgical treatment is the "macular technique" method of Meyer-Schwickerath.

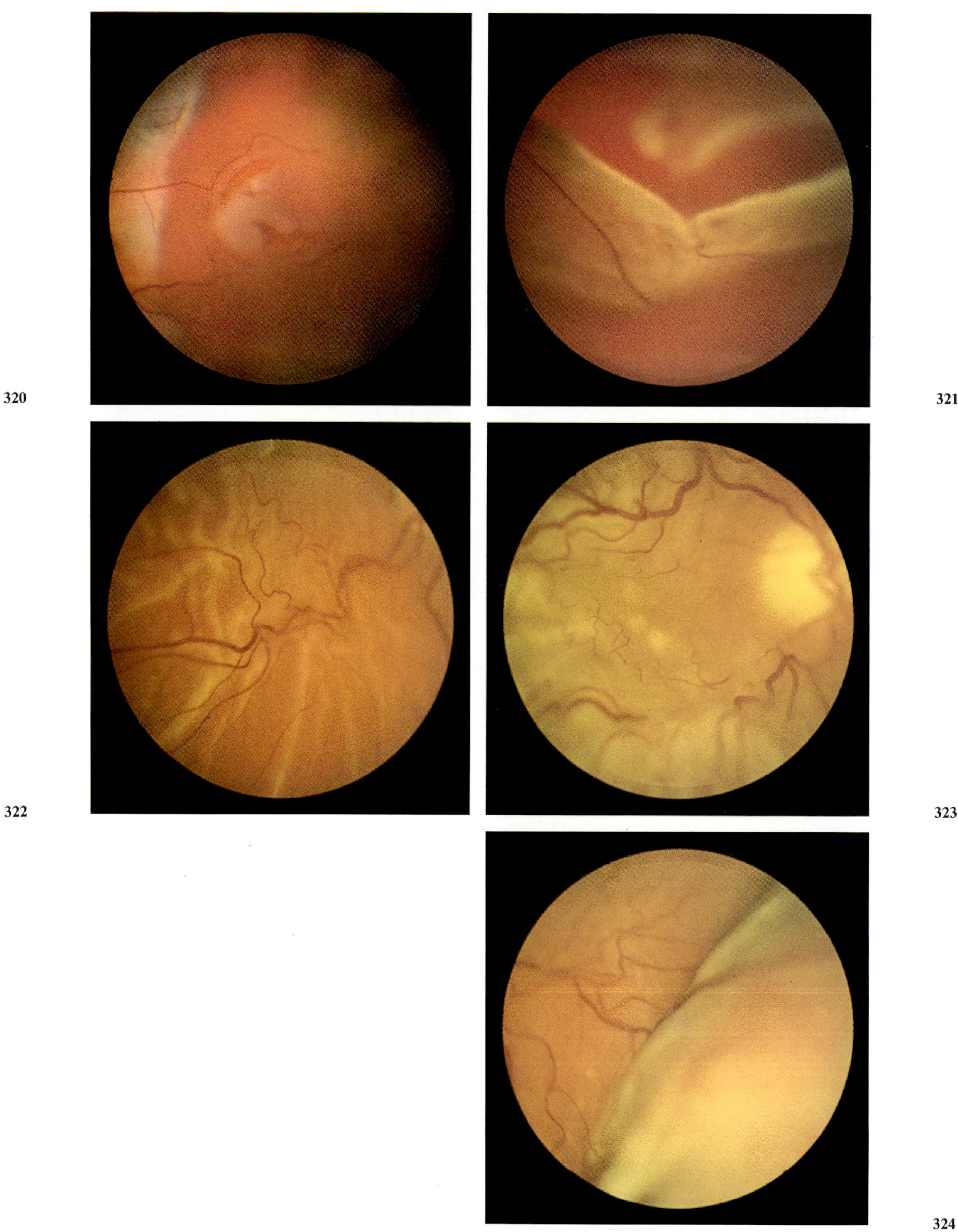

320

321

322

323

324

325

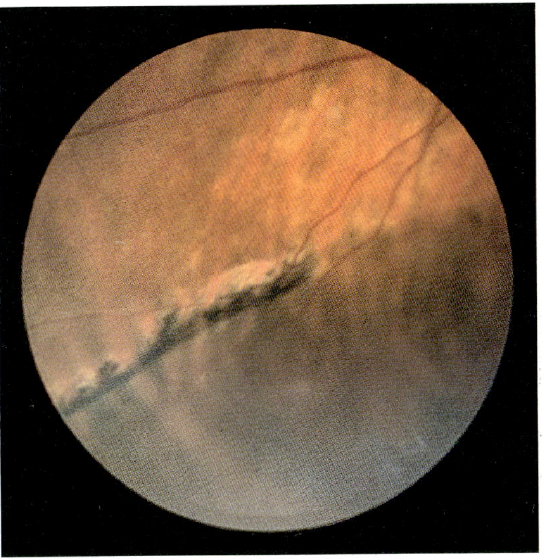

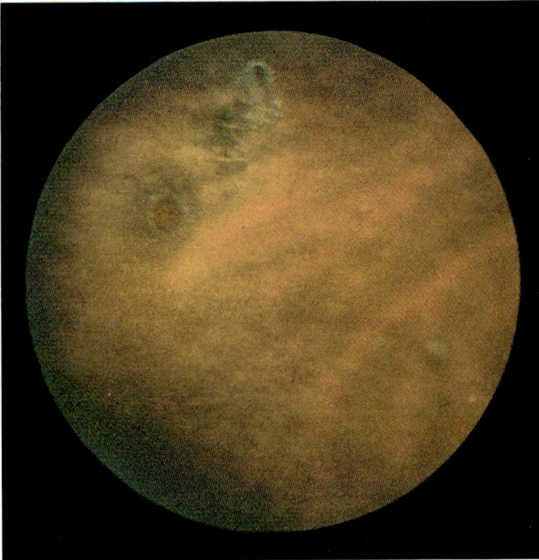

326

Figure 320. Left eye of a 68-year-old female patient with aphakic retinal detachment and a retinal horseshoe-shaped tear following cataract extraction 5 years earlier. The patient had noted photopsia 6 weeks prior to the examination.

Clinical Findings

Visual acuity was 20/200.

Clinical Course

A scleral buckling operation in combination with photocoagulation was performed. The retina reattached and visual acuity recovered to 20/50.

Figure 321. Right eye of a 40-year-old female patient with retinal detachment and a large horseshoe-shaped tear. The patient had noted gray shadows and photopsia. The central visual acuity had decreased.

Clinical Findings

Visual acuity was 20/400.

Therapy

Visual acuity recovered to 20/30 following a scleral buckling operation.

Figures 322–324. Right eye of an 80-year-old female patient with an old retinal detachment. No reattachment surgery was performed because the posterior pole was found to be severely detached at the time of the first examination. The eye became amaurotic.

Figure 325. Right eye of a 38-year-old male patient with spontaneous reattachment of a retinal detachment indicated by a darkly pigmented line. The patient did not remember any previous trauma or other cause for the detachment. The lesion was found during a routine examination. Visual acuity was 20/20.

Figure 326. Right eye of a 28-year-old female patient with peripheral retinal degeneration.

Clinical Findings

Refraction was −4.5 sphere, −2.0 cylinder, axis 15°, visual acuity 20/20. The lesion was prophylactically treated with Xenon light photocoagulation.

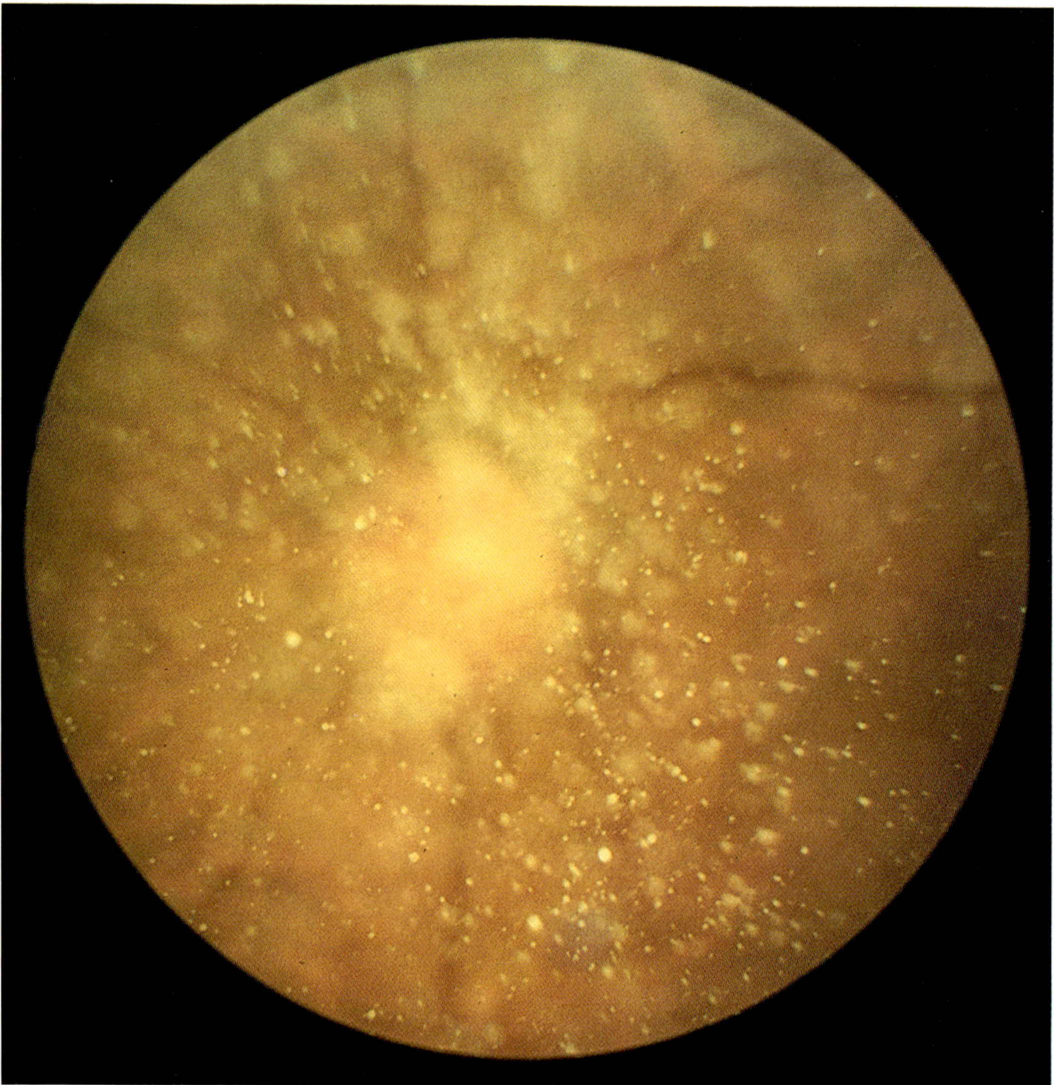

327

Figure 327. Left eye of a 53-year-old male patient with asteroid hyalosis (Benson's disease).

Clinical Findings

Visual acuity in this eye was 20/20. This deposition of light-reflecting cholesterol crystals within the vitreous does not normally cause any visual disturbance.

Fundus Changes Associated with Blood Disorders

Leukemic Retinopathy

Synonyms: Myeloic retinopathy, lymphatic retinopathy.

The retinal changes seen with leukemic retinopathy are not diagnostic for a differentiation of the type of leukemia. In other words, a chronic myeloic, a chronic lymphatic, or a nondifferentiated leukema do not show any specific retinal disorders. Furthermore, it is noteworthy that in most children no retinal abnormalities are found, even in advanced stages of the disease.

Ophthalmoscopical Appearance. The retina shows a pale yellowish discoloration. The retinal vessels, especially the arteries, are extremely light in color. The veins are tortuous and dilated and sometimes appear bead-shaped. Leukemic infiltrates within the retina are usually diffusely scattered over the fundus and appear as yellow-white round, elevated nodules surrounded by a narrow hemorrhagic rim. Perivascular hemorrhages are also seen, especially on the posterior pole.

An infiltration of the optic disc by leukemic cells usually leads to papilledema. In areas where dense, massive leukemic infiltrates accrue, severe retinal necroses with subsequent subretinal and preretinal hemorrhages ensue. Rarely, a serous retinal detachment may develop.

Fundus Associated with Paraproteinemia

The term "paraprotein" denotes a specific gamma globulin (monoclonal immunoglobulin) that is produced by a certain stem of monoclonal cells. The sera of patients with paraproteinemia (monoclonal gammopathy) show a selective excessive increase in one specific immunoglobulin fraction. Electrophoresis reveals a very steep, markedly elevated peak (M-gradient).

Depending on the immunoglobulin fraction involved, IgG, IgA, IgM, IgD, and IgE paraproteinemias must be differentiated. A quantitative analysis of the immunoglobulin fractions is possible.

Multiple myeloma is one of the most common monoclonal gammopathies. Waldenström's macroglobulinemia is characterized by an increase in a monoclonal fraction of IgM. This condition is classified today as an immunocytoma (lymphoplasmocytoid immunocytoma). Both multiple myeloma and Waldenström's syndrome increase the blood viscosity and thus may cause generalized thromboses and hemorrhages. These coagulative disorders become manifest on the ocular fundus, hence the term "fundus viscoparaproteinaemicus."

Ophthalmoscopically, thrombosis-like retinal changes may be observed. Retinal veins appear engorged and bead-like, and the arteries are narrow. These vascular abnormalities are usually found bilaterally and symmetrically. The distortion of normal blood flow and interruption of vessels results in a granular-like flow (see "Central Retinal Artery Occlusion"). The same phenomenon can be observed in the conjunctival vessels. In the literature this condition is described as a "sludged-blood" phenomenon. The optic disc has blurred margins and edema. Retinal detachments have been reported.

The Anemic Fundus

Acute Hemorrhagic Anemia

Following an acute severe blood loss, visual acuity will be reduced bilaterally. Sometimes an amaurosis (posthemorrhagic optic atrophy) may be present.

Ophthalmoscopical Appearance. The entire fundus appears pale (anemic pallor). The optic nerve head is edematous, retinal veins are engorged, and retinal arteries are deprived of blood and become narrowed. Retinal hemorrhages and cotton wool exudates may supplement this pathological condition. At first glance, anemic retinopathy resembles a central retinal artery occlusion, especially in cases in which marked retinal edema is present.

Chronic Hemorrhagic Anemia

Laboratory blood analysis for patients with chronic hemorrhagic anemia reveals a markedly reduced serum iron level. The blood hemoglobin level slowly decreases and the mean cell hemoglobin is reduced. Sideropenic anemias include such conditions as hemorrhagic anemia, pernicious anemia, nutritional anemia (especially in newborns and young children), and tumor anemia. In the latter condition, an anemic, pale fundus pattern is seen ophthalmoscopically, as well as retinal and preretinal hemorrhages, cotton wool exudates, and widely scattered drusen. All of these changes indicate a nutritional deficiency of the retina or cachexial retinopathy.

Pernicious Anemia

This type of anemia is caused by a reduced level, or a complete lack, of vitamin B_{12}. Such a deficiency is related to a lack of intrinsic factor (i.e., after a total stomach resection), or a lack of extrinsic factor (i.e., malnutrition caused by nearly exclusive uptake of carbohydrates and lack of fat and protein, as may occur in tropical regions or during wars). This type of anemia may also be associated with worm infections (*Diphyllobothrium latum*), in cases with deficient vitamin B_{12} resorption (sprue), or deficient vitamin B_{12} deposition (advanced stage of liver cirrhosis). Very specific, rare forms of this disease include pernicious anemia occurring during pregnancy (combined folic acid, iron, and vitamin B_{12} deficiency) and toxic pernicious anemia caused by such agents and/or drugs as hydantoin, primidone, phenobarbital, secobarbital, amobarbital, or lithium carbonate.

Pernicious anemia is characterized by macrocytic erythrocytes and a color index that is greater than normal. The serum concentrations of iron and bilirubin are increased. A sternal bone marrow biopsy reveals the presence of megalocytes and megaloblasts. There is a gastric achylia that does not respond to histamine. The skin appears pale and the presence of Hunter's glossitis and funicular myelosis may supplement the clinical symptoms.

Ocular symptoms of pernicious anemia may consist of a retrobulbar optic neuritis. Recurrent subconjunctival hemorrhages have also been described.

Ophthalmoscopical Appearance. The entire fundus appears pale except for the retinal and preretinal hemorrhages.

Hemolytic Anemia

One of the best described examples of hemolytic anemia is sickle cell disease. This condition was named because the erythrocytes show a typical sickle-shaped deformity that can be observed in blood cell counts after 2 to 24 hours. Skin and conjunctiva of the affected patient may show a yellowish, subicteric discoloration. Typically, splenomegaly is present. Sickle cell anemia is found more frequently in certain geographical regions (Mediterranean area, Persian Gulf area, central and west Africa, and the United States). Pathogenetically, this disease is caused by an alteration in the composition of normal adult hemoglobin (HbA).

Subgroups of this hemoglobinopathy can be differentiated by a hemogloblin eclectrophoresis. It is postulated that the S component in hemoglobin primarily causes thromboses in the coronary arteries, lung, spleen, and kidneys with subsequent hemorrhagic infarction of these areas (Rummeld, 1975). Proliferative retinopathy is seen more frequently in patients with hemoglobin C (Goldberg, 1971). The conjunctival vessels may show a sludged-blood phenomenon, similar to that associated with paraproteinemia.

Ophthalmoscopical Appearance. There are no specific retinal abnormalities associated with hemoglobinopathies. A kaleidoscope of vascular abnormalities may be found, including arterial occlusions involving the precapillary small arterioles, arterovenous shunt formations, telangiectases, fan-shaped neovascularization and vascular proliferations associated with vitreous hemorrhages, peripheral vascular sheathings, and gliositic retinal degenerations. Equatorial retinal degenerations may lead to rhegmatogenous retinal detachment. Papilledema may be present.

Another example of hemoglobinopathy is thalassemia. The normal adult hemoglobin (Hb) is replaced by a variation that is termed HbA_2. HbA_2 fraction can be analyzed using a combined electrophoretic-spectrophotometric method. Clinically, two types of thalassemia, thalassemia major (primary erythoblastic or Cooley's anemia) and thalassemia minor (target cell or Rietti's anemia), must be differentiated. Thalassemia major is found only in the Mediterreanean area and often leads to an early death in infancy. Thalassemia minor has been found in central Europe. Typical clinical findings include hepatosplenomegaly and subicteric skin and conjunctival discoloration. Other symptoms include infantilism, thinning of the inner and outer tables of the skull, and, in some cases, oxycephaly (turricephaly) with protrusio bulbi. The cell count shows target cells, poikilocytes, elliptocytes, and fragmented erythrocytes. Sideroblasts are found in the bone marrow.

Ophthalmoscopically, the disease is characterized by neovascularization, central and peripheral retinal hemorrhages, peripheral vascular sheathings, and vitreal hemorrhages.

Fundus Changes Associated with Coagulative Disorders

Most of the conditions listed below are characterized by retinal hemorrhages, neovascularization, and vascular proliferations. The fundus may resemble certain stages of Eales' disease. Most of the retinal abnormalities can be classified as examples of proliferative retinopathy. The coagulative disorder may result from a reduction or disorder of noncellular coagulation factors (hemophilia, hypoprothrombinemia, hypofibrinogenemia, overdoses of anticoagulant drugs):

Disorders of the thrombocytes: Idiopathic thrombocytopenic purpura (Werlhof's disease).

Vascular disorders: Acute vascular purpura (Henoch-Schönlein purpura), hereditary hemorrhagic telangiectasis (Osler's disease), scurvy or vitamin C deficiency.

The Rumpel-Leede test is simple and useful in examining the fragility of capillaries. For this test a tourniquet is placed on the patient's upper arm and compressed for approximately 5 minutes with a pressure that is at least 10 mm Hg higher than the patient's diastolic blood pressure. In a pathologic condition such as increased capillary fragility, if petechial hemorrhages are observed just inferior to the tourniquet, the Rumpel-Leede test is positive.

Primary Polycythemia

Synonyms: Polycythemia vera, genuine polycythemia (Figs. 331–334).

The etiology of primary polycythemia, which most often occurs in older men, is unknown. Polycythemia is caused by an irreversible proliferation of the entire myeloic system. In some cases, polycythemia is the first symptom of a developing, chronic myeloic leukemia or of an osteomyelofibrotic syndrome.

Clinical Appearance. An acute exacerbation of the disease becomes manifest clinically by cyanosis of the face and mucous membranes. Any type of physical exercise or coughing worsens the cyanosis. Patients complain of nausea, headache, and itching skin. Often splenomegaly and, less frequently, hepatomegaly can be found. Increased blood viscosity causes heart insufficiency, cerebral oxygen deficiency, and phlebothromboses. The serum uric concentrations are increased and blood pressure is elevated.

As confirmed by a laboratory diagnosis, cytopoiesis of erythrocytes, leukocytes (myelocytes), and platelets (thrombocytes) is markedly increased. The red cell count usually shows erythrocyte values between 6 and 9 million/ ml^3. Similarly, the numbers for leukocytes and platelets are also markedly elevated. Hemoglobin and hematocrit, as well as total blood volume, are also above normal.

Ophthalmoscopical Appearance. The retina is cyanotic and retinal veins appear dark blue-red and engorged. The arteries may be normal, dilated, or narrow. The optic disc is hyperemic, and papilledema that is elevated up to 3 diopters can be found. Retinal (Figs. 328–330) and preretinal hemorrhages and central vein or artery occlusions may be present.

Therapy. The therapy consists of a reduction of the cellular elements within the circulatory system, which can be achieved by removing some of the blood and subsequently reinfusing the serum only. Isovolemic hemodilution and radioactive phosphorous therapy, with or without the use of cytotoxic agents, are other therapeutic methods.

Secondary Polycythemia

As indicated by the term "secondary polycythemia," this condition represents an increase of erythrocytes and hemoglobin caused by various diseases. A secondary polycythemia may be associated with certain pulmonary and cardiac disorders, renal tumors (hypernephroma), hydronephrosis, certain cerebellar or hypophyseal tumors, liver or uterus tumors, stress, and the Pickwickian syndrome.

Ophthalmoscopical Appearance. The retinal abnormalities resemble those seen in primary polycythemia (Figs. 331 and 332).

Therapy. The therapy has to be adjusted according to the underlying disease. In certain cases, an isovolemic hemodilution may be useful.

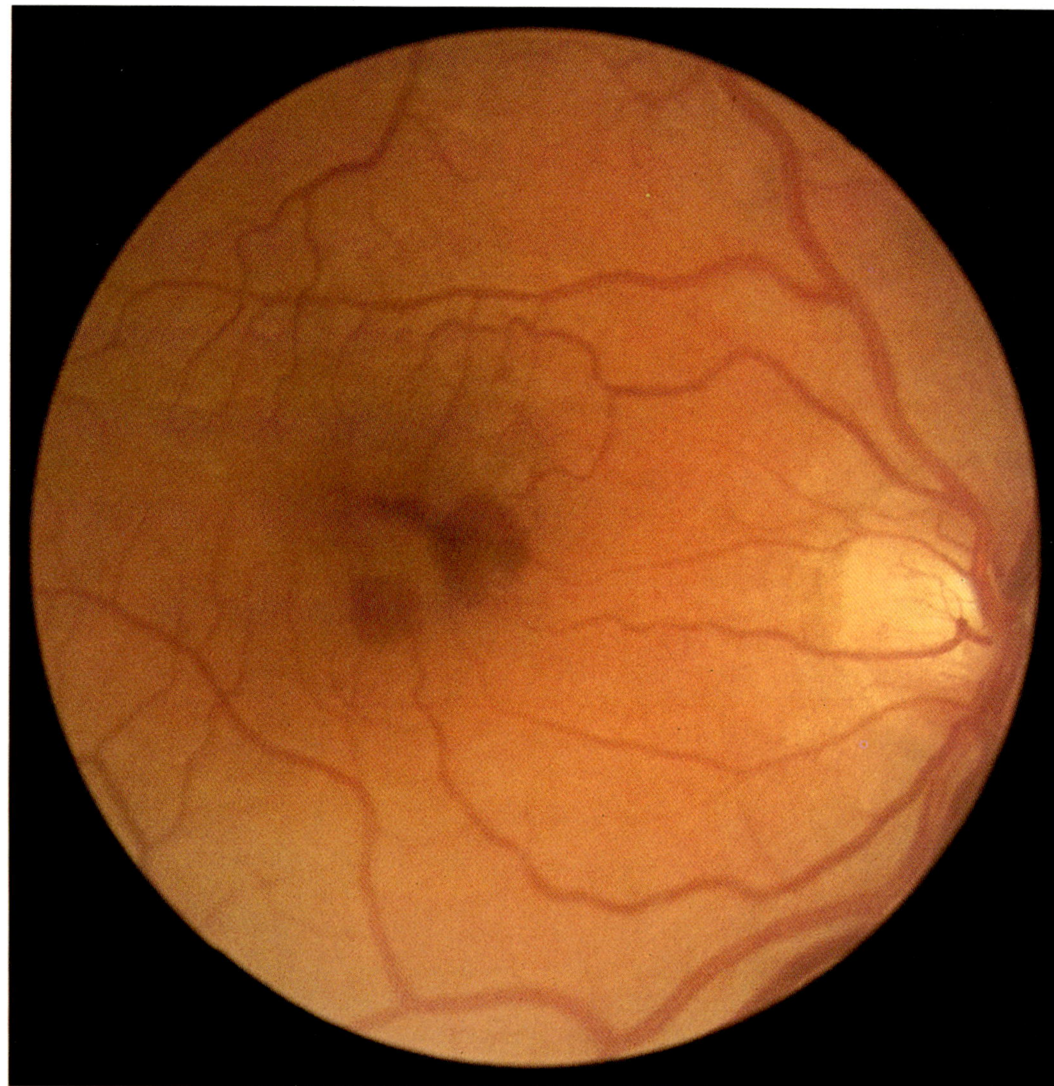

328

Figure 328. Right eye of a 24-year-old male patient with acute retinal hemorrhage in the macular region.

Clinical Findings

Visual acuity was 20/400 and intraocular pressure was 14 mm Hg. There was a central scotoma. The retinal arterioles appear tortuous. Blood pressure was 140/90 mm Hg measured on both arms and blood sedimentation rate was 4/7 mm.

Laboratory Findings

Hemoglobin 13.7%, Quick's test 82%, prothrombin time 32 seconds, erythrocytes 4.3 million, leukocytes 4900, blood platelets 253,000, Rumpel-Leede test was negative. In a consultation with an internist, a sinus tachycardia was found but all other findings were normal.

Therapy and Clinical Course

Using radiation and rheologic therapy, visual acuity completely recovered to 20/20. Familial tortuosity of the small retinal arterioles associated with macular hemorrhage (as described by Beyer, 1958) was ruled out.

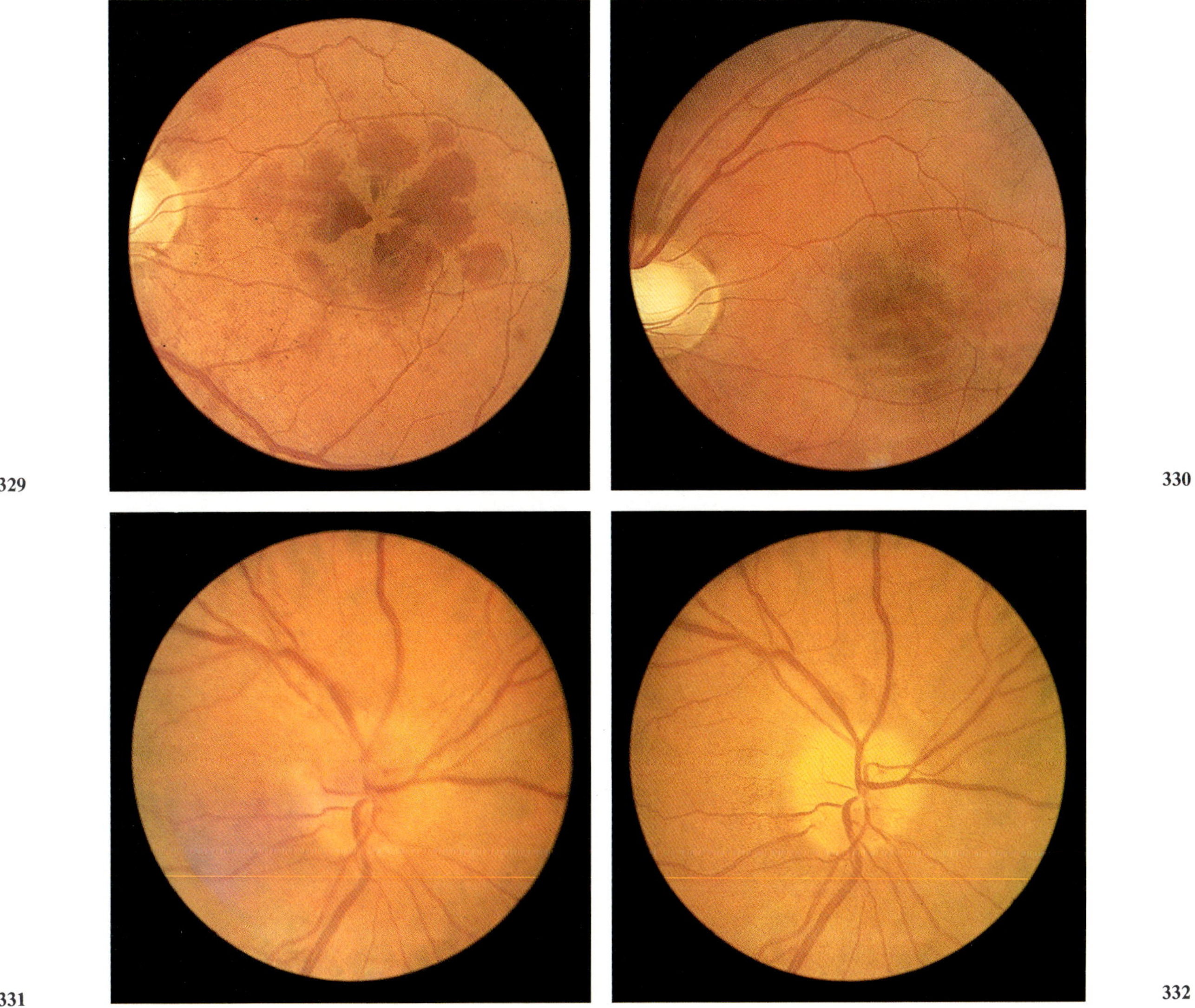

Figures 329 and 330. Left eye of a 21-year-old patient with acute retinal hemorrhage at the posterior pole.

Clinical Findings

The eye was myopic with a refraction of −3.25 sphere and visual acuity of 20/40. Intraocular pressure was 16 mm Hg. There was a central scotoma. Blood pressure measured on both arms was 180/80 mm Hg. The pulse was 124 beats per minute in a supine position and 132 beats per minute in an erect position.

Laboratory Findings

Quick's test 71%, recalcification time 176 seconds, fibrinogen 0.262 gm/100 ml, erythrocytes 4.45 million, leukocytes 5200, blood platelets 220,000, differential blood cell count normal, Rumpel-Leede test was negative. A pheochromocytoma was ruled out.

Therapy and Clinical Course

Both radiation and rheologic therapies were given. Figure 330 shows the fundus 8 days after the onset of the symptoms. Three weeks later the hemorrhages had completely resolved. Visual acuity recovered to 20/20. An acute blood pressure rise was obviously the underlying reason for the retinal hemorrhage.

Figures 331 and 332. Right eye of a 57-year-old male patient with papilledema associated with secondary polycythemia.

Clinical Findings

Refraction was +1.5 sphere for a visual acuity of 20/50. Intraocular pressure was 14 mm Hg. Visual field testing revealed a moderate enlargement of the blind spot. Blood pressure was 140/100 mm Hg measured on the right arm, and 130/100 mm Hg measured on the left arm. Blood sedimentation rate was 3/9 mm. The anterior segment was unremarkable.

Laboratory Findings

Quick's test 100%, erythrocytes 5.83 million, leukocytes 5200, blood platelets 146,000, urea 21.0 mg/100 ml, creatinine 0.8 mg/100 ml, electrolytes and liver enzymes normal, blood glucose concentration 84 mg/100 ml, cholesterol 197 mg/100 ml, triglycerides 135 mg/100 ml. There was a moderate splenomegaly present.

Clinical Course

Two weeks later (Fig. 332) the papilledema had completely resolved, the engorged venules returned to their normal caliber, and visual acuity recovered to 20/20.

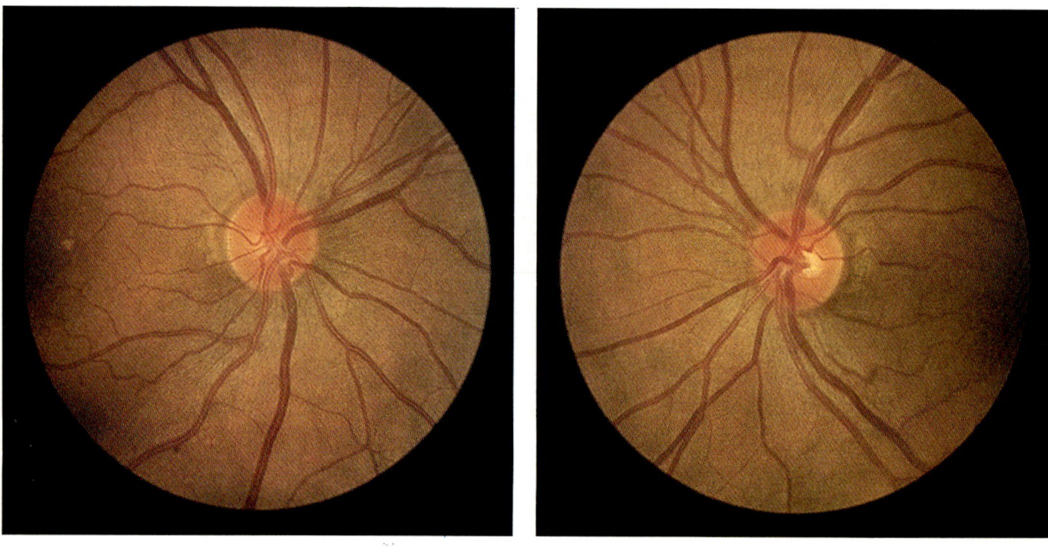

333 334

Figures 333 and 334. Right and left eyes of a 42-year-old male patient with polycythemia. The patient had brief transient visual distortions over a period of 6 weeks.

Clinical Findings

Both eyes were emmetropic and visual acuity was 20/50. Intraocular pressure was 14 mm Hg and visual fields were normal. Fundus examination revealed a bilateral dark beefy red appearance. The venules were engorged but not tortuous. The optic disc has a red appearance. Blood pressure measured on both arms was 140/90 mm Hg and blood sedimentation rate was 7/20 mm. Doppler sonography showed normal blood flow in the carotid arteries.

Laboratory Findings

Erythrocytes 6.2 million, leukocytes 5600, total serum protein 6.7 gm/100 ml, albumin 4.7 gm/100 ml, electrolytes and liver enzymes normal.

References

Aaberg, T.M., Cesarz, T.J., Rytel, M.W.: Correlation of virology and clinical course of cytomegalic retinitis. Am. J. Ophthalmol. *74:* 407 (1972).

Adams, J.E.: Trans. Ophthalmol. Soc. UK *3:* 113 (1883) (zit. nach Jaeger, W., Bischoff, E., 1977).

Aichmair, H.: Ein Knabe mit Hypoplasie der rechten Papille. Klin. Mbl. Augenheilk, *153:* 523 (1968).

Amalric, P., Schum, U.: Pigmentierte, paravenöse Netz- und Aderhautatrophie. Klin. Mbl. Augenheilk, *153:* 775 (1968).

Ammon, F.A. von: Illust. med. Z. *1:* 319 (1852) (zit. nach Duke-Elder, 1976).

Apple, D.J., Gieser, D.K., Goldberg, M.F.: Pathologische Befunde bei einem Erwachsenen mit Morbus Coats. Klin. Mbl. Augenheilk. *179:* 336 (1981).

Armaly, M.F.: Optic cup in normal and glaucomatous eyes. Invest. Ophthalmol. Vis. Sci. *9:* 425 (1970).

Arterial hypertension. Report of a WHO Expert Committee. Technical Report Series 628 (WHO, Geneva 1978).

Ashton, N., Garner, A., Peltier, S.: Experimental hypertensive retinopathy in the monkey. Trans. Ophthalmol. Soc. UK *88:* 167 (1968).

Aulhorn, E.: Über die Indikation zur Verordnung vergrössernder Sehhilfen. Augenspiegel *1:* 4 (1971).

Axenfeld, Th.: Augenerkrankungen während der Schwangerschaft, des Wochenbettes und der Stillungszeit. Mschr. Geburtsh. Gynäk. *2:* 516 (1895).

Babel, J.: Traitement des thromboses de vaisseaux rétiniens. Klin. Mbl. Augenhellk. *170:* 211 (1977).

Badtke, G. (1937), zit. bei Hollwich, F.: Das Verhalten der Netzhautgefässe in der Schwangerschaft. Ber. dt. ophthal. Ges. *63:* 117 (1960).

Badtke, G.: Neues zur Histologie und Genese der atypischen Kolobome des Fundus und der Papille. Klin. Mbl. Augenheilk. *132:* 626 (1958).

Badtke, G.: Über die Grössenanomalien der Papilla nervi optici, unter besonderer Berücksichtigung der schwarzen Megalopapille. Klin. Mbl. Augenheilk. *135:* 502 (1959).

Bailliart, P.: La pression artérielle dans les branches de l'artère centrale de la rêtine; nouvelle technique pour la déterminer. Annls Oculist. *154:* 648 (1917).

Bangerter, A.: Diskussion zu Gloor, B.P.: Epiretinale Fibroplasie und massive präretinale Retraktion. Ophthalmologica, Basel *161:* 234 (1970).

Barsewitsch, B. von: Frühgeburt und Netzhautablösung. Klin. Mbl. Augenheilk. *170:* 95 (1977).

Barsewitsch, B. von: Netzhautablösung mit spontaner Wiederanlegung. Klin. Mbl. Augenheilk. *177:* 467, 472 (1980).

Bastian, G.O., Mautner, W., Piper, H.F.: Über akute Durchblutungsstörungen des Sehnerven. Klin. Mbl. Augenheilk. *165:* 427 (1974).

Bastian, G.O., Seemann, K.B.: Erblindung bei Arteriitis cranialis vermeidbar? Dt. Ärzteblatt *42:* 2407 (1978).

Baurmann, H., Meyer, F., Oberhoff, P.: Komplikation bei der arteriovenösen Anastomose der Netzhaut. Klin. Mbl. Augenheilk. *153:* 562–571 (1968).

Beaver, P.C., Snyder, C.H., Carrera, G.M., Dent, J.H., Laferty, J.W.: Chronic eosinophilia due to visceral larva migrans. Pediatrics *9:* 7 (1952).

Becker, St. C.: Gonioskopie (Schattauer, Stuttgart 1976).

Behçet H.: Über rezidivierende aphthöse, durch ein Virus verursachte Geschwüre am Mund, am Auge und an den Genitalien. Derm. Wschr. *105:* 1152 (1937).

Belohradsky, B.H., Magret, W.: Infektionskrankheiten; in Keller, Wiskott, Lehrbuch der Kinderheilkunde (Thieme, Stuttgart 1984).

Benoit, W.: Ein Beitrag zur Kenntnis der Rindenveränderungen bei Wochenbettseklampsie. Z. ges. Neurol. Psychiat. *131:* 602 (1931).

Bergmeister (1877) zit. bei Duke-Elder, St.: Normal and abnormal development; part 1, Embryology. System of ophthalmology, vol. 3 (Kimpton, London 1963).

Bernsmeier, H.: Subretinaler Echinokokkus. Klin. Mbl. Augenheilk. *177:* 85 (1980).

Best, F.: Über eine hereditäre Maculaaffektion. Beiträge zur Vererbungslehre. Z. Augenheilk. *13:* 199 (1905).

Best, H.: Klinik der Karotisstenose und der Arteriitis temporalis. Klin. Mbl. Augenheilk, *163:* 245 (1973).

Beuningen, G.A. van: Glaukom; in Velhagen, Der Augenarzt, vol. 7 (Thieme, Leipzig 1967).

Beyer, E.V.: Familiäre Tortuositas der kleinen Netzhautarterien mit Makulablutung. Klin. Mbl. Augenheilk. *123:* 532 (1958).

Bielschowski, A.: Ein ungewöhnlicher Fall von vertikaler Heterotropie der Makula. Klin. Mbl. Augenheilk. *84:* 755 (1930).

Biesheuvel, K.: Central tapeto-retinal degeneration with peripheral involvement (differential-diagnostic difficulties). Ophthalmologica, Basel *146:* 238 (1963).

Biró, I.: Paradoxe Gefässkreuzungen am Augenhintergrund. Klin. Mbl. Augenheilk. *164:* 738 (1974).

Bjerrum, J.P.: Über die Refraktion des Neugeborenen (zit. bei Groenouw, A., 1904).

Blankenagel, A., Jaeger, W., Erste Erfahrungen mit dem Fernseh-Lesegerät für hochgradig Sehbehinderte. (Bei welchen Patienten lohnt sich ein Versuch mit diesem Gerät?) Klin. Mbl. Augenheilk. *160:* 723 (1972a).

Blankenagel, A., Jaeger, W.: Erfahrungen mit dem Fernseh-Lesegerät in einer Blindenschule. Klin. Mbl. Augenheilk. *161:* 467 (1972b).

Bleckmann, H.: Langzeitbeobachtung einer Chorioiditis striata. Klin. Mbl. Augenheilk. *166:* 668 (1975).

Bleckmann, H., Norderhus, G.: Die akute generalisierte Periphlebitis retinae. Klin. Mbl. Augenheilk. *177:* 70 (1980).

Blodi, C.: Eine Aderhautblutung, ein Melanom vortäuschend. Klin. Mbl. Augenheilk. *160:* 46 (1972).

Blodi, F.C.: Die Bedeutung der Temporalarterie in der Augenheilkunde. Klin. Mbl. Augenheilk. *155:* 318 (1969).

Bock, K.D.: Arterielle Hypertonie. Probleme der Pathogenese. Kurzmonographien Sandoz, Nr. 21 (1978).

Bock, R. (1949) zit. bei Duke-Elder, St.: Congenital deformities. System of ophthalmology, vol. 3 (Kimpton, London 1964).

Bodechtel, G.: Die Veränderungen an der Calcarina bei der Eklampsie und ihre Beziehungen zu den eklamptischen zentralen Sehstörungen. Graefes Arch. Ophthalmol. *132:* 34 (1934).

Boergen, K.-P., Lorenz, B.: Photokoagulation bei retinalen Venenastverschlüssen. Z. prakt. Augenheilk. *3:* 113 (1982).

Börner, R.: Die Erkrankungen der Uvea; in Velhagen, Der Augenarzt, vol. 4 (Thieme, Leipzig 1976).

Bonamour, G.: Le pronostic éloigné des hémorrhagies rétiniennes du nouveau-né. Bull. Soc. Ophthalmol. Fr. *62:* 277 (1949).

Bonamour, G., Bonnet, M., Grange, J.D., Pingault, C.L., Heirieis, M.: Topographische Studien über angiographisch beobachtete Läsionen bei Retinitis centralis serosa. Klin. Mbl. Augenheilk. *171:* 862 (1977).

Bonnet, M.: Beitrag zur Klinik der Maculadrusen. Klin. Mbl. Augenheilk. *162:* 326 (1973).

Bonnet, M.: "Schiessscheiben"-Makulopathie (bull's eye disease) (symptomatologische Wertung). Klin. Mbl. Augenheilk. *168:* 297 (1976).

Botzler, D.: Die Wertigkeit in der Diagnostik zerebraler Durchblutungsstörungen. Intern. Praxis *22:* 291 (1982).

Brandt, H.P., Viebig, R.: Internoretinale Fibroplasie. Klin. Mbl. Augenheilk. *155:* 804 (1969).

Braunmühl, A. von: Über Gehirnveränderungen bei puerperaler Eklampsie und ihre Entstehung durch Kreislaufstörungen. Z. ges. Neurol. Psychiat. *117:* 698 (1928).

Brégeat, P.: Traumatische Läsionen des Chiasma opticum. Klin. Mbl. Augenheilk. *170:* 374 (1977).

Brückner, R.: Augenfibel. Der Augenkranke in der Allgemeinpraxis (Thieme, Stuttgart 1966).

Bruha, H.: Zur Therapie der sogenannten Chorioretinitis centralis serosa mit dem Lasergerät. Klin. Mbl. Augenheilk. *160:* 340 (1972).

Burdin, J.C., Pierson, M., Percebois, G., Georges, J.C.: Les formes oculaires de la listériose humaine. Presse méd. *77:* 1441 (1965).

Buschmann, W., Angele, W.: Augenveränderungen bei Hypertonie und Diabetes. Therapiewoche *31:* 4397 (1981).

Busse, H., Schiffer, H.P., Unterberg, W.: Ein Fall von Retinitis septica Roth. Klin. Mbl. Augenheilk. *174:* 260 (1979).

Cagianut, B., Werner, H.: Zum Krankheitsbild der familiären Tortuositas der kleinen Netzhautarterien mit Maculablutung. Klin. Mbl. Augenheilk. *153:* 533 (1968).

Cernea, P., Constantin, F.: Die Persistenz der Bergmeister-Papille. Klin. Mbl. Augenheilk. *169:* 516 (1976).

Cherednichenko, V.M.: On the role of listrellal infections in the etiology of endogenous uveitis. Vest. Oftal. *4:* 42 (1962).

Chwastowa, A.W., Weinstein, E.S., Dimitrowskaja, I.P., Izikson, L.L., Burdjanskaja, E.I., Sorokina, M.N., Timakowa, W.I.: Behandlungsergebnisse beim beiderseitigen Retinoblastom. Klin. Mbl. Augenheilk. *176:* 758 (1980).

Clausen: Typisches, beiderseitiges hereditäres Makulakolobom. Klin. Mbl. Augenheilk. *67:* 116 (1921).

Coats, G.: Forms of retinal disease, with massive exudation. Royal London Ophthalmic Hospital Reports *XVII:* 440 (1908).

Coats, G.: Über Retinitis exsudativa (Retinitis haemorrhagica externa). Graefes Arch. Ophthal. *81:* 275 (1912).

Conrads, H., Bichmann, W.: Multiple vitelliforme Netzhautzysten. Klin. Mbl. Augenheilk. *182:* 241 (1983).

Cullen, J.F.: Occult temporal arteriitis—a common cause of blindness in old age. Br. J. Ophthalmol. *51:* 513 (1967).

Daicker, B.: Pathologische Anatomie der arteriellen und venösen Gefässverschlüsse in der Netzhaut, Klin. Mbl. Augenheilk. *170:* 198 (1977).

Daicker, B., Keller, H.H.: Riesenzellarteriitis mit endookulärer Ausbreitung und Hypotonia bulbi dolorosa. Klinisch-pathologischer Bericht. Klin. Mbl. Augenheilk. *158:* 358 (1971).

Damaske, E., Jünemann, G.: Über Spätfälle von Retinoblastom. Klin. Mbl. Augenheilk. *155:* 837 (1969).

Daxecker, F.: Partielle Evulsio nervi optici durch Pistolenschuss. Klin. Mbl. Augenheilk. *176:* 418 (1980).

Denden, A.: Über den Fundus heterotopicus. Klin. Mbl. Augenheilk. *169:* 38 (1970).

Dereani, C., Kolar, G.: Augenhintergrundsveränderungen bei jungen Diabetikern. Klin. Mbl. Augenheilk. *157:* 101 (1970).

Deutmann, A.F.: The hereditary dystrophies of the posterior pole of the eye (van Gorcum, Assen 1971).

Deutsche Liga zur Bekämpfung des hohen Blutdrucks: Normwerte des Blutdruckes und Einteilung der chronischen arteriellen Hypertonie; 2. Aufl. (Heidelberg 1980).

Doden, W.: Augensymptome bei Schädel-Hirn-Verletzten. Medsche Klin. *28:* 1216 (1962).

Doden, W.: Zur Klinik und Ätiologie der Periphlebitis retinae. Entwicklung und Fortschritte in der Augenheilkunde, pp. 152 (Enke, Stuttgart 1963).

Doden, W.: Omega-Venenbögen bei Retinopathia diabetica. Klin. Mbl. Augenheilk. *164:* 441 (1974).

Dodt, E.: Die erste Beschreibung des Knicks in der Dunkeladaptationskurve durch H. Aubert (1865). Klin. Mbl. Augenheilk. *182:* 107 (1983).

Döderlein, G.: EPH-Gestose und Augenhintergrund. Klin. Mbl. Augenheilk. *171:* 896 (1977).

Döderlein, G., Hollwich, F.: Beobachtungen bei systematischer ärztlicher Schwangerschaftsvorsorge. Zentbl. Gynäk. *83:* 413 (1961).

Doyne, R.W. (1889), zit. bei Duke-Elder, System of ophthalmology; diseases of the uvea, vol. IX, p. 721 (Kimpton, London 1966).

Drobec, P.: Das hämorrhagische Sekundärglaukom. Klin. Mbl. Augenheilk. *180:* 138 (1982).

Drobec, P.: Das hämorrhagische Sekundärglaukom nach Zentralvenenthrombose. Klin. Mbl. Augenheilk. *183:* 101 (1983).

Dubois-Poulsen, A.: Le champ visuel (Masson, Paris 1952).

Duke-Elder, St.: System of ophthalmology, vol. III, Normal and abnormal development, part I and II; vol. V, Ophthalmic optics and refraction; vol. IX, Diseases of the uveal tract; vol. X, Diseases of the retina and vitreous; vol. XI, Diseases of the lens, glaucoma; vol. XII, Neuro-ophthalmology; vol. XIV, Injuries (Kimpton, London 1976).

Egerer, I.: Die gruppierte (oder nävoide) Pigmentation des Augenhintergrundes. Klin. Mbl. Augenheilk. *168:* 672 (1976).

Eichholtz, W., Kronen, W., Mies, R., Lang, R.: Die immunsuppressive Behandlung der Behçetschen Erkrankung. Klin. Mbl. Augenheilk. *171:* 627 (1977).

Elbrechtz, H. Chr.: Über eine doppelte Papille im Auge. Klin. Mbl. Augenheilk. *166:* 389 (1975).

Elschnig. A.: Über physiologische, atrophische und glaukomatöse Exkavation. Ber. dt. ophthal. Ges. *34* (1907).

Enzmann, V., Ruprecht, K.W.: Zwischenfälle bei der Fluoreszenzangiographie der Retina. Symptomatik, Prophylaxe und Therapie. Klin. Mbl. Augenheilk. *181:* 235 (1982).

Erdmann, G., Seeliger, H.P.R.: Die Listeriose; in Gsell. Mohr, Infektionskrankheiten (Springer, Berlin 1968).

Evans, J.: Familial macular colobomata. Br. J. Ophthalmol. *21:* 503 (1937).

Fanta, H.: Die Stauungspapille; in Küchle, Almanach für die Augenheilkunde, p. 101 (Lehmann, München 1973).

Fanta, H.: Zur Pathologie okulärer maligner Melanome (primäre Tumoren, Metastasen). Klin. Mbl. Augenheilk. *170:* 440 (1977).

Ferry, A.P.: Leisons mistaken for malignant melanoma of the posterior uvea. Arch. Ophthalmol., Chicago *72:* 63 (1964).

Fink, K.: Augenstörungen im Gestationsprozess. 1. Teil. Dt. med. Wschr. *49:* 1465 (1923a).

Fink, K.: Augenstörungen im Gestationsprozess. 2. Teil. Dt. med. Wschr. *49:* 1490 (1923b).

Fischer, F.: Retinopathia diabetica simplex (vera). Klin. Mbl. Augenheilk. *157:* 110 (1970).

Flick, H., Schwab, B.: Das infiltrativ wachsende Retinoblastom—eine schwierige Differentialdiagnose. Klin. Mbl. Augenheilk. *177:* 220 (1980).

Franceschetti, A.: A curious affection of the fundus oculi, helicoid, peripapillar chorioretinal degeneration, its relation to pigmentary paravenous chorioretinae degeneration. Documenta Ophth. *16:* 81 (1962).

Franceschetti, A.: Über tapeto-retinale Degeneration im Kindesalter; in Sautter, Entwicklung und Fortschritt in der Augenheilkunde (Enke, Stuttgart 1963).

Franceschetti, A., Bock, R.: Megalopapilla: a new congenital anomaly. Am. J. Ophthalmol. *33:* 227 (1950).

Franceschetti, A., François, J., Babel, J., Rouck, A. de, Dieterle, P., Forni, G., Klein, D., Ricci, A., Verriest, G.: Les hérédo-dégénerescences chorio-rétiniennes (Masson, Paris 1963).

François, J.: Okuläre Spätrezidive bei kongenitaler Toxoplasmose. Ciba-Symposium *11:* 2 (1963).

Françcois, J.: Vaskuläre Pseudopapillitis (ischämische Optikusneuropathie). Klin. Mbl. Augenheilk. *167:* 1 (1975).

François, J.: Juvenile Makuladegenerationen. Klin. Mbl. Augenheilk. *175:* 715 (1979).

François, J., De Laey, J.J.: Biettische kristalline Fundusdystrophie. Klin. Mbl. Augenheilk. *170:* 353 (1977).

François, J., De Laey, J.J., Verbraeken, H.: Das zystoide Ödem der Macula. Klin. Mbl. Augenheilk. *162:* 125 (1973).

François, J., Rouck, A. de, Fernandez-Sasso, D.: Electrooculography on vitelliform degeneration of the macula. Arch. Ophthalmol., Chicago *77:* 726 (1967).

François, J., Neetens, A.: Physio-anatomy of the axial vascularisation of the optic nerve. Documenta Ophthal. *26:* 38 (1969).

François, J., Rabaey, M., Evans, L., Vos, E. de: Etude histo-pathologique d'une rétinite de Coats probablement toxoplasmique. Ophthalmologica, Basel *132:* 1 (1956).

Fried, M.: Prinzipien der Ablatio-Chirurgie und -Prophylaxe, Retinopathia diabetica. Z. prakt. Augenheilk. *5:* 31 (1984).

Friedburg, D.: Zusammenfassung des Round-Table-Gespräches über die Therapie der Neuritis nervi optici. Fortschr. Ophthal. *80:* 369 (1983).

Fuchs, E.: Über zwei der Retinitis pigmentosa verwandte Krankheiten (Retinitis punctata albescens und Atrophia gyrata chorioidae et retinae). Arch. Augenheilk. *32:* 111 (1896).

Fuhrmeister, H., Lohse, K.: Die moderne Diagnostik und Therapie der Chorioretinitis centralis serosa. Klin. Mbl. Augenheilk. *164:* 669 (1974).

Fuxa, G., Brandt, H.P.: Beitrag zum Ehlers-Danlos-Syndrom. Klin. Mbl. Augenheilk. *166:* 247 (1975).

Gallasch, G.: Zur Pathogenese des Papillenödems bei Polyzythämie. Klin. Mbl. Augenheilk. *182:* 94 (1983).

Gamringer, H., Schreck, E., Wollensak, J.: Zur Pathogenese und Therapie der Cyclitis anularis exsudativa pseudotumorosa. Klin. Mbl. Augenheilk. *135:* 638 (1959).

Gass, D.M.: Stereoscopic atlas of macular diseases (Morsby, St. Louis 1970).

Gasteiger, H.: Über Anzeigen zur Unterbrechung der Schwangerschaft aufgrund von Augenveränderungen. Dt. GesundhWes. *11:* 319 (1953).

Gasteiger, H.: Über augenärztliche Indikationen zur Unterbrechung der Schwangerschaft. Wiss. Z. Karl-Marx-Univ. Leipzig, Math.-naturwiss. Reihe, Heft 1, 3. Jahrg. (1953/54).

Gasteiger, H.: Augenheilkunde. Leitfaden für Studium und Praxis (de Gruyter, Berlin 1963).

Gerke, E., Meyer-Schwickerath, G.: Proliferative diabetische Retinopathie und Schwangerschaft. Klin. Mbl. Augenheilk. *182:* 170 (1982).

Gernet, H.: Achsenlänge und Refraktion lebender Augen von Neugeborenen. Graefes Arch. Ophthal. *166:* 530 (1964).

Gilbert, W.: Über chronische Verlaufsformen der metastischen Ophthalmie («Ophthalmia lenta»). Arch. Augenheilk. *96:* 119 (1925).

Glees, M.: Über zilioretinale und optikoziliare Gefässe als allgemein diagnotischer Hinweis. Klin. Mbl. Augenheilk. *128:* 580 (1956).

Gloor, B., Werner, H.: Postkoagulative und spontan auftretende internoretinale Fibroplasie mit Makuladegeneration. Klin. Mbl. Augenheilk. *151:* 822 (1967).

Gloster, J.: The value of optic disc photography in the diagnosis and management of glaucoma. Recent advances in glaucoma, p. 155 (Springer, Berlin 1977).

Goder, G.: Durchblutungsstörungen des Auges und Biopsie der Arteria temporalis. Abh. Geb. Augenheilk., vol. 36 (Edition Leipzig 1968).

Goldberg, M.F.: Natural history of untreated proliferative sickle retinopathy. Arch. Ophthalmol., Chicago *85:* 428 (1971).

Goldmann, H.: Zwei Vorlesungen über Biomikroskopie des Auges (Rösch, Vogt & Co., Bern 1954).

Goodner, E.K., Okumoto, M.: Intraocular listeriosis. Am. J. Ophthalmol. *64:* 682 (1967).

Graefe, A. von: Wiederanlelgung der abgelösten Netzhaut bei Retinitis albuminurica. Arch. Ophthalmol. *2(1):* 222 (1855).

Graefe, A. von: Über zentrale rezidivierende Retinitis. Graefes Arch. Ophthal. *12:* 211 (1866).

Graefe, A. von: Beitrag zur Pathologie und Therapie des Glaukoms. Arch. Augenheilk. *15:* 108 (1869).

Green, W.R.: Bilateral Coats' disease. Massive gliosis of the retina. Arch. Ophthalmol., Chicago *77:* 378 (1967).

Grehn, F., Schmidt, D.: Papillenrandblutung beim Glaukom. Z. prakt. Augenheilk. *4:* 131 (1983).

Greither, A.: Krankheiten der Schleimhäute: der Morbus Behçet (aphthose Touraine); in Grottron, Schönfeld, Dermatologie und Venerologie, vol. 4, p. 649 (Thieme, Stuttgart 1960).

Groenouw, A.: Schwangerschaft, Geburt, Wochenbett und Laktation; in Graefe, Saemisch, Hess, Handbuch der gesamten Augenheilkunde, vol. 11, *1* (Springer, Berlin 1920).

Grote, W.: Extradurale spinale Tumoren. Diagnostik und Therapie. Dt. Ärztebl. *29:* 2101 (1975).

Grüner, H.J., Fechner, P.U.: Die Megalopapille, eine seltene kongenitale Anomalie, Klin. Mbl. Augenheilk. *171:* 611 (1977).

Grüner, H.J., Fechner, P.U.: Über das Morning-glory-Syndrom. Klin. Mbl. Augenheilk. *172:* 114 (1978).

Grüntzig, J., Leide, E., Tillmann, W.: Ein Fall von monolateraler Retinopathia pigmentosa? Klin. Mbl. Augenheilk. *167:* 737 (1975).

Grützner, P.: Macula-Ektopie nach oben. Klin. Mbl. Augenheilk. *161:* 114 (1972).

Guist, G.: Z. Augenheilk. *73:* 232 (1931); zit. b. Duke-Elder, St.: System of ophthalmology: diseases of the retina; vol. X (Kimpton, London 1976).

Gunn, M.: Trans. ophthal. Soc. UK *12:* 124 (1882); *18:* 356 (1898); *24:* 119 (1904); zit. b. Duke-Elder, St.: System of ophthalmology: diseases of the retina; vol. X (Kimpton, London 1976).

Haase, W., Hellner, K.A.: Über familiäre bilaterale sektorenförmige Retinopathia pigmentosa. Klin. Mbl. Augenheilk. *147:* 365 (1965).

Hagen, S.: Die seröse postoperative Chorioidalablösung und ihre Pathogenese. Klin. Mbl. Augenheilk. *66:* 161 (1921).

Hager, G., Lommatzsch, P.: Strahlentherapie in der Ophthalmologie. Aktuelle Ophthalmologie, Fachalmanach für die Augenheilkunde, p. 242 (Lehmanns, München 1976).

Hager, H.: Ophthalmologisch-diagnostische Möglichkeiten bei der Hypertonie und Hypertoniebehandlung. Schriften Bayr. Landesärztekammer, vol. 2, Vorträge der 14. wissenschaftl. Ärztetagung Nürnberg 1963a.

Hager, H.: Die Ophthalmo-Dynamographie als Methode zur Beurteilung des Gehirnkreislaufes. Klin. Mbl. Augenheilk. *142:* 827 (1963b).

Hager, H.: Differentialdiagnose des Schlaganfalles durch die Ophthalmodynamographie. Triangel *6:* 259 (1964).

Hager, H.: Zur Behandlung arterieller Durchblutungsstörungen der Netzhaut und des Sehnerven. Ber. 68. Vers. dt. ophthal. Ges., p. 382 (Bergmann, München 1968).

Hager, H.: Probleme bei der Behandlung okularer Durchblutungsstörungen. Klin. Mbl. Augenheilk. *165:* 127 (1974).

Haller, P., Patzold, U., Schliack, H.: Arteriitis cranialis. Dt. Ärztebl. *52:* 3035 (1977).

Hallum, A.V.: Changes in retinal arterioles associated with the hypertensions of pregnancy. Arch. Ophthalmol., Chicago *37:* 472 (1947).

Hammerstein, W., Berger, M., Hennekes, R.: Die Bedeutung des erhöhten Hämoglobin A_{1c} für die Pathogenese der diabetischen Retinopathie. Klin. Mbl. Augenheilk. *182:* 298 (1983).

Hammerstein, W., Bischof, G., Leide, E.: Chorioideremie im Kindesalter. Klin. Mbl. Augenheilk. *174:* 599 (1979).

Hammerstein, W., Kramp, A., Kramp, H.: Fluoreszenzangiographische Befunde von Venenthrombosen der Retina. Klin. Mbl. Augenheilk. *177:* 319 (1980).

Hammerstein, W., Scheja, J., Brüster, H., Trobisch, H., Bischof, G., Kramp, H.: Retinabefunde bei der Thalassämie. Klin. Mbl. Augenheilk. *179:* 191 (1981).

Handmann, M.: Erbliche, vermutlich angeborene zentrale gliöse Entartung des Sehnerven mit besonderer Beteiligung der Zentralgefässe. Klin. Mbl. Augenheilk. *83:* 145 (1929).

Hanselmayer, H.: Fundusveränderungen beim Grönblad-Strandberg-Syndrom aus fluoreszenzangiographischer Sicht. Klin. Mbl. Augenheilk. *159:* 478 (1971).

Hanselmayer, H.: Zur Laserkoagulation bei Makulaschichtlöchern. Klin. Mbl. Augenheilk. *169:* 231 (1976).

Hanselmayer, H., Werner, W.: Netzhautarterienspasmus nach oraler überdosierter DHE-Medikation. Klin. Mbl. Augenheilk. *162:* 807 (1973).

Hartmann, M.G.: Leitsymptom: Fieber mit Ikterus; in Heisig, Innere Medizin in der ärztlichen Praxis (Thieme, Stuttgart 1981).

Hayreh, S.S.: Blood supply and vascular disorders of the optic nerve. Ann. Inst. Barraquer *4:* 7 (1963).

Hayreh, S.S.: Blood supply of the optic nerve head and its role in optic atrophy, glaucoma, and oedema of the optic disc. Br. J. Ophthalmol. *53:* 721 (1969).

Hayreh, S.S.: Anterior ischemic optic neuropathy (Springer, Berlin 1975).

Hayreh, S.S.: So-called 'central retinal vein occlusion.' I. Pathogenesis, terminology, clinical features. Ophthalmologica, Basel *172:* 1 (1976a).

Hayreh, S.S.: So-called 'central retinal vein occlusion.' II. Venous stasis retinopathy. Ophthalmologica, Basel *172:* 14 (1976b).

Heilmann, K.: Ophthalmoskopie. Grundlagen, Untersuchungstechnik, Anwendungsmöglichkeiten, Befunde (Enke, Stuttgart 1973).

Heinz, K.: Eine Methode zur Vermessung der Stauungspapille; zit. bei Huber, Augensymptome bei Hirntumoren (Huber, Bern 1956).

Heinzel, K.: Über vorübergehende Erblindung während der Laktationsperiode. Beitr. Augenheilk. *2:* 235 (1894).

Heisig, N.: Innere Medizin in der ärztlichen Praxis (Thieme, Stuttgart 1981).

Helbron, J.: Über Netzhautablösung bei Schwangerschaftsnephritis. Berl. klin. Wschr. *4:* 69, 103 (1902).

Hentsch, R., Külz, J.: Beitrag zur sekundären Pigmentdegeneration der Netzhaut nach Masern. Klin. Mbl. Augenheilk. *154:* 706 (1969).

Herrmann, W.: Erkrankungen durch grampositive sporenlose Stäbchen. Corynebacteriaceae; in Reploh, Otte, Lehrbuch der medizinischen Mikrobiologie und Infektionskrankheiten (Fischer, Stuggart 1961).

Herzau, V., Aulhorn, E., Wiethölter, H.: Diagnose und Therapie bei Pseudotumor cerebri aus augenärztlicher Sicht. Fortschr. Ophthal. *80:* 26 (1983).

Heydenreich, A.: Zur Frage der Schwangerschaftsunterbrechung bei der Retinopathia gravidarum. Zentbl. Gynäk. *77:* 1 (1955).

Heydenreich, A.: Lichtkoagulation bei Erkrankungen der Netzhautmitte. Klin. Mbl. Augenheilk. *160:* 146 (1972).

Heydenreich, A.: Spätkomplikationen bei Venenverschlüssen am Augenhintergrund und ihre Behandlung mit der Lichtkoagulation. Klin. Mbl. Augenheilk. *165:* 259 (1974).

Heydenreich, A.: Innere Erkrankungen und Auge (Enke, Stuttgart 1979).

Heydenreich, A., Lemke, L., Jütte, A.: Differentialdiagnose von Papillenveränderungen mit Fluorescein. Klin. Mbl. Augenheilk. *163:* 131 (1973).

Hiller, H.: Morbus Coats—Miliaraneurysmenretinitis Leber. Klin. Mbl. Augenheilk. *158:* 225 (1971a).

Hiller, H.: Zur spontanen internoretinalen Fibroplasie. Klin. Mbl. Augenheilk. *159:* 22 (1971b).

Hippel, A. von (zit. bei Groenouw, 1904): Pathologisch-anatomische Befunde am Auge des Neugeborenen. Arch. Ophthalmol. *XLV:* 313 (1898).

Hockwin, O., Koch, H.R.: Arzneimittelnebenwirkungen am Auge (Fischer, Stuttgart 1977).

Höpping, W.: Das Retinoblastom. Dt. Ärztebl. *38:* 2265 (1977).

Höpping, W.: Das Retinoblastom: Derzeitiger Stand der Diagnostik und Therapie. Klin. Mbl. Augenheilk. *181:* 63 (1982).

Hövener, G.: Lichtkoagulation bei Zentralvenenverschluss. Klin. Mbl. Augenheilk. *173:* 392 (1978).

Hollwich, F.: Der Einfluss des Lichtes über das Auge auf den Farbwechsel des Frosches. Klin. Mbl. Augenheilk. *133:* 784 (1958).

Hollwich, F.: Das Verhalten der Netzhautgefässe in der Schwangerschaft. Ber. dt. ophthal. Ges. *63:* 117 (1960).

Hollwich, F.: Die Bedeutung der Augenhintergrundsveränderungen in der Schwangerenvor- und -für-Sorge. Mbl. Gynäk. *83:* 41 (1961).

Hollwich, F.: Familiäres Auftreten von Fundus flavimaculatus. Klin. Mbl. Augenheilk. *143:* 817 (1963a).

Hollwich, F.: Das klinische Bild der Augentoxoplasmose. Med. Mschr. *10:* 638 (1963b).

Hollwich, F.: Augenlicht und vegetative Funktionen. Nova Acta Leopoldina *31:* 189 (1966).

Hollwich, F.: Erkrankungen der Netzhaut; in Velhagen, Der Augenarzt, vol. 8 (Thieme, Leipzig 1982).

Hollwich, F., Glitz, S.: Zur vitelliformen Makuladegeneration (Bestsche infantile Makuladegeneration). Klin. Mbl. Augenheilk. *179:* 264 (1981).

Hollwich, F., Krebs, W.: Erkrankungen der Papille; in Velhagen, Der Augenarzt, vol. 8 (Thieme, Leipzig 1982).

Hollwich, F., Lemke, L.: Karzinommetastasen in der Aderhaut. Dt. med. Wschr. *90:* 329 (1965).

Hollwich, F., Schiffer, H.P., Weihmann, J.: Arteriitis temporalis. Klinisches Bild, Prognose und Therapie. Klin. Mbl. Augenheilk. *167:* 62 (1975).

Holzbach, E.: Über Amaurose in der Schwangerschaft. Zentbl. Gynäk. *21:* 709 (1908).

Honegger, H.: Der Augenhintergrund bei Neu- und Frühgeborenen. Ber. Versamm. dt. ophthal. Ges. *69:* 156 (1969).

Horay, G.: Beitrag zur Klinik der sog. Laktationsneuritis. Klin. Mbl. Augenheilk. *71:* 473 (1923).

Hornicker, E.: Über eine Form von zentraler Retinitis auf angioneurotischer Grundlage (Retinitis centralis angioneurotica). Graefes Arch. Ophthal. *123:* 286 (1930).

Horton, B.I., Magath, I.B., Brown, G.E.: An undescribed form of arteritis of the temporal vessels. Proc. Staff Meet. Mayo Clin. *7:* 700 (1932).

Huber, A.: Augensymptome bei Hirtumoren (Huber, Bern 1956).

Huber, A.: Augensymptome nach akutem Schädel-Hirn-Trauma. Ärztl. Prax., Wien *93:* 3173 (1966).

Huber, A.: Tumoren der Sella und ihrer Umgebung. Klinik, Diagnostik und Differentialdiagnose. Aktuelle Ophthalmologie, Fachalmanach für die Augenheilkunde, pp. 151–187 (Lehmanns, München 1976).

Huck, D., Meythaler-Radek, B.: Gefässverschlüsse der Netzhaut im jüngeren Lebensalter. Klin. Mbl. Augenheilk. *164:* 398 (1974).

Huismans, H.: Vorgetäuschter Tumor cerebri durch Ovulationshemmer. Klin. Mbl. Augenheilk. *165:* 344 (1974a).

Huismans, H.: Intoxikationsamblyopie nach Chinin-Abusus. Medsche Mschr., Stuttg. *28:* 540 (1974b).

Huismans, H.: Cysta vitelliformis—Bericht über ein seltenes heredodegeneratives Makulaleiden. Klin. Mbl. Augenheilk. *166:* 252 (1975a).

Huismans, H.: Bericht über eine *Toxocara-canis*-Infestation (Hundespulwurm) im menschlichen Auge unter dem Bild des Solitärgranuloms. Klin. Mbl. Augenheilk. *167:* 113 (1975b).

Huismans, H.: Zur Therapie des Posner-Schlossmann-Syndroms. Klin. Mbl. Augenheilk. *167:* 881 (1975c).

Huismans, H.: Spontane Rekanalisation einer beidseitigen Zentralvenenthrombose im dritten Schwangerschaftsmonat. Klin. Mbl. Augenheilk. *168:* 423 (1976a).

Huismans, H.: Spätamotio chorioidae nach Cataract-Extraktion. Klin. Mbl. Augenheilk. *168:* 732 (1976b).

Huismans, H.: Vaskuläre retinale Komplikation nach Langzeittherapie mit hormonalen Kontrazeptiva. Klin. Mbl. Augenheilk. *169:* 505 (1976c).

Huismans, H.: Kolobom (Dysplasie) der Makula. Klin. Mbl. Augenheilk. *169:* 605 (1976d).

Huismans, H.: Über das okulare Solitägranulom bei Larva migrans (*Toxocara canis,* Hundespulwurm). Klin. Mbl. Augenheilk. *169:* 260 (1976e).

Huismans, H.: Miopos-Augensalbe »stark« in der Behandlung des akuten Glaukoms. Klin. Mbl. Augenheilk. *169:* 770 (1976f).

Huismans, H.: Case report on *Toxocara canis* infection of human eye. Ophthalmol. Dig. *40:* 3 (1967g).

Huismans, H.: Weitere Mitteilung einer Komplikation unter einer Langzeittherapie oraler hormonaler Kontrazeptiva. Klin. Mbl. Augenheilk. *171:* 781 (1977a).

Huismans, H.: Akute intraokulare *Toxocara-canis*-Infektion unter dem klinischen Bild einer juxtapapillären Choriorentinitis. Klin. Mbl. Augenheilk. *170:* 39 (1977b).

Huismans, H.: Über das Solitärgranulom bei okular *Toxocara-canis*-Infektion. Ophthalmologica, Basel *174:* 10 (1977c).

Huismans, H.: Epikritische Bewertung einer venösen Anastomosenbildung der Netzhaut. Klin. Mbl. Augenheilk. *170:* 738 (1977d).

Huismans, H.: Intraokulare (subretinale) Echinokokkose. Klin. Mbl. Augenheilk. *171:* 601 (1977e).

Huismans, H.: Akute Ischämie des Nervus opticus. Ophthalmologica, Basel *176:* 69 (1978a).

Huismans, H.: Zum Alport-Syndrom. Klin. Mbl. Augenheilk. *172:* 775 (1978b).

Huismans, H.: Makulaforamen als retinale Komplikation bei kongenitaler Papillen- und Netzhaut-Aderhaut-Anomalie. Klin. Mbl. Augenheilk. *175:* 832 (1979a).

Huismans, H.: Tierische Parasiten des menschlichen Auges. Bücherei des Augenarztes, Heft 80 (Enke, Stuttgart 1979b).

Huismans, H.: Diagnostische Problematik bei tapeto-retinaler Pigmentdegeneration. Klin. Mbl. Augenheilk. *177:* 506 (1980a).

Huismans, H.: Larva migrans visceralis und ZNS. Nervenarzt *51:* 51 (1980b).

Huismans, H.: Larva migrans visceralis aus auganärztlicher Sicht. Klin. Mbl. Augenheilk. *177:* 584 (1980c).

Huismans, H.: Zur Frage eines Einflusses von Neo-Synephrine-Augentropfen auf den Blutdruck beim jugendlichen Hypertoniker mit Blutdruckkrisen. Klin. Mbl. Augenheilk. *176:* 852 (1980d).

Huismans, H.: Wie kommen Hundespulwurmlarven ins Auge? Ärztl. Prax., München *32:* 2373 (1980c).

Huismans, H.: Adapter für das Dynamometer nach H.K. Müller für die Routineuntersuchung in der Praxis. Klin. Mbl. Augenheilk. *179:* 51 (1981).

Huismans, H.: Monolaterale rezidivierende Neuritis n. optic unter Langzeittherapie mit dem hormonalen Kontrazeptivum Anacyclin 28. Klin. Mbl. Augenheilk. *180:* 173 (1982a).

Huismans, H.: Bilaterales (toxisches?) Papillenödem bei Chloroquintherapie wegen primär chronischer Polyarthritis. Klin. Mbl. Augenheilk. *181:* 36 (1982b).

Huismans, H.: *Toxocara canis* (Werner 1782). Sitzber. 142. Vers. Rhein.-Westf. Augenärzte, p. 53 (1982c).

Huismans, H.: *Toxocara canis,* Augenspiegel *10:* 9 (1983a); *11:* 14 (1983b); *12:* 14 (1983c).

Huismans, H.: Ultraschall-Doppler-Sonographie in der augenärztlichen Praxis ("Retina-Doppler"). Klin. Mbl. Augenheilk. *183:* 138 (1983d).

Huismans, H.: Angiopathia retinae syphilitica bei Lues latens seropositiva. Klin. Mbl. Augenheilk. *184:* 48 (1984a).

Huismans, H.: Retinale Punktblutung. Ein spezifisches Zeichen für eine EPH-Gestose? Klin. Mbl. Augenheilk. *185:* 138 (1984b).

Huismans, H.: Rezidivierende Iritis als Initialsymptom beim Plasmozyton (IgG-Typ). Klin. Mbl. Augenheilk. *187:* 126 (1985).

Hutchinson, J. (1875), zit. bei Duke-Elder, St.: System of ophthalmology, vol. X, p. 568 (Kimpton, London 1967).

Hutchinson, J.: Diseases of the arteries. On a peculiar form of thrombotic arteritis of the aged which is sometimes productive of gangrene. Arch. Surg. *1:* 323 (1890).

Imre, G.: Coats' disease and hyperlipemic retinitis. Am. J. Ophthalmol. *64:* 726 (1967).

Irinoda, K.: Farbatlas der Fundusveränderungen bei Hypertonie (Urban & Schwarzenberg, München 1972).

Ivandic, T.: Sektorenförmige tapetoretinale Degenerationen. Klin. Mbl. Augenheilk. *160:* 98 (1972).

Jacobsohn, E.: Ein Fall von Retinitis pigmentosa atypica. Klin. Mbl. Augenheilk. *26:* 202 (1888).

Jaeger, E. von: Beiträge zur Pathologie des Auges; Wein 1855 (zit. b. Doden, W., Klin. Mbl. Augenheilk. *164:* 441, 1964).

Jaeger, W.: Ermittlung der wahren Papillengrösse (Beitrag zur Diagnose der Mikropapille). Fortschr. Ophthal. *80:* 527 (1983).

Jaeger, W., Bischoff, E.: Vitelliforme Makuladegeneration und Bestsche Makuladegeneration sind dasselbe Krankheitsbild. Klin. Mbl. Augenheilk. *170:* 890 (1977).

Jaeger, W.: Blankenagel, A.: Lesegeräte für Blinde. Technische Möglichkeiten, bisherige Erfahrungen und künftige Entwicklung. Klin. Mbl. Augenheilk. *168:* 613 (1976).

Jaeger, W.: Blankenagel, A.: Neueste Entwicklungen auf dem Gebiet optischer und elektronischer Sehhilfen für hochgradig Sehbehinderte und Blinde. Klin. Mbl. Augenheilk. *186:* 251 (1985).

Jaeger, W., Käfer, O.: Erkennung, Klassifikation und Differentialdiagnose der heredodegenerativen Erkrankungen des Augenhintergrundes durch Chromatoophthalmoskopie. Klin. Mbl. Augenheilk. *175:* 148 (1979).

Janert, H., Mohnike, G., Günther, L.: Ophthalmologische Diabetesstudien. II. Mitteilung. Augenhintergrundsbefunde bei 2600 stationär kontrollierten Zuckerkranken. Klin. Wschr. *34:* 807 (1956).

Janku, J. (1959), zit. bei Jírovec, Parasitologie für Ärzte (Fischer, Jena 1960).

Jensen, V.A.: Studies of the branching of the retinal blood-vessels. Acta Ophthal. *14:* 100 (1936).

Jordan, W.M.: Pulmonary embolism. Lancet *ii:* 1146 (1961).

Jünemann, G., Reich, H., Huismans, H.: Zum Behçet-Syndrom. Klin. Mbl. Augenheilk. *159:* 274 (1971).

Junge, J.: Über eine doppelte Papille im Augenkolobom. Klin. Mbl. Augenheilk. *172:* 748 (1978).

Käfer, O.: Die Macula lutea beim Zentralarteienverschluss. Klin. Mbl. Augenheilk. *164:* 733 (1974).

Karcher, H.: Zum Morning Glory Syndrom. Klin. Mbl. Augenheilk. *175:* 835 (1979).

Keith, N.M., Wagener, H.P., Barker, M.W.: Some different types of essential hypertension. Trans. Am. Ophthalmol. Soc. *45:* 57 (1947); Am. J. Med. Sci. *197:* 332 (1939).

Kennedy, S.T.J., Schwartz, B., Takamoto, T., Eu, J.K.T.: Interference fringle scale for absolute ocular fundus measurement. Invest Ophthal. Vis. Sci. *24:* 169 (1983).

Kindler, P.: Morning glory syndrome: unusual congential optic disc anomaly. Am. J. Ophthalmol. *69:* 376 (1970).

Kitihara, S.: Über klinische Beobachtungen bei der in Japan häufig vorkommenden Chorioretinitis centralis serosa. Klin. Mbl. Augenheilk. *97:* 345 (1936).

Kleberger, E.: Beobachtungen seröser Netzhaut- und Aderhautablösungen nach Lichtkoagulation der diabetischen Retinopathie. Klin. Mbl. Augenheilk. *174:* 725 (1979).

Klein, S., Marré, E., Koza, K.-D., Heidelmann, G.: Retinale Thrombosen bei metabolischen Störungen. Klin. Mbl. Augenheilk. *173:* 501 (1978).

Klemen, U.M., Freyler, H.: Diabetische Retinopathie: 10 Jahre nach Lichtkoagulation. Klin. Mbl. Augenheilk. *174:* 489 (1979).

Knapp, H. (1892), zit. bei Duke-Elder, System of ophthalmology; diseases of the uvea, vol. IX, p. 721 (Kimpton, London 1966).

Königstein: Untersuchungen an den Augen neugeborener Kinder. Wien. med. Jahrb. *47* (1881).

Kolin, J.: Netzhautpigmentepithelstörungen bei der sekundären Polyzythämie im Fluoreszensbild. Klin. Mbl. Augenheilk. *153:* 517 (1968).

Kommerell, G.: Binasale Refraktionsskotome. Klin. Mbl. Augenheilk. *154:* 85 (1969).

Kommerell, G.: Schlängelung der Netzhautarterien durch die Pulswelle. Eine stereo-chronoskopische Demonstration. Klin. Mbl. Augenheilk. *173:* 486 (1978).

Kommerell, G., Castrillón-Oberndorfer, W.L.: Tabak-Amblyopie. Beitrag zur Pathogenese und Therapie. Klin. Mbl. Augenheilk. *153:* 551 (1968).

Komoto, J.: Über die sogenannte Atrophia gyrata chorioideae et retinae. Klin. Mbl. Augenheilk. *52:* 416 (1914).

Korting, G.W.: Behçet-Krankheit; Haut und Auge (Thieme, Stuggart 1969).

Kramp, H., Ebell, W.: Fundusveränderungen bei einem Patienten mit akuter lymphatischer Leukämie. Klin. Mbl. Augenheilk. *179:* 194 (1981).

Kranenburg, E.W.: Crater-like holes in the optic disc and central serous retinopathy. Arch. Ophthalmol., Chicago *64:* 912 (1960).

Krebs, W., Jäger, G.: Netzhautblutungen bei Neugeborenen und Geburtsverlauf, Klin. Mbl. Augenheilk. *148:* 483 (1966).

Kreibig, W.: Optikomalazie, die Folge eines Gefässverschulsses im retrobulbären Abschnitt des Sehnerven. Klin. Mbl. Augenheilk. *122:* 719 (1953).

Krieglstein, G.K., Langham, M.E.: Glaukon ohne Hochdruck. Ein Beitrag zur Ätiologie. Klin. Mbl. Augenheilk. *166:* 18 (1975).

Kröner, B.: Multiple ischämische Infarkte in der Retina und Uvea durch kristalline Kortikosteroid-Embolie nach subkutaner Injektion im Gesicht. Klin. Mbl. Augenheilk. *178:* 121 (1981).

Kropp, R., Neubauer, H., Heimsoth, V., Heimann, K.: Der Augenhintergrund bei jugendlichen Hypertonikern. Klin. Mbl. Augenheilk. *156:* 479 (1970).

Krückmann, E.: Über ophthalmologische Indikationen zur Unterbrechung der Schwangerschaft. Zentbl. Geburtsh. *95:* 340 (1929).

Krzystkowa, K., Mirkiewicz-Sierdzka, B., Bryk, E.: Kongenitale Hypoplasie der Papillae nervi optici. Klin. Mbl. Augenheilk. *167:* 333 (1975).

Küchle, H.J.: Augenveränderungen und typische Augenerkrankungen des höheren Lebensalters. Kassenarzt *21:* 31 (1981).

Küchle, H.J., Richard, G.: Zur Therapie arterieller Gefässverschlüsse von Netzhaut und Sehnerv. Ophthalmologica, Basel *179:* 291 (1979).

Kyrieleis, W.: Über die Bedeutung der Augenhintergrundsuntersuchung bei den Schwangerschaftstoxikosen. Geburtsh. Frauenheilk. *10:* 869 (1954).

Kyrieleis, W., Schroeder, C.: Über funktionelle Veränderungen am Netzhautgefässsystem normaler Schwangerer während der letzten Schwangerschaftsmonate. Arch. Augenheilk. *105:* 110 (1932).

Laffers, Z., Brehm, H.: Intraorbitale, extrabulbär gelegene Projektilverletzungen. Klin. Mbl. Augenheilk. *176:* 413 (1980).

Landesberg: Contribution to the pathology of childbed. A case of imaginary blindness in childbed. Philadelphia Med. Times 1887. VII, No. 253.

Langenbeck, K.: Neuritis retrobulbaris und Allgemeinveränderungen. Graefes Arch. Ophthal. *87:* 226 (1914).

Laux, U., Eckert, G.: Assoziationen anomaler Makulavenen mit einer Deuteranopie. Klin. Mbl. Augenheilk. *174:* 722 (1979).

Laux, U., Marquardt, R.: Das Farbstoff-Füllungsmuster im normalen Serienangiogramm. Klin. Mbl. Augenheilk. *175:* 786 (1979).

Leber, Th.: Über eine durch Vorkommen multipler Mikroaneurysmen charakterisierte Form von Retinaldegeneration. Graefes Arch. Ophthal. *81:* 1 (1912).

Legerlotz, C.: Geburtseinleitung nach Netzhautablösung. Klin. Mbl. Augenheilk. *158:* 597 (1971).

Leiber, B., Olbrich, G.: Die klinischen Syndrome, vol. 1 (Urban & Schwarzenberg, München 1981).

Lemmingson, W.: Abortivformen bei retrolentaler Fibroplasie. Ber. 69. Vers. dt. ophthal. Ges. Heidelberg, p. 343 (1959).

Lemmingson, W.: Zur Behandlung der Retinitis Coats mit Lichtkoagulation. Klin. Mbl. Augenheilk. *139:* 600 (1961).

Lennartz, H., Piesbergen, H.: Klinik und Diagnostik der Zytomegalie des Erwachsenen. Dt. med. Wschr. *108:* 1403 (1983).

Lenz, W.: Medizinische Genetik (Thieme, Stuttgart 1976).

Leuenberger, A.E., Jeker, J.: Bemerkenswerte Fälle von Arteriitis temporalis. Klin. Mbl. Augenheilk. *174:* 496 (1979).

Leydhecker, W.: Eine neue Definition der okulären Hypertension. Z. prakt. Augenheilk. *4:* 173 (1983a).

Leydhecker, W.: Frühdiagnostische Methoden bei Verdacht auf Glaucoma simplex. Z. prakt. Augenheilk. *4:* 177 (1983b).

Leydhecker, W., Krieglstein, G.K., Brunswig, D.: Indikation und Grenzen der Fibrinolysetherapie bei Verschluss der Zentralarterie. Klin. Mbl. Augenheilk. *172:* 43 (1978).

Leydhecker, W., Milanow, M.: Zwei ungewöhnliche Fälle von Vasculitis transsudativa retinae. Klin. Mbl. Augenheilk. *160:* 154 (1972).

Liebreich, R. (1868), zit. bei Duke-Elder, St., System of ophthalmology; neuroophthalmology, the optic nerve, vol. XII, p. 199 (Kimpton, London 1971).

Liegl, O., Werner, H., Janitschke, K.: Echinokokkus-Zyste in der Orbita. Klin. Mbl. Augenheilk. *177:* 80 (1980).

Liesenhoff, H.: Über die Behandlung präretinaler Gewesbsproliferationen (Sternfalten-Retinitis) mit subkonjunktivalen Injektionen von Prednisolon-21-Hemisuccinat-Natrium. Klin. Mbl. Augenheilk. *153:* 507 (1968).

Lisch, K.: Hydrophthalmie und Papillenkonfiguration. Klin. Mbl. Augenheilk. *168:* 330 (1976).

Lisch, W., Bolsinger, A.: Leimenkühler, G.: Autosomal dominante Drusen. Klin. Mbl. Augenheilk. *175:* 274 (1979).

Littan, K.E.: Multiple vitelliforme Netzhautzysten. Ber. dt. Ophthal. Ges. *67:* 442 (1965).

Littmann, H.: Zur Bestimmung der wahren Grösse eines Objektes auf dem Hintergrund des lebenden Auges. Klin. Mbl. Augenheilk. *180:* 286 (1982).

Lommatzsch, P.: Ein Vorschlag zur mikrochirurgischen Behandlung des persistierenden hyperplastischen primären Glaskörpers. Klin. Mbl. Augenheilk. *172:* 55 (1978).

Lommatzsch, P.K.: Erfahrungen bein der Behandlung des Retinoblastoms in der DDR. Klin. Mbl. Augenheilk. *175:* 641 (1979).

Lüllwitz, W.: Zum natürlichen Verlauf der temporalen Astvenenverschlüsse. Klin. Mbl. Augenheilk. *172:* 325 (1978).

Lund, O.E.: Vaskuläre Augenerkrankungen und ihre Bedeutung für generalisierte Gefässleiden. Klin. Mbl. Augenheilk. *176:* 16 (1980).

Lund, O.E., Förster, Ch., Bise, K.: Zerebral bedingte Sehstörungen als Erstsymptom bei subakuter sklerosierender Panenzephalitis. Klin. Mbl. Augenheilk. *182:* 290 (1983).

Lutz, G.: Augenerkrankungen während der Gravidität und im Puerperium. Mitt. ophthal. Klin. Tübingen. *1:* 1 (1884).

Mailáth, L., Nagy, Gy., Gat, Gy., Racz, M.: Über das Augenhintergrundsbild bei Polycythaemia vera. Klin. Mbl. Augenheilk. *169:* 343 (1976).

Maijáth, G., Fülöp, E., Pajor, R.: Die Bedeutung des Pseudoxanthoma elasticum für die Augenheilkunde. Klin. Mbl. Augenheilk. *159:* 632 (1971).

Makabe, R.: Retinitis punctata albescens—eine Beobachtung mit Fluoreszenz-Fundusangiographie. Klin. Mbl. Augenheilk. *157:* 114 (1970).

Makabe, R.: Fluoreszenz-Fundusangiographie und Laserkoagulation bei Chorioretinitis centralis serosa. Klin. Mbl. Augenheilk. *176:* 157 (1980).

Mann, I.: On certain abnormal conditions of the macular region usually classes as colobomata. Br. J. Ophthalmol. *11:* 99 (1927).

Manschot, W.A., Daamen, C.B.F.: A case of cytomegalic inclusion disease with ocular involvement. Ophthalmologica, Basel *143:* 137 (1962).

Manschot, W.A., De Bruijn, W.C.: Coats's disease: definition and pathogenesis. Br. J. Ophthalmol. *51:* 145 (1967).

Manz, W. (1876), zit. bei Duke-Elder, St., System of ophthalmology; diseases of the retina, vol. X, p. 150 (Kimpton, London 1967).

Mauthner (1871), zit. bei Duke-Elder, St., System of ophthalmology; congenital deformities. vol. III/2, p. 619 (Kimpton, London 1964).

Mautner, W.: Ablatio fugax nach Lichtkoagulation am hinteren Pol bei Retinopathia diabetica. Klin. Mbl. Augenheilk. *164:* 807 (1974).

Mayer, A.: Über Amaurose im Status prae-eclampticus. Zentbl. Gynäk. *49:* 3490 (1931).

McIntyre, N., Phillips, M.J., Voigt, J.C.: Two cases of thromboembolic disease associated with oral contraceptives. Br. Med. J. *iv:* 1029 (1962).

Mennig, H.: Geschwülste der Augenhöhle und ihre operative Behandlung (Thieme, Leipzig 1970).

Merté, H.-J., Heilmann, K.: Glaukom. Aktuelle Ophthalmologie. Fachalmanach für die Augenheilkunde, pp. 188 (Lehmanns, München 1976).

Meunier, A.P., Boursin, P.: La pigmentation groupée de la retine. Bull. Soc. Belge Ophthalmol. *99:* 470 (1951).

Mewe, L.: Zur Problematik der Schwangerschaftsunterbrechung aus der Sicht des Augenarztes. Klin. Mbl. Augenheilk. *178:* 219 (1981).

Mewe, L., Busse, H.: Augenhintergrundsveränderungen bei Arteriosklerose und chronisch arterieller Hypertonie. Klin. Mbl. Augenheilk. *174:* 493 (1979).

Meyer, H.J.: Grubenpapille mit zentraler Netzhautablösung. Klin. Mbl. Augenheilk. *154:* 797 (1969).

Meythaler, H.: Über die Verschlüsse von Blutgefässen der Netzhaut. Klin. Mbl. Augenheilk. *149:* 32 (1966).

Meythaler, H., Herold, M.: Zur Klinik und Histologie von Tumormetastasen der Aderhaut. Klin. Mbl. Augenheilk. *175:* 654 (1979).

Mifka, P.: Die Augensymptomatik bei der frischen Schädel-Hirn-Verletzung (de Gruyter, Berlin 1968).

Miller, G.R., Smith, J.L.: Ischemic optic neuropathy. Am. J. Ophthalmol. *62:* 103 (1966).

Minning, W.: Die Infektionskrankheiten des Menschen und ihre Erreger, vol. 2 (Thieme, Stuttgart 1969).

Mittelstrass, H., Wolfshaegen, O.: Die Bedeutung der Augenhintergrundsuntersuchung für die Klinik der eklamptischen Schwangerschaftserkrankungen. Berich über die Erfahrungen der Klinik seit 1920. Geburtsh. Frauenheilk. *10:* 671 (1948).

Mönckeberg, C.: Graviditätsretinitis und eklamptische Amaurose. Zentbl. ges. Ophthal. *27:* 726 (1931).

Morgan, G.: Diffuse infiltrating retinoblastoma. Br. J. Ophthalmol. *55:* 600 (1971).

Moser, E.: Reversibler Visusabfall durch Fundusveränderungen bei Leukämie. Klin. Mbl. Augenheilk. *174:* 240 (1979).

Müller, F., Pietruschka, G.: Lehrbuch der Augenheilkunde (Thieme, Leipzig 1976).

Müller-Limmroth, W.: Elektrophysiologie des Gesichtssinnes. Theorie und Praxis der Elektroretinographie (Springer, Berlin 1959).

Mumenthaler, M.: Neurologie (Thieme, Stuttgart 1976).

Mylius, K.: Funktionelle Veränderungen am Gefässsystem der Netzhaut. Z. Augenheilk. *10:* suppl., pp. 1-49 (1928).

Naumann, G.: Intraokulare Tumoren beim Kinde. Ber. Vers. dt. ophthal. Ges. *69:* 179 (1968).

Naumann, G.: Persönliche Mitteilung zur Infrarotfundusphotographie (1984).

Naumann, G., Hamann, K.U., Garbrecht, M.: Zur ophthalmologischen Diagnose der Zytomegalie-Retinitis. Klin. Mbl. Augenheilk. *164:* 328 (1974).

Naumann, G., Völcker, H.: «Primäres» Retikulumzellsarkom der Retina. II. Klinische Diagnose und Verlauf nach Strahlentherapie. Klin. Mbl. Augenheilk. *171:* 499 (1977).

Naumoff; zit b. Groenouw: Über einige pathologisch-anatomische Veränderungen im Augergrunde bei neugeborenen Kindern. Arch. Ophthal. *36(3):* 180 (1890).

Neubauer, H.: Progressive Aderhautatrophie. Graefes Arch. Ophthal. *156:* 577 (1955).

Neubauer, H.: Die gegenwärtigen diagnostischen Möglichkeiten bei Retinopathia hypertonica. Sber. Vers. Rhien.-Westf. Augenärzte *116:* 73 (1967).

Nichorlis, St.: Demonstration eines Falles von rezidivierender Aderhautabhebung nach kombinierter Katarakt-Glaukom-Operation. Klin. Mbl. Augenheilk. *155:* 303 (1969).

Niesel, P.: Zur Hämodynamik der retinalen Venenastthrombose (eine fluoreszenzangiographische Studie). Klin. Mbl. Augenheilk. *173:* 189 (1978).

Nolan, J.: Chronic toxocaral endophthalmitis. Successful treatment of a case with subconjunctival depot corticosteroids. Br. J. Ophthalmol. *52:* 276 (1968).

Noorden, G.K. von, Khodadoust, A.: Retinal hemorrhage in newborns and organic amblyopia. Arch. Ophthalmol., Chicago *89:* 91 (1973).

Nover, A.: Der Augenhintergrund. Untersuchungstechnik und typische Befunde (Schattauer, Stuttgart 1980).

Nyfeldt, A.: Etiologie de la mononucléose infectieuse. C.r. Séanc. Soc. Biol. *101:* 590 (1929).

Otto, J.: Lehrbuch und Atlas der Orthoptik (Huber, Wien 1975).

Pape, R.: Abgrenzungsschwierigkeit zwischen dem postoperativen Spätödem und dem sog. spontanen Ziliarkörper und Aderhautödem. Klin. Mbl. Augenheilk. *154:* 760 (1969).

Pau, H.: Über die Amotio chorioideae (Spongiosis chorioideae). Klin. Mbl. Augenheilk. *130:* 347 (1957).

Pau, H.: Angiomatosis retinae im Alter. Klin. Mbl. Augenheilk. *164:* 61 (1974a).

Pau, H.: Differentialdiagnose der Augenkrankheiten (Thieme, Stuttgart 1974b).

Pau, H.: Netzhaut-Glaskörper-Anomalien als Urasche der idiopathischen Netzhautablösung. Klin. Mbl. Augenheilk. *170:* 469 (1977).

Pau, H.: Verlauf einer Netzhautarterienastembolie. Klin. Mbl. Augenheilk. *173:* 279 (1978).

Pau, H.: Die zentrale seröse Retinitis oder Chorioretinitis (Retinopathie oder Chorioretinopathie) und die zentrale hämorrhagische Chorioretinitis (juvenile disciforme Makulaablösung; fokale hämorrhagische Chorioitidis, presumed histoplasmosis). Klin. Mbl. Augenheilk. *175:* 634 (1979a).

Pau, H.: Massive subretinale Lipoideinlagerungen. Klin. Mbl. Augenheilk. *174:* 13 (1979b).

Pau, H.: Handmannsche Sehnervenanomalie und Morning Glory Syndrom ("Windenblüten-Syndrom"). Klin. Mbl. Augenheilk. *176:* 745 (1980).

Pau, H.: Aderhautmetastase eines hyperneophroiden Karzinoms. Klin. Mbl. Augenheilk. *178:* 206 (1981).

Pau, H., Graeber, W.: Physiologische Chemie—Linse; in Velhagen, Der Augenarzt, vol. 1, p. 289 (Thieme, Leipzig 1969).

Paulmann, H.: Beitrag zur Behandlung parazentraler Venenastverschlüsse. Klin. Mbl. Augenheilk. *168:* 501 (1976).

Paulmann, H., Heimann, K.: Beitrag zum Problem der serösen Netzhautablösung. Klin. Mbl. Augenheilk. *167:* 324 (1975).

Perkin, G.D., Rose, F.C.: Optic neuritis and its differential diagnosis (Oxford University Press); zit. b. Friedburg, D.: Zusammenfassung des Round-Table-Gesprächs über die Therapie der Neuritis nervi optici. Fortschr. Ophthal. *80:* 369 (1983).

Pflüger, E.: Neuritis optica. Graefes Arch. Ophthal. *24:* 169 (1878).

Pietruschka, G.: Über klinische Beobachtungen bei Iridozyklitis, insbesondere hinsichtlich der Fundusveränderungen. Klin. Mbl. Augenheilk. *124:* 309 (1954).

Pietruschka, G., Priess, G.: Zur klinischen Bedeutung und Prognose der Drusenpapille. Klin. Mbl. Augenheilk. *162:* 331 (1973).

Pillat, A.: Die senile Pigmentierung der Netzhaut (senile Pigmententartung). Graefes Arch. Ophthal. *150:* 1 (1950).

Polte: Augenuntersuchungen bei Schwangeren und Wöchnerinnen. Klin. Mbl. Augenheilk. *43:* 531 (1905).

Pommer, H.: Die Geburt als Ursache von kindlichen Netzhautblutungen. Klin. Mbl. Augenheilk. *160:* 203 (1972).

Prammer, G.: Veränderungen der Netzhautgefässe nach Retinopathia traumatica Purtscher. Klin. Mbl. Augenheilk. *168:* 840 (1976).

Prop, F.J.A., Prop-Arnold, G.C.B., Eijgenstein, L.H.: Gewebezüchtungsuntersuchungen zur Unterscheidung des erblichen vom sporadischen Retinoblastom. Klin. Mbl. Augenheilk. *176:* 396 (1975).

Pülhorn, G.: Augenbeteiligung bei der subakut sklerosierenden Panenzephalitis. Klin. Mbl. Augenheilk. *168:* 808 (1976).

Purtscher, O.: Angiopathia retinae traumatica. Lymphorrhagie des Augengrundes. Graefes Arch. Ophthal. *82:* 347 (1912).

Radda, T.M., Binder, S.: Larvierte Arteriitis temporalis. Wien. klin. Wschr. *92:* 293 (1980).

Radda, T.M., Binder, S.: Zur Differentialdiagnose der ischämischen Optikusneuropathie. Klin. Mbl. Augenheilk. *179:* 352 (1981).

Raistrick, E.R., Dean-Hart, J.C.: Adult toxocaral infection with focal retinal lesion. Br. Med. J. *iii:* 416 (1975).

Raitta, Ch.: Der Zentralvenen- und Netzhautvenenverschluss. Acta Ophthal., suppl. 83 (1965).

Rau, H.: Stauungspapillen bei Spinaltumoren. Beitrag zur Klinik der Liquorzirkulationsstörungen. Dt. med. Wschr. *99:* 351 (1974).

Reese, A.B.: Teleangiectasis of the retina and Coats' disease. Am. J. Ophthalmol. *42:* 1 (1965).

Rehn, K.: Klinik der Kollagenosen. Dt. Ärzteblatt *79:* 21 (1982).

Reich, M.: Verlust des Sehvermögens wegen Papillitis bel einer Schwangeren; rasche Genesung bei ärztlichem Eingreifen. Klin. Mbl. Augenheilk. *20:* 349 (1882).

Reinbach, W.: Entwicklungsgeschichte des Auges. Z. prakt. Augenheilk. *4:* 139 (1983).

Reiss, H.J., Potel, J., Krebs, A.: Granulomatosis infantiseptica (eine Allgemeininfektion bei Neugeborenen und Säuglingen mit miliaren Granulomen). Z. ges. inn. Med. *6:* 451 (1951).

Remky, H., Kölbl, I.: Multiple vitelliforme Zysten. Klin. Mbl. Augenheilk. *159:* 322 (1971).

Remky, H., Rix, J., Klier, H.F.: Dominant-autosomale Maculadegeneration (Best, Sorsby) mit zystichen und vitelliformen Stadien (Huysmans, Zanen). Klin. Mbl. Augenheilk. *146:* 473 (1965).

Reuscher, A., Chromek, W., Kommerell, G.: Gesichtsfeldausfälle und Fluoreszenzangiographie bei Apoplexia papillae. Klin. Mbl. Augenheilk. *172:* 69 (1978).

Riaskoff, S., zit. bei Doden (1974): Die diabetische Retinopathie und ihre Behandlung mit Lichtkoagulation (1972).

Riaskoff, S.: Therapeutische Konsequenzen der diabetischen Retinopathie. Klinikarzt *7:* 40 (1978).

Richard, G.: Die Anwendung der Videoangiographie der Retina. Klin. Mbl. Augenheilk. *185:* 119 (1984).

Rieger, G.: Atrophia gyrata chorioideae et retinae. Demonstration eines Falles. Klin. Mbl. Augenheilk. *161:* 577 (1972).

Rieger, G.: Zum Krankheitsbild der Handmannschen Sehnervenanomalie. "Windenblüten"-("Morning Glory"-) Syndrom? Klin. Mbl. Augenheilk. *170:* 697 (1977).

Riehm, E.: Differentialdiagnostische Erwägungen bei der sog. Arteriitis temporalis und arteriosklerotischen Gefässverschlüssen. Ber. 64. Vers. dt. ophthal. Ges., p. 477 (1961).

Rintelen, F.: Möglichkeiten und Grenzen der ophthalmoskopischen Beurteilung bei Hypertonie und Arteriosklerose. Ciba Symposium *5:* 34 (1957).

Rintelen, F.: Zur Kenntnis der Leitungsstörungen des Fasciculus opticus, insbesondere der "Apoplexia papillae". Ophthalmologica, Basel *141:* 283 (1961).

Rintelen, F.: Pathogenese und Differentialdiagnose des Papillenödems. Klin. Mbl. Augenheilk. *164:* 1 (1974).

Rix, R., Meythaler, H., Emmerich, F.: Eine Familie mit tapetoretinaler Degeneration und Morbus Coats. Klin. Mbl. Augenheilk. *181:* 303 (1982).

Rochels, H., Trevino, E., Brand, M.: Aplasia vasorum retinae bei konnataler Zytomegalie. Klin. Mbl. Augenheilk. *182:* 237 (1983).

Rohrschneider, W.: Schwangerschaft und Auge. Zentbl. ges. Ophthal. *35:* 225 (1936).

Rossochowitz, W., Metze, G.: Beitrag zum Adamantiades-Behçet-Syndrom. Klin. Mbl. Augenheilk. *157:* 414 (1970).

Roth, M.: Beiträge zur Kenntnis der varicösen Hypertrophie der Nervenfasern. Virchows Arch. path. Anat. Physiol. *55:* 197 (1872).

Rummeld, R.: Hämoglobinanomalien in der ophthalmologischen Praxis. Klin. Mbl. Augenheilk. *166:* 644 (1975).

Sachsenweger, R.: Die Augenkrankheiten im Kindesalter (Enke, Stuttgart 1973).

Sachsenweger, R.: Neuroophthalmologie (Thieme, Stuttgart 1975).

Sachsenweger, R.: Die Sehnervenpapille. Ein Atlas für Ophthalmologen, Neurologen und Internisten (Fischer, Stuttgart 1979).

Sallmann, L. von: Zur Anatomie der Gefässkreuzung am Augenhintergrund. Z. Augenheilk. *91:* 322 (1937).

Saraux, H., Murat, J.P.: Les pseudopapillites d'origine vasculaire. Annl Oculist. *200:* 1 (1967).

Sautter, H.: Die Arteriosklerose des Augenhintergrunds. Klin. Mbl. Augenheilk. *127:* 641 (1955).

Sautter, H.: Korrelationen zwischen Augenbefund und allgemeiner Pathologie bei der Arteriosklerose. Ber. dt. ophth. Ges., 2. Vers., 1959, pp. 4–10 (Bergmann, München 1959).

Sautter, H.: Arteriosklerose des Augenhintergrundes; in Schettler, Arteriosklerose. Ätiologie, Pathologie, Klinik und Therapie (Thieme, Stuttgart 1961).

Sautter, H.: Ein "arteriosklerotisches Frühsyndrom" am Auge. Ber. 65. Vers. dt. Ophthal. Ges., p. 379 (1963).

Sautter, H., Demeler, U., Naumann, G.: Tektonische "Minkeratoplastik" zur Behandlung des persistierenden Hypotonie-Syndroms nach Elliott-Trepanation. Klin. Mbl. Augenheilk. *161:* 629 (1972).

Sautter, H., Lerche, W.: Zur Pathogenese degenerativer Veränderungen der Macula lutea der menschlichen Netzhaut. Eine klinische, histologische und elektronenmikroskopische Untersuchung. Materia Medica Nordmark *21(10):* 549 (1969).

Sautter, H., Lüllwitz, W., Naumann, G.: Die Infrarot-Photographie in der Differentialdiagnose pigmentierter tumorverdächtiger Fundusveränderungen. Klin. Mbl. Augenheilk. *164:* 597 (1974).

Sautter, H., Lüllwitz, W.: Altersveränderungen der Funduspheripherie. Ber. 74. Vers. dt. Ophthal. Ges., p. 446 (Bergmann, München 1977).

Sautter, H., Straub, W.: Atlas of the ocular fundus. Photographs of typical changes in ocular and systemic disease (Urban & Schwarzenberg, München 1977).

Sautter, H., Straub, W., Turss, R., Rossmann, H.: Atlas des Augenhintergrundes; 3. Aufl. (Urban & Schwarzenberg, München 1984).

Sautter, H., Utermann, D.: Der Pseudotumor der Macula. Klin. Mbl. Augenheilk. *145:* 1 (1964).

Sautter, H., Utermann, D.: Weiterer Beitrag zur Klinik und Pathogenese des "arteriosklerotischen Frühsyndroms" am Auge. Ber. 68. Vers. dt. Ophthal. Ges. 1967, p. 44 (Bergmann, München 1968).

Sautter, H., Utermann, D.: Arteriosklerotische Veränderungen am Augenhintergrund. Manifestationsarten arteriosklerotischer Fundusveränderungen, ihre Beziehungen zur allgemeinen Gefässsklerose und therapeutische Gesichtspunkte. Dt. Ärzteblatt *16:* 1259 (1984).

Schäfer, W.D., Tenner, A.: Atrophia gyrata mit Nystagmus und Strabismus. Klin. Mbl. Augenheilk. *156:* 377 (1970).

Scheler, F., Gröne, H.J.: Hypertonie in Klinik und Praxis (Schattauer, Stuttgart 1980).

Scheschy, H., Benedikt, O.: Optikusatrophie durch indirekte Traumen. Klin. Mbl. Augenheilk. *161:* 309 (1972).

Schiek, W.: Hämoglobin A_{lc} bie Diabetes mellitus. Persönl. Mitteilung (1984).

Schiffer, H.P., Busse, H.: Beitrag zum Krankheitsbild des Fundus flavimaculatus mit Makuladegeneration. Klin. Mbl. Augenheilk. *166:* 365 (1975).

Schiffer, H.P., Busse, H., Weihmann, J.: Karzinommetastasen in der Aderhaut. Klin. Mbl. Augenheilk. *173:* 195 (1978).

Schildberg, P., Wessing, A.: Die fokale hämorrhagische Chorioiditis. Eine klinische und fluoreszenzangiographische Studie. Klin. Mbl. Augenheilk. *166:* 651 (1975).

Schiötz, I.: Netzhautablösung während der Schwangerschaft. I. Drei Fälle von Netzhautablösung bei Schwangerschaftsniere. II. Ein Fall nicht-albuminurischer Netzhautablösung bei einer Gravida mit Myopie. Klin. Mbl. Augenheilk. *62:* 234 (1919).

Schirmer, K.E.: Photogrammetrie der Sehnervenpapille. Klin. Mbl. Augenheilk. *164:* 688 (1974).

Schleich: Die Augen von 150 neugeborenen Kindern ophthalmoskopisch untersucht. Mitt. ophth. Klinik Tübingen II, p. 44.

Schlieter, F., Szepan, B., Polenz, B.: Über das Wyburn-Mason-Syndrom. Klin. Mbl. Augenheilk. *168:* 788 (1976).

Schmaltz, B., Schürmann, K.: Traumatische Optikusschäden. Probleme der Ätiologie und der operativen Behandlung. Klin. Mbl. Augenheilk. *159:* 33 (1971).

Schmidt, B.: Überlegungen zur Therapie des Netzhautvenenverschlusses mit Enzyminhibitoren. Klin. Mbl. Augenheilk. *158:* 273 (1971).

Schmidt, D., Faulborn, J.: Retinopathia pigmentosa mit Coats-Syndrom. Klin. Mbl. Augenheilk. *157:* 643 (1970).

Schmidt, D., Faulborn, J.: Familiäres Vorkommen von Coats-Syndrom kombiniert mit Retinopathia pigmentosa. Klin. Mbl. Augenheilk. *160:* 158 (1972).

Schmidt-Martens, F.W.: Die diabetische Retinopathie. Dt. Ärzteblatt *35:* 2233 (1972).

Schoeler: Jahresbericht der Augenklinik, Berlin 1881.

Schofeld, P.B.: Diffuse infiltrating retinoblastoma. Br. J. Ophthal. *44:* 35 (1960).

Schott, K.: Über das sogenannte Kolobom der Makula. Klin. Mbl. Augenheilk. *67:* 415 (1921).

Schrader, K.: Auge und Allgemeinleiden (Schattauer, Stuttgart 1966).

Schreck, E.: Veränderungen des Sehorgans bei Haut- und Geschlechtskrankheiten; in Gottron, Schöfeld, Dermatologie und Venerologie, vol. 4, p. 831 (Thieme, Stuttgart 1960a).

Schreck, E.: Syndroma uveo-aphthosum (oculo-bucco-genitale) (Morbus Gilbert-Behçet); in Gottron, Schönfeld, Dermatologie und Venerologie, vol. 4, p. 874 (Thieme, Stuttgart 1960b).

Schreck, E.: Differentialdiagnose in der Ophthalmologie (Enke, Stuttgart 1977).

Schubert, T., Koch, H.R., Seitz, H.M.: Chorioretinitis durch *Toxocara canis.* Sitzber. 140. Vers. Rhein.-Westf. Augenärzte (1981).

Schürmann, P., MacMahon, H.E.: Die maligne Nephrosklerose, zugleich ein Beitrag zur Frage der Bedeutung der Blutgewebsschranke. Virchows Arch. path. Anat. Physiol. *291:* 47 (1933).

Schwarzhuber, A.: Untersuchungen über die Möglichkeit des serologischen Nachweises von Larva migrans visceralis mit dem Peroxydase-Test. Inaug.-Diss. München (1978).

Seeliger, H.P.R., Potel, G.: Listeriose; in Grunbach, Bonin, Die Infektionskrankheiten des Menschen und ihre Erreger (Thieme, Stuttgart 1969).

Seidel, E.: Weitere experimentelle Untersuchungen über die Quelle und den Verlauf der intraokularen Saftströmung. Graefes Arch. Ophthal. *104:* 158 (1921).

Seitz, H.M.: Persönliche Mitteilung (1984).

Seitz, R.: Die Genese und Ätiologie des Kreuzungsphänomens und seine Bedeutung für die Diagnostik von Netzhautgefässerkrankungen. Klin. Mbl. Augenheilk. *139:* 491 (1961).

Seitz, R.: Klinik und Pathologie der Netzhautgefässe (Enke, Stuttgart 1968).

Seitz, R.: Die essentielle Hypertonie. Materia Medica Nordmark *21/8:* 451 (1969).

Seitz, R., Kersting, G.: Die Drusen der Sehnervenpapille und des Pigmentepithels. Klin. Mbl. Augenheilk. *140:* 75 (1962).

Shafey, S., Scheinberg, P.: Neurological syndromes occurring in patients receiving synthetic steroids (oral contraceptives). Neurology, Minneap. *16:* 205 (1966).

Siam, A.L.: Toxocaral chorioretinitis. Treatment of early cases with photocagulation. Br. J. Ophthalmol. *57:* 700 (1973).

Siegenthaler, W., Siegenthaler, G.: Arteriitis temporalis Horton. Dt. med. Wschr. *86:* 425 (1961).

Sjörgen, H.: Dystrophia reticularis laminae pigmentosae retinae. Acta Ophthal. *28:* 279 (1950).

Slezak, H.: Über Atrophia gyrata centralis chorioideae sed non retinae. Graefes Arch. Ophthal. *170:* 117 (1966).

Slezak, H.: Zur Differentialdiagnose tumorähnlicher Veränderungen des Augenhintergrundes. Klin. Mbl. Augenheilk. *153:* 465 (1968).

Slezak, H.: Makulazyste bei angeborener Grubenpapille. Diskussionsbemerkung. Klin. Mbl. Augenheilk. *154:* 754 (1969).

Slezak, H., Hommer, K.: Funds pulverulentus. Graefes Arch. Ophthal. *178:* 177 (1969).

Small, G.: Coats' disease and muscular dystrophies. Trans. Am. Acad. Ophthalmol. Otolaryngol. *72:* 225 (1968).

Smith, M.E., Zimmermann, L.E., Harley, R.D.: Ocular involvement in congenital cytomegalic inclusion disease. Arch. Ophthalmol., Chicago *76:* 696 (1970).

Smith, M.S., Kreiger, A.: Visual loss associated with oral contraceptives. Am. J. Ophthalmol. *69:* 874 (1970).

Sommer, P., Kunze, P.: Pseudo-Uveitis durch Retinoblastom. Beitrag zur Klinik und Pathologie. Klin. Mbl. Augenheilk. *155:* 844 (1969).

Sorsby, A.: Congenital coloboma of the macula together with an account of the familial occurrence of bilateral macular coloboma in association with apical dystrophy of hands and feet. Br. J. Ophthalmol. *19:* 65 (1935).

Sorsby, A., Crick, R.P.: Central areolar chorioidal sclerosis. Br. J. Ophthalmol. *37:* 129 (1953).

Sorsby, A., Mason, M.E.: Fundus dystrophy of unusual features. Br. J. Ophthalmol. *33:* 67 (1949).

Soyka, D.: Kurzklehrbuch der klinischen Neurologie (Schattauer, Stuttgart 1975).

Speiser, P.: Die Hämangiome des Augenhintergrundes. Klinisches Bild und Behandlung. Klin. Mbl. Augenheilk. *178:* 313 (1981).

Spirig, R., Bosshard, Ch.: Arteriitis temporalis Horton—aussergewöhnliche Verlaufsformen. Klin. Mbl. Augenheilk. *176:* 719 (1980).

Spitznas, M.: Makulablutung bei Dengue-Fieber. Klin. Mbl. Augenheilk. *172:* 105 (1978).

Spitznas, M., Joussen, F., Wessing, A., Meyer-Schwickerath, G.: Coats' disease. An epidemologic and fluorescein angiography study. Graefes Arch. Ophthal. *195:* 241 (1975).

Stärk, N.: Papillenschwellungen bei Kindern. Ber. Vers. dt. ophthal. Ges. 1968, p. 165 (Bergmann, München 1968).

Stangler-Zuschott, E.: Fusionsstörungen nach ausgedehnten Netzhautblutungen bei Neugeborenen. Klin. Mbl. Augenheilk. *172:* 209 (1978).

Stargardt, K.: Über familiäre progressive Degeneration in der Maculagegend des Auges. Graefes Arch. Ophthal. *71:* 534 (1909).

Starzycka, M., Byrk, E.: Schmetterlingsförmige Dystrophie der Makula. Klin. Mbl. Augenheilk. *169:* 454 (1976).

Stefani, F.H.: Maligne Tumoren bei Angehörigen von Retinoblastompatienten. Klin. Mbl. Augenheilk. *168:* 716 (1976).

Stefani, F.H.: Das Retinoblastom. Augenärztl. Fortbildg *4:* 396 (1977).

Stefani, F.H., Greite, J.-H., Schramm, W.: Rezidivierende Netzhautblutungen bei Tortuositas der Netzhautarteriolen. Klin. Mbl. Augenheilk. *167:* 608 (1975).

Stein, R., Godel, V., Nemet, P.: Die Chloroquin-Retinopathie. Das eigenartige Verhalten des Lichtsinnes. Klin. Mbl. Augenheilk. *161:* 183 (1972).

Stempel, I., Straub, W.: Diabetische Augenerkrankungen. Internist. Welt *4:* 243 (1981).

Stewart-Wallace, A.M.: Cerebrovascular accidents and oral contraception. Br. Med. J. *ii:* 1528 (1964).

Stieber, W.: Venenbogen bei Retinopathia diabetica. Klin. Mbl. Augenheilk. *166:* 695 (1975).

Stoye, M.: Helmintheninfektionen und Spielplatzhygiene. Notabene medici *11:* 214 (1981).

Stoye, M.: Askariden- und Ankylostomideninfektionen des Hundes. Tierärztl. Praxis *11:* 229 (1983).

Stoye, M., Bosse, M.: Humanhygienische Bedeutung und Bekämpfung von Nematoden der Kleintiere. Prakt. Tierazt *62:* 62 (1981).

Straub, W.: Metastatisches Aderhautkarzinom beim Brustkrebs des Mannes. Klin. Mbl. Augenheilk. *116:* 61 (1950).

Straub, W.: Augenspiegelkurs. Untersuchungstechnik und Befunde (Urban & Schwarzenberg, München 1971).

Straub, W., Remmler, O.: Fehler bei Untersuchungsmethoden. Diagnostische Irrtümer. Bücherei des Augenarztes. vol. 73 (Enke, Stuttgart 1978).

Streicher, T., Krčméry, K.: Das fluoreszenzangiographische Bild der hereditären Drusen. Klin. Mbl. Augenheilk. *169:* 22 (1976).

Streiff, B.: Über Megalopapille. Klin. Mbl. Augenheilk. *139:* 824 (1961).

Sugar, H.S.: Congenital pits in the optic disc. Am. J. Ophthalmol. *63:* 298 (1967).

Tenner, A., Kraus, E.: Das fluoreszenzangiographische Bild der Aderhautmetastasen einer Struma Langhans. Klin. Mbl. Augenheilk. *158:* 844 (1971).

Tenner, A., Pape, R., Genée, E.: Fluoreszenzangiographie und Ophthalmodynamographie beim Spätbild des Morbus Purtscher. Klin. Mbl. Augenheilk. *160:* 109 (1972).

Terry, Th.L.: Extreme prematurity and fibroblastic overgrowth of persistent vascular sheath behind each crystalline lens. Am. J. Ophthalmol. *24:* 203 (1942).

Thaler, A.: Sektorenförmige Retinopathia pigmentosa. Klin. Mbl. Augenheilk. *166:* 369 (1975).

Theodossiadis, G.: Die Anwendung von Argon-Laserkoagulation bei aktiver Toxoplasmose-Chorioretinitis. Klin. Mbl. Augenheilk. *178:* 466 (1981).

Theodossiadis, G., Charamis, J., Velissaropoulos, P.: Behandlungsergebnisse der Lichtkoagulation bei Ast- und Zentralvenenverschluss. Klin. Mbl. Augenheilk. *164:* 713 (1974).

Theil, H.-J., Behnke, H.: Klinik und Vererbung der vitelliformen Maculadegeneration. Klin. Mbl. Augenheilk. *158:* 235 (1971).

Thiel, H.-J., Wiedemann, H.R.: Der "kirschrote Fleck der Macula" als Ausdruck einer Speicherkrankheit. Klin. Mbl. Augenheilk. *161:* 174 (1972).

Thiel, R.: Augenhintergrundsveränderungen bei arterieller Hypertonie und Nierenkrankheiten. Dt. med. Wschr. *75:* 1495 (1950).

Thiel, R.: Atlas der Augenkrankheiten; 6. Aufl. (Thieme, Stuttgart 1963).

Thumm, H.W.: Diagnostische und therapeutische Irrtümer bei Arteriitis temporalis. Klin. Mbl. Augenheilk. *174:* 732 (1979).

Tillmann, W.: Fluoreszenzangiographie bei Optikomalazie. Klin. Mbl. Augenheilk. *158:* 247 (1971).

Tillmann, W., Antoniadis, A.: Periphere Netzhautablösung bei Grubenpapille. Klin. Mbl. Augenheilk. *162:* 234 (1973).

Tillmann, W., Rummeld, R.: Zilioretinale Arterienverschlüsse. Klin. Mbl. Augenheilk. *166:* 392 (1975).

Tillmann, W., Ufermann, K.: Papillenschwellung bei Uveitis. Klin. Mbl. Augenheilk. *161:* 42 (1972).

Timm, G.: Augenveränderungen bei der subakuten sklerosierenden Leukoenzephalitis van Bogaert. Klin. Mbl. Augenheilk. *140:* 434 (1962).

Uhthoff, W.: Untersuchungen über den Einfluss des chronischen Alkoholismus auf das menschliche Sehorgan. Graefes Arch. Ophthal. *23:* 257 (1887).

Usher, C.H.: The Bowman Lecture. On a few hereditary eye affections. Trans. Ophthal. Soc. UK *55:* 164 (1953).

Utermann, D.: Senile Makuladegeneration. Klinik und Therapie. Dt. Ärzteblatt *10:* 619 (1973).

Utermann, D., Ziemssen, M.: Zur Therapie der senilen Makuladegeneration mit Herzglycosiden. Klin. Mbl. Augenheilk. *158:* 847 (1971).

Varga, M., Gáil, J.: Behandlung der proliferativen Veränderungen des Augenhintergrundes mit Photokoagulation. Ophthalmologica, Basel *157:* 154–160 (1969).

Valude, M.: Atrophie optique durant la grossesse, accouchement prématuré artificiel. Ann. Ocul. *57:* 271 (1892).

Vannas, S., Raitta, C.: Die Prognose der Zentralvenenverschlüsse. Klin. Mbl. Augenheilk. *153:* 457 (1968).

Vasella, F.: Diagnostische Massnahmen bei Zytomegalie. Dt. med. Wschr. *38:* 1818 (1968).

Velhagen, K.: Schwangerschaftsunterbrechung und Auge. Dt. Gesundh Wes. *13:* 17 (1940).

Velhagen, K.: Zur prophylaktischen Operation des Makulaloches. Klin. Mbl. Augenheilk. *146:* 516 (1965).

Velický, J.: Iridozyklitische Retinopathie. Bücherei des Augenarztes, vol. 51 (Enke, Stuttgart 1968).

Verderame, Ph.: Über nichtalbuminurische und albuminurische Netzhautablösung und ihre Wiederanlegung bei Schwangeren. Klin. Mbl. Augenheilk. *49:* 452 (1911).

Vodovozov, A.M.: Reflexe des Augenhintergrundes bei Stauungspapillen. Vest. oftal. *81/3:* 18 (1965).

Vodovozov, A.M.: Unterlagen zur Muskelreflexhypothese des Schielens (die Bedeutung der Asymmetrie im Bau der Augen für die Pathogenese des Begleitschielens). Klin. Mbl. Augenheilk. *168:* 655 (1976a).

Vodovozov, A.M.: Das zentrale vitreo-retinale fibroplastische (ödematös-fibroplastische) Syndrom. Klin. Mbl. Augenheilk. *169:* 212 (1976b).

Vodovozov, A.M.: Ophthalmochromoskopie; in Velhagen, Der Augenarzt, vol. 5, p. 203 (Thieme, Leipzig 1978).

Vodovozov, A.M.: Über die Klassifikation der Lichtreflexe des Augenhintergrundes. Klin. Mbl. Augenheilk. *179:* 145 (1981).

Völcker, H.E., Naumann, G., Rentsch, F., Wollensak, J.: "Primäres" Retikulumzellsarkom der Retina. I. Eine klinisch-pathologische Studie und Literaturübersicht. Klin. Mbl. Augenheilk. *171:* 489 (1977).

Voge, M.H., Wessing, A.: Makulaveränderungen bei Grubenpapille. Klin. Mbl. Augenheilk. *164:* 90 (1974).

Vogelsang: Beitrag zur Pathologie des Auges bei eineiigen Zwillingen. Klin. Mbl. Augenheilk. *97:* 117 (1936).

Volhard, F.: Handbuch der Inneren Medizin; 2 Aufl.; vol. 6, p. 373 (Springer, Berlin 1931).

Waldeyer, A.: Anatomie des Menschen (de Gruyter, Berlin 1957).

Wallow, I.: Nekkrotisierende Retinitis bei schwerer Allgemeinerkrankung. Ber. Vers. dt. Ophthal. Ges. *70:* 55 (1969).

Walsh, J.B., Clark, D.B., Thompson, R.S., Nicholson, D.H.: Oral contraceptives and neuro-ophthalmological interest. Arch. Ophthalmol., Chicago *74:* 628 (1965).

Waubke, Th.: Ein Beitrag zur Pathogenese der Chorioiretinitis Jensen und die Möglichkeit einer therapeutischen Beeinflussung. Klin. Mbl. Augenheilk. *134:* 627 (1959).

Weiden, H.: Über Netzhautblutungen bei Neugeborenen mit unterschiedlichem Geburtsablauf. Klin. Mbl. Augenheilk. *156:* 363 (1970).

Weigelin, E., Lobstein, A.: Ophthalmodynamometrie (Krager, Basel 1963).

Weigelin, S.: Sehnervenerkrankung bei Schwangerschaft. Arch. Augenheilk. *61:* 1 (1908).

Weinstein, P.: Ophthalmologische Differentialdiagnose bei Gehirntumoren. Bücherei des Augenarztes, vol. 60 (Enke, Stuttgart 1972).

Weller, T.H.: The cytomegaloviruses; ubiquitous agents with protean clinical manifestations. New Eng. J. Med. *285:* 267 (1971).

Weller, T.H., Hanshaw, J.B.: Virologic and clinical observations on cytomegalic inclusion disease. New Eng. J. Med. *266:* 1233 (1962).

Welter, S.L.: Naevus pigmentosus des Augenhintergrundes. Klin. Mbl. Augenheilk. *78:* 682 (1927).

Wessing, A.: Fluoreszenzangiographie der Retina. Lehrbuch und Atlas (Thieme, Stuttgart 1968).

Wessing, A.: Diabetische Retinopathie und Lichtkoagulation. Klin. Mbl. Augenheilk. *159:* 692 (1971).

Wessing, A.: Über Technik und Indikation für die Lichtkoagulation bei diabetischer Retinopathie. Klin. Mbl. Augenheilk. *160:* 274 (1972).

Wessing, A.: Die Bedeutung der Fluoreszenzangiographie für die praktische Augenheilkunde. Aktuelle Ophthalmologie, Almanach für die Augenheilkunde, p. 59 (Lehmanns, München 1973).

Wessing, A.: Die exsudative senile Makulopathie, klinisches Bild, Pathogenese, Prognose und Therapie. Klin. Mbl. Augenheilk. *171:* 371 (1977).

Wessing, A.: Senile Makuladegeneration: Gibt es eine Therapie? Sitzber. 65. Tag. Württemb. augenärztl. Verein. Tübingen 1981. Klin. Mbl. Augenheilk. *181:* 66 (1982).

Wessing, A., Spitznas, M.: Morbus Coats und Lebersche Miliaraneurysmenretinitis. Ber. dt. Ophthal. Ges., vol. 74, p. 199 (Bergmann, München 1977).

Wiederholt, M., Leonhardt, H., Schmid-Schönbein, H., Hager, H.: Die Behandlung von Zentralvenenverschlüssen und Zentralarterienverschlüssen mit isovolämischer Hämodilution. Klin. Mbl. Augenheilk. *177:* 157 (1980).

Wilder, H.C.: Nematode endophthalmitis. Trans. Am. Acad. Ophthalmol. Otolaryngol. *55:* 99 (1950).

Wissmann, R.: Die Beurteilung der Augenveränderungen in der Schwangerschaft, mit besonderer Berüksichtigung der Eklampsie. Ber. Vers. dt. Ophthal. Ges. *43:* 263 (1922).

Witmer, R.: Arteriitis temporalis. Ophthalmologica, Basel *121:* 160 (1951).

Witmer, R.: Neuritis optica. Klin. Mbl. Augenheilk. *160:* 29 (1972).

Witmer, R.: Uveitis. Aktuelle Ophthalmologie, Fachalmanach für die Augenheilkunde, p. 23 (Lehmanns, München 1976).

Witmer, R.: Sekundärglaukom und Uveitis, hypertensive Uveitis. Klin. Mbl. Augenheilk. *170:* 837 (1977).

Witschel, H.: Retinopathia pigmentosa und "Morbus Coats". Klin. Mbl. Augenheilk. *164:* 405 (1974).

Witschel, H., Grehn, F.: Das Osteom der Aderhaut. Klin. Mbl. Augenheilk. *180:* 524 (1982).

Wobmann, P.: Angioid streaks und Drusenpapille. Klin. Mbl. Augenheilk. *161:* 191 (1972).

Wodowosow, A.M., Sverdlin, S.M.: Tiefe und verborgene Drusen des Sehnervs als Urasche einter scheinbaren Stauungspapille. Klin. Mbl. Augenheilk. *176:* 367 (1980).

Wollensak, J.: Weiteres zur Klinik und Differentialdiagnose der Cyclitis anularis exsudativa pseudotumorosa. Klin. Mbl. Augenheilk. *141:* 559 (1962).

Wutz, W., Bartl, G., Rodler, H., Hiti, H.: Frontotransversaler Durchschuss beider Orbitae mit beidseitiger Bulbusberstung bei Suizidversuch. Klin. Mbl. Augenheilk. *176:* 409 (1980).

Zanen, J., Rausin, G.: Kyste vitelliforme congénital de la macule. Bull. Soc. Belge Ophtal. *96:* 544 (1950).

Zehetbauer, G.: Zur Zeitdauer der Entwicklung einer Stauungspapille bei Hirndrucksteigerung. Klin. Mbl. Augenheilk. *171:* 613 (1977).

Zeidler, E.: Kernspintomographie. Einführung für Ärzte und Medizinstudenten (Deutscher Ärzteverlag, Köln 1984).

Zielinski, H.W.: Die diabetische Retinopathie in der augenärztlichen Praxis. Klin. Mbl. Augenheilk. *167:* 715 (1975).

Zinn, J.G. (1755), zit. bei Duke-Elder, St., Diseases of the uveal tract: cilio-chorioidal detachments, vol. IX, p. 939 (Kimpton, London 1966).

Suggested Readings

Albert, D.M.: Jaeger's Atlas of Diseases of the Ocular Fundus (WB Saunders, Philadelphia 1972).

Apple, D.J., Rabb, M.F.: Ocular Pathology. Clinical Applications and Self-Assessment (ed 3) (CV Mosby, St. Louis 1985).

Apple, D.J., Rabb, M.F. (ed): Anatomy and histopathology of the macular region. Int. Ophthalmol. Clin. *21(3):* 1-9 (1981).

Apple, D.J., Kivlin, J.D. (ed): New aspects of colobomas and optic nerve anomalies. Int. Ophthalmol. Clin. *24:* 109-121 (1984).

Apple, D.J., Pfeffer, B.R., McFarland, S.T., Isenberg, R.A.: Diabetes and eye disease: Histopathological correlations (Chap. 19). In Benson, W.E., Brown, G.C., Tasman, W. (eds): Diabetes and Its Ocular Complications pp. 179-189 (WB Saunders, Philadelphia 1988).

Ballantyne, A.J., Michaelson, I.C.: Textbook of the Fundus of the Eye (ed 2) (Williams & Wilkins, Baltimore 1970).

Benson, W.E. Retinal Detachment: Diagnosis and Management (Harper & Row, New York 1980).

Blodi, F.C., Apple, D.J. (translators): Vogt's Atlas of Slit Lamp Biomicroscopy (Wayenbourgh, Bonn 1979).

Fine, B.S., Brucker, A.J.: Macular edema and cystoid macular edema. Am. J. Ophthalmol. *92:* 466 (1981).

Fine, S.L., Owens, S.L., Haller, J.A., Knox, D.L., Patz, A.: Choroidal neovascularization as a late complication of ocular toxoplasmosis. Am. J. Ophthalmol. *91:* 318 (1981).

Finkelstein, D., Clarkson, J., Diddie, K., Hillis, A., Kimball, A., Orth, D., Trempe, C.: Branch vein occlusion: Retinal neovascularization outside the involved segment. Ophthalmology *89:* 1357 (1982).

Friedman, E.A., L'Esperance, F.A., Jr.: Diabetic Renal-Retinal Syndrome (Grune and Stratton, New York 1980).

Green, J.L., Rabb, M.F.: Degeneration of Bruch's membrane and retinal pigment epithelium. Int. Ophthalmol. Clin. *21(3):* 27 (1981).

Hayreh, S.S.: Classification of central retinal vein occlusions. Ophthalmology *90:* 458 (1983).

Henkind, P. (ed): The First International Cystoid Macular Edema Symposium. Surv. Ophthalmol. *28* (suppl): 431 (1984).

Hilton, G., Machemer, R., Michels, R., Okun, E., Schepens, C., Schwartz, A.: The classification of retinal detachment with proliferative vitreoretinopathy. Ophthalmology *90:* 121 (1983).

Horn, G., Rabb, M.R., Lewicky, A.O.: Retinal telangiectasis of the macula: A review and differential diagnosis. Int. Opthalmol. Clin. *21(3):* 139 (1981).

Landers, M.B., III, Wolbarsht, M.L., Dowling, J.E., Laties, A.M. (eds): Retinitis Pigmentosa: Clinical Implications of Current Research (Plenum Publishing Corp., New York 1977).

L'Esperance, F.A. Jr. (ed): Current Diagnosis and Management of Chorioretinal Diseases (CV Mosby, St. Louis 1977).

Michaelson, I.C. (ed): Textbook of the Fundus of the Eye (ed 3) (Churchill Livingstone, New York 1981).

Mohler, C.W., Fine, S.L.: Long-term evaluation of patients with Bests' vitelliform dystrophy. Ophthalmology *88:* 688 (1981).

Molony, J.B.M., Drury, M.I.: The effect of pregnancy on the natural course of diabetic retinopathy. Am. J. Ophthalmol. *93:* 745 (1982).

Naumann, G.O.H., Apple, D.J.: Pathology of the Eye (Springer-Verlag, New York 1986).

Peyman, G.A., Apple, D.J., Sanders, D.R. (eds): Intraocular Tumors (Appleton-Century-Crofts, New York 1977).

Peyman, G.A., Sanders, D.R., Goldberg, M.R. (eds): Principles and Practice of Ophthalmology (WB Saunders, Philadelphia 1981).

Rosner, L.J., Ross, S.: Multiple Sclerosis. pp. 46-47 (Prentice Hall Press, New York 1987).

Schwatz, B. (ed): Perspective on ocular hypertension. Surv. Ophthalmol. *25:* 124 (1980) (special edition).

Shields, J.A.: Diagnosis and Management of Intraocular Tumors (CV Mosby, St. Louis 1983).

Shields, J.A., Stephens, R.F., Sarin, L.K.: The differential diagnosis of retinoblastoma. In Harley RD (ed): Pediatric Ophthalmology (ed 2, vol 2) (WB Saunders, Philadelphia 1983).

Shimizu, K.: Fluorescein Microangiography of the Ocular Funds (Williams & Wilkins, Baltimore 1973).

Tasman, W.: Retinal Diseases in Children (Harper & Row, New York 1971).

Tasman, W., Shields, J.A.: Disorders of the Peripheral Fundus (Harper & Row, New York 1980).

Index

Page numbers in *italics* denote figures; those followed by "t" denote tables.

Acetazolamide (Diamox)
  for acute glaucoma, 140
  for ischemic optic neuropathy, 135
  for retinal artery occlusion, 36, *71*
Adrenocorticotropic hormone (ACTH), 50
AK-Dilate. *See* Phenylephrine hydrochloride
AK-Penlolate. *See* Cyclopentolate hydrochloride
Akarpine. *See* Pilocarpine
Amaurosis, eclamptic, 168
Amaurosis fugax,
  with retinal artery occlusion, 36
  with temporal arteritis, *153*
Amblyopia of intoxication, 128, *142–143*
Ampicillin, 55t
Anatomy, 1–5
Anemia, 193–194
  acute hemorrhagic, 193
  chronic hemorrhagic, 193
  Cooley's, 194
  hemolytic, 194
  pernicious, 194
  Rietti's, 194
Aneurysms, Leber's miliary, 48
Angiography, retinal fluorescein, 9–10, 10t, *11*, 53, *143*, *147–149*, 179
Angioid streaks, 45–46, *98–99*
Angiopathia retinae traumatica Purtscher, 178–179
Anomalies. *See* Developmental anomalies
Anterior cerebral artery, 4
Anterior chamber tap, for retinal artery occlusion, 36
Anthelmintic drugs, 56–57
Aphthous ulcers, 49–50, *104*
Apoplexia retina. *See* Retinal vein occlusion
Argon laser coagulation, 38, 54
Argyll Robertson pupil, 137
Arteriosclerotic retinopathy, 40, 40t–41t, 42, *84–91*
Arteriovenous crossings, 33, *63–64*
Arteritis, temporal, 135–136, *153–156*
Asteroid hyalosis, *192*
Astrocytoma, *145*
Atlas, 1
Atrophy
  Behr's optic, 128
  central progressive choroidal, 61–62, *97*
  gyrate, 61, *125*
  Leber's optic, 127, 128, 137
  optic, 136–138, 137t, 138t, *143*
  pigmented paravenous chorioretinal, 46
Atropine, 50, 180

Behçet's syndrome, 49–50, *104–105*
Behr's optic atrophy, 128
Benson's disease, *192*
Bergmeister's papilla, persistent, 14–16, *23*
Berlin's edema, 178, *183*
Best's disease, 42–43, *92–93*
Birth trauma, 178
  congenital papilledema, 178
  congenital retinal hemorrhage, 178
Blind spot, 3
Blood pressure. *See also* Hypertension
  adult ranges of, 34t
  classifications of, 34t–35t
Bonnet-Dechaume-Blanc syndrome, 162–163
"Box-car" effect, 36
Brachial artery pressure, 9
Bridge coloboma, 13, *20, 24*
Bruch's membrane, 5
  anatomy of, 5
  drusen of, 44–45, *96*
  ruptures in, 17, *31*
"Bull's eye" dystrophy, *152*

Carotid artery examination, 4
Casoni's skin test, 57, *118*
Cataracts, diabetic, 40
Cat's-eye reflex, 160
Cellophane macula, 12
Central progressive choroidal atrophy, 61–62
Central retinal artery
  anatomy of, 3
  branches of, 3, 4
  occlusion of, 35–36, *69–72*
  spontaneous pulsation of, 4
Central retinal vein, 3
  occlusion of, 37, *73–77, 176*
Central serous chorioretinopathy, 50, *106–107*
Central tapetoretinal dystrophy, 43–44, *94–95*
Chemotherapy, 163
Cherry-red spot, 2, 36
Children, fundus of, 173
  birth trauma of, 178
  developmental anomalies of, 13–32. *See also* Developmental anomalies
  full-term newborn, 173
  premature newborn, 173
  retinopathy of prematurity, 173–174
Chloroquine therapy, papilledema due to, 134, 134t, *151–152*
Choriocapillaris, 1–3, 5
Chorioretinitis, 52, *108–112*
  Jensen's juxtapapillary, *111*
  listeriosis and, 54–55, 55t, *115*
  of optic disc, 53
  serpiginous, *99*
  sclopetaria, 179, *183–184*
Chorioretinopathy
  arteriosclerotic, 40, 40t–41t, 42, *84–91*
  central serous, 50, *107*
Choroid, 1, 4–5
  central sclerosis of, 45, *97*
  coloboma of, 13, *20*
  detachment of, 179–180, *185*
  hemorrhage of, 179
  layers of, 5
  nevi of, 44, *95*
  rupture of, 179, *184*
  tumors of
    benign, 162
    malignant melanoma, 161–162, *165*
    metastases of extraocular tumors, 163, *167*
    metastatic, 162
Choroideremia, 61–62
Choroiditis, 51–52
  central hemorrhagic, 53, *112*
  central localized, 52
  disseminated, 52, *108*
  focal macular, 53, *112*
Chromatoophthalmoscopy, 8
Ciliary body, 1
Ciliochoroidal detachment, 179–180, *185*
Cilioretinal arteries, 16, *27*
  occlusion of, *177*
Circinate retinopathy, 50–51, *107–108*
Closed-circuit television reader, 41–42
Coagulation disorders, 194–195, *196–198*
Coats' disease, 48–49, *103–104*
  secondary, 49
Colloid bodies, 131, 133, *146–148*
Colloid degeneration, 44–45, *96*
Colobomas
  bridge (rudimentary), 13, *20, 24*
  Fuchs', 13, *21, 24*
  juxtapapillary, 14
  macular, 13, *21*
  optic disc, 13, 14, *20, 24*
  of retina and choroid, 13, *20*
Color vision, in central sclerosis of choroid, 45
Commotio retinae, 178, *182–183*
Contraceptive drugs, oral
  extraocular complications of, 175
  ocular complications of, 175, *176–177*
Contusio retinae, 178, *182–183*
Cooley's anemia, 194

Copper wire arteries, 33, *64*
Copper wire reflex, 12, *65*
Cornea, 1
Corticosteroids. *See also* specific steroids
  for Behçet's syndrome, 50
  for central serous chorioretinopathy, 50
  for choroidal detachment, 180
  for epiretinal membranes, 48
  for ischemic optic neuropathy, 135
  for ischemic papilledema, *152*
  for retinopathy of prematurity, 174
  for temporal arteritis, *156*
Cotton wool exudates, 34, *67, 69, 176, 178*
Cranial arteritis, 135–136, *153–156*
Crystal reflex, 12
Cyclodialysis, 5
Cyclopentolate hydrochloride (Cyclogyl), 8t
Cytomegalic inclusion disease, 57–58, *118*

Dawson's subacute sclerosing leukoencephalitis, 58–59
Deuteranomaly, *95*
Developmental anomalies, 13–32
  bridge coloboma, 13, *20*
  cilioretinal arteries, 16, *27*
  colobomas of retina and choroid, 13, *20*
  congenital central glial dysplasia of optic nerve head, 15
  duplication of optic disc, 14–15
  ectopia of macula, 19
  enlargement of optic disc, 15, *25*
  epipapillary glial membrane, 14–16, *23*
  hyperopia, 18, *32*
  hypoplasia/aplasia of optic disc, 15, *25*
  macular colobomas, 13, *21*
  medullated retinal nerve fibers, 13–14, *21–22*
  myopia, 16–18, *29–31*. *See also* Myopia
  optic disc coloboma, 13, *20*
  optic pit, 14, *24*
  opticociliary artery or vein, 16, *27*
  persistent Bergmeister's papilla, 14–16, *23*
  persistent hyaloid artery, 16, *26–27*
  staphyloma-like ectasia of posterior fundus, 18–19
Dexamethasone, 48
Dextran 40 or 70
  for retinal artery occlusion, 36, *75*
  testing reaction to, 36
Diabetic retinopathy, 39–40, *79–83*
  classification of, 39t
  hemoglobin A_{1c} in diabetics, 40
  optic changes, due to, 40
Diamox. *See* Acetazolamide
Dilatair Solution. *See* Phenylephrine hydrochloride
Ditch reflex, 12
Doppler sonography, 10–11, *11*
Dot reflex, 12
Drugs. *See* specific names
Drusen
  of Bruch's membrane, 44–45, *96*
  optic disc, 131, 133, *147–148*
Dystrophy. *See* specific types

Eales' disease, 46–47, *99, 101*
Echinococcus granulosus infection, 56–57, *118*
Ectopia, macular, 19
  primary, 19
  pseudoectopia, 19
  secondary, 19
Edema
  Berlin's, 178, *182–183*
  retinal, 34
Encephalomyelitis, disseminated, 127–128
Enucleation 162, *165*
Epipapillary glial membrane, 14–16, *23*
Epiretinal membranes, 47–48, *102*
Estrogen, effects of, 175
Evulsio nervi optici, 181
Examination methods, 7–11
  chromatoophthalmoscopy, 8
  direct ophthalmoscopy, 7
  doppler sonography, 10–11, *11*
  indirect ophthalmoscopy, 7
  infrared fundus photography, 8
  ophthalmodynamography, 8–9, *11*
  ophthalmodynamometry, 9
  retinal fluorescein angiography, 9–10, 10t, *11*, 53, *143, 147–149*, 179
Exudates
  cotton wool, 34, 37, *67, 69*
  hard, 34, 37, *69*
Exudative external retinitis, 48–49, *103*

Familial macular cerebral degeneration, 43–44, *95*
Fibrinolytic therapy
  contraindications to, 36
  for retinal artery occlusion, 36
  for retinal vein occlusion, 38
Fibroplasia, retrolental, 173–174
Fleck reflex, 12
Flecked retina syndrome, 44–45, *96*
Flexner-Wintersteiner rosettes, 160
Fluorescein angiography, retinal, 9–10, 10t, *11*, 53, *143, 147–149*, 179
Focal reflexes, 12
Foerster-Fuchs' spot, 17
Foreign body, in optic disc, 181
Fovea centralis retinae, 1, 2
Foveolar reflex, 12
Fuchs' circinate retinitis, 50–51, *107–108*
Fuchs' coloboma, 13, *21, 24*
Fundus
  albipunctate, *177, 182*
  anemic, 193–194
  of children, 173
  coloration of, 5, *6*
  hypertensive changes in, 33–34, *67–69*
  light reflexes of, 12
  "pepper and salt", 44
Fundus albinoticus, 5
Fundus albipunctatus, 60
"Fundus astigmatism", 19
Fundus flavimaculatus, 60–61
  in Stargardt's disease, 43
Fundus pulverulentus, 61
Fundus scleroticus, 40, 40t–41t, *84–86, 88–89, 91*

Gamma globulin, 50
Geniculocalcarine tract, 5
Giant cell arteritis, 135–136, *153, 155–156*
Giant cell inclusion disease, 57–58, *118*
Glaucoma, 138–140, *157, 159*
  acute, 139–140
  angle-closure, *159*
  axial hyperopia and, 18
  cupping of disc in, 138
  diagnostic criteria for, 139
  hints for non-ophthalmologists, 139–140
  low-tension, *159*
  myopia and, 17–18
  neovascular, 39
  open-angle, *157, 159*
  pigmentary, *157*
  staging of excavations in, 139, 139t
Glial hamartoma, 162, *166*
Glial membrane, epipapillary, 14, *23*
Glioblastoma, *143, 145*, 160
Glioma retinae, 160–161, *164*
Gold reflex, 12
Gruber's syndrome, 13
Guist's sign, 33, 35t, *63*
"Gun barrel" visual field, 137
Gunn's dots, 12
Gunn's sign, 33, 35t, *63*
Gyrate atrophy, 61, *125*

Haller's layer, 5
Hamartoma, glial, 162, *167*
Harada's syndrome, 52
Hemangiomas, arteriovenous, 162, *167*
Hemoglobin A_{1c}, in diabetics, 40
Hemorrhage, 34, *196–197*
Hemorrhage, congenital retinal, 178
Henle's fiber layer, 2, 3
Homatropine hydrobromide, 8t
Horner's syndrome, 4
Horton's arteritis, 135–136, *153, 155–156*
Hyaline bodies, 131, 133, *147–148*
Hyaline dystrophy, 44–45, *96*
Hyaloid artery, persistent, 16, *26–27*
Hyperbaric oxygen therapy, 174
Hyperopia, 18
  axial, 18
  index, 18
  refractive, 18
Hyperornithinemia, 61
Hypertension
  arterial, 33–34, *72–74*
  benign intracranial, 131
  blood pressure classifications, 34t–35t
  fundus changes in, 33–34, *63, 67–69, 118*
  myopia and, 17
  ocular, 139
  renal induced, *67, 172*
  retinal vessels in, 33, *63–65, 67*
Hypopyon iritis, 49
Hypopyon neuritis, *104*

I-Homatrine 5% Ophthalmic Solution. *See* Homatropine hydrobromide
I-Pilocarpine. *See* Pilocarpine
Infrared fundus photography, 8
Insulin *79, 81–82*

Intoxications, affecting optic nerve, 128, *143*
Intramacular reflex, 12
Intraocular pressure. *See also* Glaucoma
  normal, 139
  ocular hypertension, 139
Iridocyclitis, papilledema and, 133–134, *151*
Iris, 1
Isopto Carpine. *See* Pilocarpine
Isopto Homatropine. *See* Homatropine hydrobromide
Isovolemic hemodilution, 38, 195

Jensen's juxtapapillary retinochoroiditis, 52–53, *111*
Juvenile exudative macular retinitis, 53, *112*
Juvenile macular degeneration, 42
  classification of, 42t
  diagnosis of, 42
  Stargardt's, 43–44, *95*

Kimmelstiel-Wilson disease, *81*
Kuhnt-Junius degeneratio maculi luteae disciformis, 41t, *86, 87–89*

"Lacquer cracks", 17
Lamina basalis, 5
Lamina cribrosa sclerae, 3, 4
Lamina elastica, 5
Lamina vitrea, 5
Laser coagulation
  for Coats' disease, 49
  for *Echinococcus granulosus* infection, 57
  for retinal vein occlusion, 38
Late ocular recidivation, 53–54
"Lattice degeneration", 188
Leber's miliary aneurysms, 48
Leber's optic atrophy, 127, 128, 137
Leukemic retinopathy, 193
Light coagulation
  for Toxocariasis, 56
  for Wyburn-Mason syndrome, 163
Light reflexes of fundus, 12
Linear reflexes, 12
Listeriosis, chorioretinitis and, 54–55, 55t, *115*
Low-vision aids, 41–42
Lupus erythematosis, *152*

Macula, 1–3
  cellophane, 12
  cherry-red spot of, 2, 36
  coloboma of, 13, *21*
  degeneration of
    age-related (senile), *99*
    disciform, 41t
    juvenile, 42, 42t
    vitelliforme, 42–43, *92–93*
  dysplasia of, 13
  ectopia (heterotropia) of, 19
    primary, 19
    pseudoectopia, 19
    secondary, 19
  holes in, 189
  light or radiation trauma of, 180
  papillomacular bundle of, 3
  serous-hemorrhagic disciform detachment of, 53, *112*
Macular reflex, 12
Macular star figure, 3, 34, 37, 50–51, *67, 69, 107–108*
Malignant melanoma, of choroid, 161–162, *165*
Mannitol, for retinal artery occlusion, 36
Marcus-Gunn pupillary sign, 127
Mariotte's spot, 3
Mebendazole, for *Echinococcus granulosus* infection, 57
Medullated retinal nerve fibers, 13–14, *21–22*
Megalopapilla, 15, *25*
Membrane(s)
  Bruch's, 5
    drusen of, 44–45, *96*
    ruptures in, 17, *31*
  epipapillary glial, 14–16, *23*
  epiretinal, 47–48, *102*
Ménière's syndrome, *85*
Metallic reflexes, 12
Miotic drugs, parasympathomimetic, 8t
Monoclonal gammopathy, 193
Morbus Coats, 48–49, *103*
Morbus Gilbert-Adamantiades-Behcet, 49–50, *104–105*
Morning glory syndrome, 15
Müller cells, 1, 2
Müller dynamometer, 9
Multiple myeloma, 193
Multiple sclerosis, 127–128
Muscae volitantes, 188
Mydfrin. *See* Phenylephrine hydrochloride
Mydriacyl. *See* Tropicamide
Mydriatic drugs
  parasympatholytic, 8t
  sympathomimetic, 8t
Myopia, 16–18
  axial, 16–17
  glaucoma and, 17–18
  hypertension and, 17
  index, 16
  malignant (excessive), 17, *29, 31*
  papilledema and, 17
  refractive, 16
  refractive error and, 17, 17t
  "school", 17
  simple (stationary), 16–17

Neo-Synephrine. *See* Phenylephrine hydrochloride
Neuritis. *See* Optic neuritis
Neuroepithelioma, 160–161, *164*
Neuroretinoangiomatosis, 162–163
Nevi, choroidal, 44, *95*
Nervoid pigmentation, *95*
Nitroglycerin, for retinal artery occlusion, 36

Occlusion
  branch arteriolar, 36–37
  retinal artery, 35–36, *69–72*
  retinal vein, 37–38, *73–79*
Ocular recidivation, late, 53–54
Oculobuccogenital syndrome, 49–50, *104*
Omega branching, 33, *64*
Ophthalmic artery, 4
  pressure in, 9
Ophthalmochromoscopy, 8
Ophthalmodynamography, 8–9, *11*
Ophthalmodynamometry, 9
Ophthalmoscopy, 7
Optic atrophy, *85,* 136–138
  causes of, 137t
  differential diagnosis of, 138, 138t
  Leber's, 127, 128, 137
  traumatic, 180–181, *186*
Optic disc
  anatomy of, 3
  chorioretinitis of, 53
  coloboma of, 13, *20*
  congenital excavation of, 14, *24*
  drusen of, 131, 133, *147–148*
  duplication of, 14–15
  enlargement of, 15, *25*
  foreign body in, 181
  hypoplasia/aplasia of, 15, *25*
  vascular supply of, 3–4
Optic nerve trauma, 180–181
  foreign body in optic disc, 181
  hematoma of optic nerve sheath, 181
  nerve disruption, 181
  optic atrophy, 180–181, *186*
Optic neuritis, 126, *141*
  differential diagnosis of, 132t–133t
  etiology of, 126t
  ischemic, 134–135, *152*
  during pregnancy, 169
  prelaminar, 126
  retrolaminar (retrobulbar), 126–127, *141*
  terminology of, 126
  toxic, 128, *143*
Optic neuropathy
  acute ischemic, 134–135, *152*
  hereditary, 128
  toxic, 128, *143*
Optic pit, 14, *24*
Optic radiation, 5, 50
Opticociliary artery, 16
Opticociliary vein, 16, *27*
Ora serrata, 1, 174
Oral antidiabetic drug, *79–81*
Oral contraceptives
  extraocular complications of, 175
  ocular complications of, 175, *176–177*
"Owl eye cells", 58

Pandy's reaction, *85, 116*
Papilla, 3
  persistent Bergmeister's, 14–16, *23*
Papillary plethora, 129
Papillary reflexes, 12
Papilledema, 34, *68,* 128–130, *143–145*
  brain tumor and, 128, *145*
  chronic atrophic, 129–130
  congenital, 178
  differential diagnosis of, 130, 132t–133t
  due to chloroquine therapy, 134, 134t, *151–152*

Papilledema—*continued*
early, 129
fully developed, 129
iridocyclitis and, 133–134, *151*
ischemic, 134–135, *152*
myopia and, 17
terminology of, 128
vascular changes, 130
Papillitis, 126, 132t–133t
Papillomacular bundle, 3
Paramacular reflex, 12
Paraproteinemia, 193
Parasympatholytic (mydriatic) drugs, 8t
Parasympathomimetic (miotic) drugs, 8t
Pars ceca retinae, 1
Pars optica retinae, 1
Penicillin, *76*
Pentolair 1% Solution. *See* Cyclopentolate hydrochloride
Pentoxifylline (Trental) for retinal artery occlusion, 36
"Pepper and salt" fundus, 44
Periarteritis segmentalis superficialis, 135–136, *153, 155–156*
Perimacular reflex, 12
Pette-Döring disease, 58–59
Phenylephrine hydrochloride, 8t
Pigment epithelium, 1
Pigmentary retinopathy, 59–60, *120–121, 123, 125*
Pigmented paravenous chorioretinal atrophy, 46
Pilocarpine, 8t
for acute glaucoma, 140
Polycythemia, 195, *196–198*
primary, 195, *198*
secondary, 195, *197*
Polymyalgia arteritica, 135–136, *153, 155–156*
Polysclerosis, 127–128
Posterior fundus ectasia, 18–19
Prednisolone
for corneal edema, 140
for epiretinal membranes, 48
for glaucoma, 140
for listeriosis, 55t
for retinal artery occlusion, 36
for temporal arteritis, 136
for toxocariasis, 56
Pregnancy
cesarean section, 169
eclamptic amaurosis of, 168
nomenclature of gestosis, 168t
optic neuritis during, 169
proteinura (preeclampsia), 168, *170–171*
retinal detachment during, 169
subconjunctival hemorrhage, 168, *170*
toxemia, *171–172*
Prethrombosis, 34
Progressive albipunctate dystrophy, 60
Proliferative retinopathy, 47, *101*
Pseudocoloboma, macular, 53
Pseudopapilledema, *149*
Pseudopapillitis, 132t–133t, 133, 134t, *148–149*
vascular, 134–135, *152*
Pseudoretinitis pigmentosa, 61, *124–125*, 179, *183–184*
Pseudotumor cerebri, 131
Purtscher's disease, 178–179
Purtscher-Fuchs' spot, *31*
Pyrimethamine, for toxoplasmic retinochoroiditis, 54

Radiation therapy
for central serous chorioretinopathy, 50, *71, 75, 77, 196–197*
for choroidal metastases, 163
for malignant melanoma, 162
Reflexes, light, 12
Rete mirabile, 37
Retina
anatomy of, 1–3, *2*
cerebral layer, 1
neuroepithelial layer, 1
coloboma of, 13, *20*
congenital hemorrhage of, 178
contusion of, 178, *182–183*
detachment of, 188–189, *191–192*
during pregnancy, 169
primary, 188–189
secondary, 189
spontaneous reattachment, *191*
edema of, 34
microscopic structure of, 1
types of holes in, 188, *191*
vascular supply of, 3
Retinal artery occlusion, 35–37
branch, 36–37
central, 35–36, *69–72*
Retinal ischemia, *177*
Retinal pigment epithelium
reticular dystrophy of, 61
hyperplasia of, *95, 176*
Retinal vein occlusion, 37–38
branch, 38, *77–79*
central, 37, *73–77*
Retinitis
cytomegalic inclusion, 57–58, *118*
exudative external, 48–49, *103*
Fuchs' circinate, 50–51, *107–108*
juvenile exudative macular, 53, *112*
pigmentosa, 59–60, *120–121, 123, 125*
mimics of, 60–61
without pigment, 60
punctata albescens, 60
sclopetaria, 179, *183–184*
septic, 51
Retinoblastoma, 160–161, *165*
endophytic growth of, 161
hereditary, 161
Retinochoroiditis
Jensen's juxtapapillary, 52–53
toxoplasmic, 53–54
acquired infection, 54
congenital infection, 53
late ocular recidivation, 53–54
Retinopathia sclopetaria, 179, *183–184*
Retinopathy
arteriosclerotic, 40–41
circinate, 50–51, *107–108*
diabetic, 39–40, *79, 81–82*
hemorrhagic, 37–38, *73–77, 79*
hypertensive. *See* Hypertension
ischemic, 35–37, *69–74*
leukemic, 193
lymphatic, 193
myeloic, 193
of prematurity, 173–174
proliferative, 47, *101*
pseudopigmentosa, 61, *125*
solar or eclipse, 180
traumatic, 178–179, *183*
venous stasis, 38
Retrolental fibroplasia, 173–174
Rheologic agents
for central sclerosis of choroid, 45
for Sorsby's pseudoinflammatory dystrophy, 44
for temporal arteritis, *156*
Rhodopsin, 1
Ribavirin (Virazole), for subacute sclerosing panencephalitis, 59
Rietti's ("target cell") anemia, 194
Rumpel-Leede test, 195, *196*

Salus' sign, 33, 35t, *64*
Sattler's layer, 5
Schimmelpennig-Feuerstein-Mims' syndrome, 13
Sclera, 1
Sclerectasia, 17
eccentrical posterior, 18–19
Scotomas
Bjerrum 8, *159*
central or pericentral, 179
Senile fundus tabulatus, 41t
Septic retinitis, 51
Sickle cell disease, 194
Silver wire arteries, 33
Silver wire reflex, 12, 33, *64*
Skip lesions, 136
Sludged blood phenomenon, 36, *156*
"Snail track degeneration", 188
Sonography, doppler, 10–11, *11*
Sorbitrate, *75*
Sorsby's pseudoinflammatory dystrophy, 44
Spongiosis chorioideae, 179–180, *185*
Staphyloma-like ectasia of posterior fundus, 18–19
Staphyloma posticum verum, 17
Stargardt's disease, 43–44, *95*
Stargardt's spots, 17
Strabismus
axial hyperopia and, 18
macular pseudoectopia and, 18
Subacute sclerosing panencephalitis, 58–59
Sulfamethoxazole for toxoplasmic retinochoroiditis, 54
Sulfonamide for toxocariasis, 56
Supertraction, 17
Suprachoroidal layer, 5
Sympathomimetic (mydriatic) drugs, 8t
Syphilitic retinal angiopathy, *76*

Tapetal reflexes, 12
Tapetoretinal degeneration, 12, 59–60, *120–125*

Telescopic devices, 41
Temporal arteritis, 135–136, *153, 155–156*
Terry's retrolental fibroplasia, 173–174
Tetracycline
for cytomegalic inclusion disease, 58
for listeriosis, 55t
for toxocariasis, 56
Thalassemia (major, minor), 194
Thiabendazole, for toxocariasis, 56
Thrombosis, central retinal vein, 37, *73–77*
Tilted disc syndrome, 13
Toxemia of pregnancy, *170, 172*
Toxocariasis, 55–56, *112, 115–117*
Toxoplasmic retinochoroiditis, 53–54
acquired infection, 54
congenital infection, 53
late ocular recidivation, 53–54
Trauma
of birth
congenital papilledema, 178
congenital retinal hemorrhage, 178
blunt, *184, 186*
choroidal detachment, 179–180, *185*
choroidal rupture, 179, *184*
commotio retinae, 178, *182–183*
contusio retinae, 178, *182–183*
light or radiation trauma of macula, 180
optic nerve trauma
foreign body in optic disc, 181
hematoma of optic nerve sheath, 181
optic atrophy, 180–181, *186*
optic nerve disruption, 181
perforation, *184*
retinopathia sclopetaria, 179, *183–184*
retinopathy, 178–179
Triangular reflex, 12
Tropicamide (Tropicacyl), 8t
Tumors, 130
associated with papilledema, *145*
choroidal
benign, 162
gliobastoma, *143, 145*
hypophyseal, 169, 195
malignant melanoma, 161–162, *165*
meningioma, *165*
metastases of extraocular tumors, 163, *167*
metastatic, 162–163
retinoblastoma, 160–161, *165*
Tunica fibrosa, 1
Tunica interna, 1
Tunica vasculosa, 1

Ulcers, aphthous, 49–50, *104*
Uvea, 1
Uveitis, posterior, 51–52
Uveo-encephalitic syndrome, 49–50, *104*

Van Bogaert's disease, 58
Vasculature
anatomy and physiology of, 4
of prelaminar optic nerve, 3–4
of retina, 3
in hypertension, 33, *63–67*
of retrolaminar optic nerve, 4
Vascular retinal ischemia, *176–177*
Vein pulsation, spontaneous, 4
Venoarterial crossings, 33
Venous stasis retinopathy, 38, *75*
Vidarabine (Vira-A)
for cytomegalic inclusion disease, 58
for subacute sclerosing panencephalitis, 59
Visual aids, 41–42
Visual field test, 139, 180
Visual field defects
losses due to choriodal detachment, 128
losses due to glaucoma, 139t
Visually evoked potentials, 128
Visual system, 5
optic pathways, 2t
Vitelliforme macular degeneration, 42–43, *92–93*
Vodovozov's classification of light reflexes, 12
Vogt-Koyanagi syndrome, 52

Waldenstrom's macroglobulinemia, 193
Weiss reflex, 12
Widal listeriosis test, 55, 55t
Wiedemann's syndrome, 13
Wyburn-Mason syndrome, 162–163

Xenon laser coagulation, 38, 49

Zinn's circle, 4, 5